ANABOLIC STEROIDS

DEMYSTIFIED

THOMAS D FAHEY

FRANK I KATCH

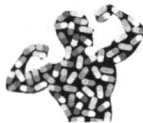

Anabolic Steroids. Demystified

9 8 7 6 5 4 3 2 1

Authors: Fahey, Thomas D. and Katch, Frank I. Title: *Anabolic Steroids. Demystified* Description: First edition. [2021] | Includes bibliographical references and index.

Identifiers: ISBN: 978-0-9640591-5-3

Subjects: MeSH: Testosterone, Anabolic Steroids, Steroids, Olympic Games, Exercise, Sport, Muscle, Hormones, Athletics, Physical Fitness, Sports Medicine, Bodybuilding, hormone replacement therapy

FOREWORD

Anabolic Steroids Demystified presents an insider's view of anabolic steroids by two world-class sports scientists and athletes: Thomas Fahey and Frank Katch. Their experiences as scientists, coaches, and athletes help you separate the street news from the street noise about these controversial drugs. The ebook version includes direct access to over 1600 original source journal articles and abstracts. Topics include:

- Who takes these drugs and why.
- How world-class athletes and bodybuilders use anabolic steroids.
- Steroid use by recreational bodybuilders and physically active people.
- Effects of anabolic steroids on strength, power, endurance, and sports skills.
- The biochemistry of anabolic steroids
- The effects of anabolic steroids on sports performance in men, women, and children.
- Anabolic steroids and motor control.

- Side effects of anabolic steroids and their effects on the cardiovascular system, longevity, cancer, liver, kidneys, skin, blood, and soft tissue.
- Sexual effects of anabolic steroids
- Psychological effects of anabolic steroids, including "roid rage."
- Medical uses of anabolic steroids.
- Supplemental testosterone in middle-aged and older adults.
- History of anabolic steroids, including steroid use during the cold war and Russian steroid scandals. The book includes stories about steroid use in sport revealed for the first time.
- The ethics and legal considerations of anabolic steroid use.
- Drug testing by the World Anti-Doping Agency. How countries and athletes try to beat the tests.
- Controversies about steroid use in Russia, USSR, and East Germany.
- Long term steroid effects on performance, health, and lifespan.

This is must reading for athletes, researchers, coaches working with athletes who might take steroids, the media, sports fans, parents of athletes, and politicians.

INTRODUCTION

It is challenging to discuss performance at the Olympic Games or the local gym without mentioning anabolic steroids. They have captured the imagination of people throughout the world. Steroids are bigger, better, and louder than similar things in popular lexicon, so it seems exaggerated and unreal. For example, "The cityscape is spectacular, *like Manhattan on steroids*." They have profoundly affected big-time amateur and professional sport and dominated the headlines during every Olympics.

Anabolic steroids are drugs that resemble the hormone testosterone. Anabolic refers to the tissue-building property of the drugs. They are a leading topic of conversation every time an athlete breaks a record or does something extraordinary. While coaches and trainers should never recommend these drugs to clients, they should thoroughly understand their use and abuse.

Not all steroids are anabolic. Steroids help control metabolism, inflammation, immunity, salt and water balance, sexual development, and resistance to illness and injury. Anabolic-androgenic steroids—such as testosterone, build muscle and promote male sex characteristics (i.e., hair growth, deep voice, sex organ growth). Steroids called glucocorticoids—such as cortisone or prednisone, suppress inflammation or exaggerated immune responses and treat swelling, rashes, asthma, bronchitis, and altitude sickness.

Contrary to widespread belief, athletes are not the principal users of these drugs. The average user is a recreationally active thirty-year-old man or woman trying to improve body composition or a middle-aged or older adult attempting to prevent aging.

Middle-age and older adults consider testosterone an *elixir vitae*. Druggists filled over 5,500,000 testosterone prescriptions in 2018 (https://clincalc.com/DrugStats/Drugs/Testosterone). Athletes continue to use these drugs secretly, but they receive severe athletic and even legal penalties if caught. Most strength coaches and personal trainers will work with people taking these drugs and answer questions without recommending them.

Why we wrote this book: We wrote this book for people who want a thorough introduction to anabolic steroids but lack physiology, chemistry, and medical training. It is thoroughly referenced and based on evidence-based research. Contents include sections on history, mechanism of action, effects on performance, use patterns of athletes and recreational adults (type, dosage, polydrug use), side effects— including longevity, sexual physiology, cardiovascular function, cancer, liver and kidney, women and children, psychology, and aging. The book includes extensive discussions of steroids and ethics, doping control, steroids and the law, and state-sponsored doping in the former Soviet Union and Russia.

Unique features: This book's unique and revolutionary feature is direct access to over 1600 full-page articles and abstracts. Click on the URL at the end of each reference to get access to the article or abstract. This feature will help non-scientists understand the science behind these drugs and provide further in-depth information for serious researchers in 15 areas of interest.

About the Authors

Together, the authors have over 100 years of experience in the sports sciences between them. They've seen it all. Both are noted textbook authors and have extensive experience in sport science research, athletics, coaching, and sports consulting. They know the behind the scene secrets and will help you separate the street noise from the street news about anabolic steroids.

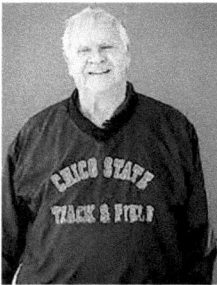

Thomas Fahey is a Professor Emeritus of Kinesiology at California State University, Chico. He received his doctorate from the University of California, Berkeley, in 1972, specializing in exercise physiology, motor development, and biomechanics. In 2006, he was named outstanding professor at California State University, Chico. Dr. Fahey authored 31 books on exercise physiology, wellness, and strength, including Exercise Physiology: Human Bioenergetics and its Applications, 5th edition, Fit & Well (McGraw Hill, 15th edition), and two courses for International Sports Science Association. He published hundreds of articles for scientific journals and bodybuilding and fitness magazines. He wrote monthly research reviews and articles for *Muscular Development, Fitness RX for Men,* and *Fitness RX* for Women magazines. He collaborates with researchers from Puerto Rico and Mexico on the genetic basis of athletic performance.

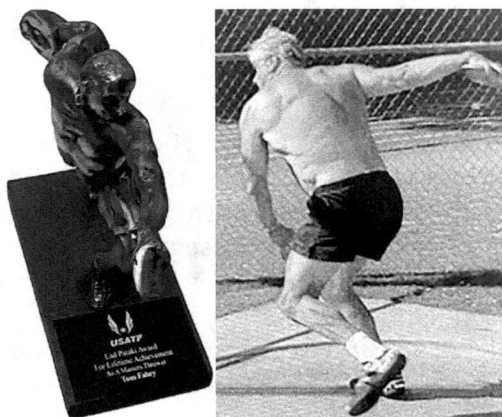

Fahey was an All-American track and field athlete in college in the discus throw. He continued to pursue athletic excellence after graduation. He was master's world champion in the discus throw (won medals in five consecutive world championships, including the gold in 2003), eleven-time US master's national discus champion (consecutive), and four-time gold medal winner in Master's World Games (consecutive). In 2008, USA Track and Field (USATF) named him the outstanding master's field athlete of the year and awarded him the Lad Pataki Lifetime Achievement honor in 2018.

He volunteered as a track and field coach (throws) for over 35 years. He had a total knee replacement in 2018 but plans to continue competing in master's throwing events. He also enjoys golf, skiing, horseback riding, cycling, hiking, weightlifting, and fishing. He lives in Chico and Fort Jones, California.

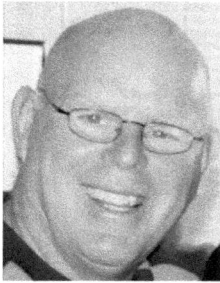

Frank Katch took early retirement as Professor of Exercise Science at the University of Massachusetts, Amherst (1977-2001). He moved to Santa Barbara, CA, where he lives with his wife Kerry (married 1970, with three grown children and four grandchildren). At UMass, he served as Department Head (1977-1990) and Graduate Program Director (1977-1986). Before UMass, his first teaching job after completing graduate studies at the University of California Santa Barbara and Berkeley was at Queens College of the City University at New York (1970-1977). He has published over 150 articles in peer-reviewed scientific and professional journals, presented over 250 invited lectures at national and international conferences, including opening ceremonies or plenary talks at health, business, and fitness meetings in the United States, South America, Europe, and Asia. His college texts with Lippincott, Williams & Wilkins (lww.com) include English, French, Spanish, German, Italian, Portuguese, and Japanese translations, including International European editions): *Exercise Physiology: Energy, Nutrition, and Human Performance*. (First prize in medicine category from the British Medical Association). 9th ed., in production scheduled publication Spring, 2022; *Sports and Exercise Nutrition*. 5th ed., 2019; *Essentials of Exercise Physiology*. 5th ed., 2016, and *Introduction to Nutrition, Exercise and Health*. 4th ed., 1992.

Other collaborations include three consumer books; *Getting in Shape* (Houghton Mifflin, 1979), *Fitness Walking* (Putnam, 1985), and *The Fidget Factor* [Andrews McMeel, 2000]). He has contributed over 160 feature articles in popular consumer magazines (*Mademoiselle, Vogue, Harper's, Woman's Day, Reader's Digest, Weight Watcher's, Muscle and Fitness, Shape, Self,* and *American Health*); consulted with professional football teams (NFL Cowboys, Jets, Dolphins, Saints, Redskins), professional baseball (Boston Red Sox), NBA, US Olympic Team, corporations, and appeared on major TV news networks—ESPN, CBS, NBC, ABC, Real Sports, and QVC home shopping network, and two national fitness infomercials.

Dr. Katch makes time to exercise 60 min daily most days of the week (beach walking with his wife, training for strength and balance), enjoy being with his grandkids and adult kids, play golf often, BBQ, maintain a succulent garden, travel, and eat exotic flavor ice cream and anything chocolate!

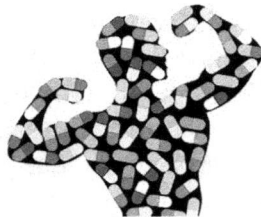

CONTENTS

ANABOLIC STEROIDS: HISTORICAL PERSPECTIVE

Anabolic steroids include testosterone and chemical modifications of testosterone. They have anabolic (tissue building) and androgenic (masculinizing) effects, so they are often called anabolic-androgenic steroids. A long and controversial history has continued to this day. The reference section on the epidemiology of anabolic steroids contains several excellent full-text articles on the history of these drugs (Kanayama & Pope (2018); Dodson et al. (2007); Kochakian (2010); Morgentaler & Traish, 2020; Bhasin, et al., 2021). If you have the ebook version, click on the URLs to retrieve the articles.

How to Books: Dozens of "how-to" books and websites on anabolic steroids are available on the Internet.

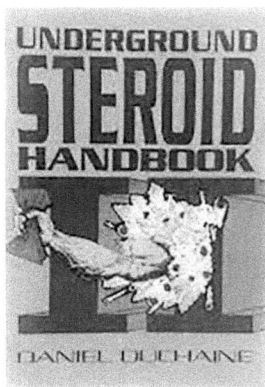

Figure 1-1 *The Underground Steroid Handbook* by
Dan Duchaine was the first "how to" books on
anabolic steroids.

The Underground Steroid Handbook by Dan Duchaine,
initially published in 1981, was the first of many books
on steroids based largely on personal experience and
word of mouth from bodybuilders and weight-trained
athletes (Figure 1-1). This is understandable because
little research existed on the effects of these drugs on
performance or health. The existing studies used low
doses that did not improve performance.

Unreliable Information on the Internet: Information
on the Internet or the popular press is unreliable.
When I (Fahey) wrote articles for *Muscular Development*
magazine, a reader asked about clearance rates of various anabolic steroids. Charts showing this were
readily available on many sites. However, when I wrote
to the authors asking for sources, they could not provide them. They made up the clearance rates based on
personal experience (e.g., "I know a guy who got

popped when tested 30-days after taking drug X."). None of the authors presented data or measured clearance rates. Draw your conclusions about steroids based on evidence— not someone's opinion.

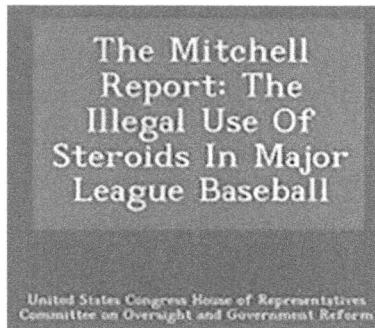

The Mitchell Report: The Illegal Use Of Steroids In Major League Baseball

United States Congress House of Representatives Committee on Oversight and Government Reform

Figure 1-2: The Mitchell report summarized a congressional investigation on the use of anabolic steroids in Major League Baseball.

We know a lot about the risks and benefits of anabolic steroids and their use patterns. Thousands of studies and research reviews give us a clearer picture of these drugs and their side effects. Historical documents from the former Soviet Union and East Germany, the *Mitchell Report* on drug use in Major League Baseball in the United States (2007, Figure 1-2), and anecdotal reports from athletes and coaches from throughout the world show widespread anabolic steroid use was instituted in sport before comprehensive doping control. This book will help scientists, coaches, athletes, and health professionals understand this controversial subject's science and history.

· · ·

THOMAS D FAHEY & FRANK I KATCH

Most Sport Governing Bodies Ban Anabolic Steroids: The World Anti-Doping Agency (WADA), established in November, 1999, oversees the World Anti-Doping Code adopted by over 600 sports organizations. Athletes, active people, coaches, and scientists should understand banned substances in sport. They should understand training, nutrition, and supplements to maximize performance without resorting to drugs.

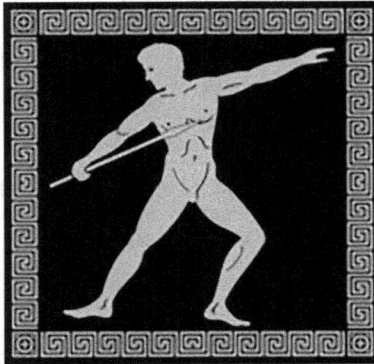

Figure 1-3: Ancient athletes used performance-enhancing drugs. Source: Shutterstock.

Research on testosterone began over 125 years ago. Specialization in sport has made these drugs a significant issue. Drug use to improve performance is almost as old as sport itself. Ancient Greek athletes used a variety of concoctions to enhance performance (Figure 1-3). Inca warriors in South America chewed coca leaves before doing battle in the rarified air of the Andes mountains. At the turn of the 20th century, athletes often breathed supplemental oxygen to improve endurance. Athletes, such as boxers and soccer players, got a boost by drinking a cocktail composed of strychnine, brandy, and cocaine.

Early Research on Testosterone

The roots of testosterone research reach back to ancient times. Farmers learned that castrated animals had reduced sex drives and were more docile. Royalty in Persia employed castrated men called eunuchs to guard the harem because they had reduced sex drives and could not conceive.

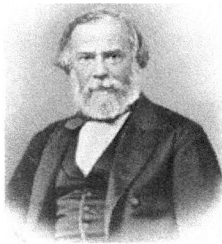

Figure 1-4: Charles-Édouard Brown-Séquard (1817-1894) was an early testosterone researcher. Source: Wiki Commons.

Charles-Édouard Brown-Séquard: Modern scientific research on testosterone began in 1889 when 72-year-old Charles-Édouard Brown-Séquard, (1817-1894), pioneer French neurologist, endocrinologist, and physiologist, reported that testicular extracts of dogs and guinea pigs made him feel younger and more virile (Figure 1-4). He injected one-part testicular venous blood, one-part semen, and one-part testicular fluid from dog or guinea pig testes to trigger sexual effects in animal models, so it's conceivable the treatment affected him (Morgentaler and Traish, 2020).

His report on the topic started widespread testicular extract use in Europe and North America for the next 30 years. No reports stated that athletes of that era formally used the extracts but were widely heralded in the popular press as health tonics, so they might

5

have used them to enhance performance. Even then, critics attributed improvements in mood and energy levels to the placebo effect— the power of suggestion. No reports suggest that athletes used the preparations. The media heralded them as a health tonic, so perhaps some athletes used them to improve performance.

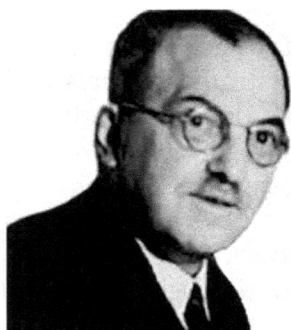

Figure 1-5: Ernst Laqueur (1880-1947) isolated a tiny amount of crystalline testosterone from bull testes in 1934. Source: Wiki Commons.

Steroid Chemistry's Golden Age: The 1930s have been called steroid chemistry's golden age. A Polish-born pharmacologist and physician Ernst Laqueur (1880-1947; Figure 1-5) isolated a tiny amount of crystalline testosterone from bull testes in 1934. He also did notable research on insulin and estrogen. University of Chicago scientists isolated 20 milligrams of testosterone from 40 pounds of bull testicles obtained from the Chicago stockyards. These studies promoted research and development programs on testosterone by European drug companies Schering, Organon, and Ciba.

Butenandt and Ružička won the 1939 Nobel Prize in Chemistry for synthesizing testosterone from cholesterol. This started an on-going lively debate in the medical community regarding testosterone replacement therapy. The early interest in testosterone centered on its effect on libido and sexual performance in men and women. A report by Huggins and Hodges involving eight men suggested that testosterone therapy promoted prostate cancer put a damper on testosterone's clinical use (Morgentaler and Traish, 2020).

World War II and the Cold War

During World War II, the media reported that German and American armies experimented with testosterone (testosterone propionate) to improve performance, and Adolf Hitler was supposedly an early user of the drug. Historians Marcel Reinold and John Haberman (2014) said this is a myth stemming from speculation by a journalist. While steroid-crazed Nazis appeal to popular perceptions, there is little evidence this happened. Athletes first noticed the benefits of anabolic steroids in the late 1940s.

The Male Hormone, by Paul de Kruif (New York: Harcourt Brace & Co., 1945) mentioned that testosterone boosts muscle strength, which caught the eye of bodybuilders and strength athletes. Word spread quickly in the athletic community that testosterone increased lean muscle mass, making it a serious candidate as a performance-enhancing drug.

Steroids and International Sports Competitions.

After World War II, international athletic competitions became cold war surrogates to the battlefield. Eastern and Western bloc countries squared off on the playing fields, ice rinks, basketball courts, and running tracks. Governments poured money into athletics hoping to promote their political agendas. Victory was the only acceptable outcome for both sides (Figure 1-6). In this climate, widespread drug use to improve performance was almost inevitable. Athletes discovered testosterone affected aggressiveness and mood, contributing to the drug's ergogenic (performance-enhancing) effects.

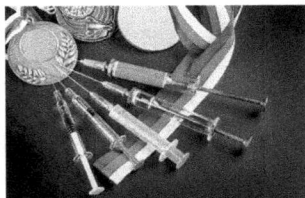

Figure 1-6 Performance-enhancing drugs became political tools in the East-West Block rivalry.

The first purported use of anabolic steroids in sport occurred at the 1952 Helsinki Olympics. Athletes from the Soviet Union dominated weightlifting. U.S. weightlifting coach Bob Hoffman told the Associated Press he suspected that Soviet athletes were using synthetic testosterone (Kremenik, et al., 2006). A Soviet physician confirmed this to Dr. John Ziegler (team physician for USA Weightlifting) at the World Weightlifting Championships in Vienna in 1954. Ziegler became an advocate for anabolic steroids and administered it to elite bodybuilders and strength and power athletes (Kanayama and Pope, 2017).

The World Learns about Anabolic Steroids: Testosterone propionate, the available form of the drug, produced significant masculinizing effects. Zeigler worked with the Swedish pharmaceutical company Ciba to develop methandrostenolone (Dianabol) to reduce testosterone's side effects (Figure 1-7). Most strength athletes knew this drug by the early 1960s. Athletes openly discussed how many "blues" they had to take to lift more "blues." Dianabol pills and 20 kg bumper plates are both blue!

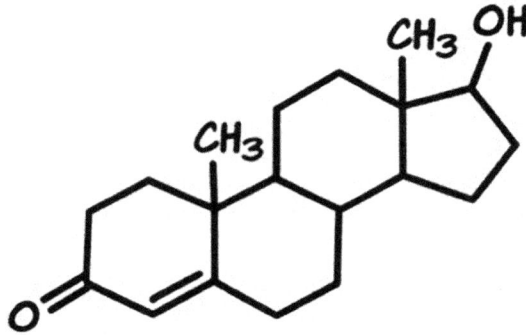

Figure 1-7: chemical structure of testosterone.
Source: Shutterstock.

Widespread Dianabol use was commonplace in the 1960s among athletes in the West and Eastern Block. The Western athletic community and news media widely suspected drug use by Eastern athletes. While Western athletes used steroids unsystematically, Eastern athletes' drug use was institutionalized. Steroid use was systematic in the German Democratic Republic and Soviet Union. *Faust's Gold: The East German Doping Machine (MacMillan, 2001)*, a noteworthy book by Steven Ungerleider, documented the systematic anabolic steroids and other drug use by East German athletes— particularly in women.

Co-author Fahey was the director of an exercise performance lab in the San Francisco Bay Area in the mid-1970s until the mid-1980s. Several times, elite American swimmers' fathers approached him to get their daughters on an anabolic steroid program. He explained the severe side effects their daughters would experience and refused to recommend them. American anxiety about steroids by Americans was understandable. Between 1956 and 1988, East Germany— a country of only 17 million— won 203 gold, 192 silver, and 177 bronze medals in the Summer and Winter Olympics.

Soviet Scientists and Steroids: Dr. Fahey visited the Research Institute of Physical Culture in Leningrad (now St. Petersburg) in the mid-1980s. The scientists were open about state-sponsored doping in the Soviet Union. Several Soviet scientists and coaches emigrated to the West. Of interest, in the late 1990s, Fahey was collaborating on a paper about world doping activities with Victor Rogozkin (Director of the Leningrad lab) and Michael Kalinski (Chairman of Biochemistry, University of Kyiv and later professor and Chair of Kinesiology at Kent State and Murray State Universities in the U.S.).

Rogozkin abruptly pulled out of the project claiming that things had changed in Russia and were going back the way they were. The Russian Olympic program took state-sponsored doping to new levels with systematic doping of elite athletes and dishonest doping control tests at the Sochi Olympics. These actions resulted in bans of Russian Olympians at the Rio and Tokyo Olympics. Some Russian athletes still competed in Tokyo under the Russian Olympic Committee flag.

Anabolic Steroids and Anti-Doping Policies

Excesses in drug use in sport caught up with the athletes. Between 1960 and 1963, the public became disgusted with drug-related deaths in cycling, boxing, and track and field. Many people believed that athletic drug use threatened all sports, undermining the foundations of the Olympic ideal. Anabolic steroid use increased throughout the 1960s because many physicians promoted that anabolic steroids had few side effects, and sports governing bodies issued no sanctions.

First Anti-Doping Regulations: The International Olympic Committee (IOC) formulated its anti-doping policies beginning in 1964. Their basic philosophy was to:

- Protect the athletes' health,
- Defend medical and sports ethics, and
- Provide equal chance competitions.

In 1968, the International Olympic Committee (IOC) began the first large-scale drug-testing program at the Grenoble Winter Olympics and the Mexico City Summer Olympics. Testing occurred at competitions rather than random testing used today. The IOC banned anabolic steroids in 1968, with the first steroid drug tests at the 1976 Montreal Olympic Games.

The early history of athletic drug testing was controversial and inconsistent. During the early years, amphetamines and anabolic steroids were the most commonly banned drugs used by athletes. While amphetamines were easily measured, anabolic steroid assays were more difficult and expensive.

Gradually, anabolic steroid detection became more sophisticated. Drug testing methods lacked sensitivity, specificity, and predictability. Drug testing was only scheduled at major championships. Oral anabolic steroids cleared the body quickly, so athletes could easily avoid detection. State drug labs contributed to the problem because they followed a policy of evasion and deceit. East German labs conducted 12,000 tests a year between 1978 and 1988 but did not report any positive tests (deMondenard, J-P, 2000).

Doping Control Gets Serious: While the first steroid doping tests occurred at the 1976 Montreal Olympics, it was not until the 1983 Pan American Games in Caracas, Venezuela that things became serious. Scientists developed an accurate test for anabolic steroids and secretly unveiled it at the games. At least 38 athletes tried to sneak out of the athletes' village at night only to be confronted by the waiting press at the airport.

In the 1988 Seoul Olympics, Ben Johnson failed a steroid test following a gold medal-winning performance. Johnson was a two-time bronze medal winner at the 1984 Los Angeles Olympics (100-meters and 4 x 100-m relay) and won gold medals in the 1987 World Championship, 1986 Moscow Goodwill Games, and the 1986 Edinburgh Commonwealth Games. Officials stripped Johnson of his Olympic and World Championship gold medals. Of interest, six of the eight finalists in the Seoul Olympics were later involved in drug scandals.

• • •

Anabolic Steroid Control Act: In 1990, the U.S. Congress passed the Anabolic Steroid Control Act, which classified anabolic steroids as a separate drug class and listed 24 anabolic drugs as controlled substances. The Act contained enough flexibility to control newly developed anabolic steroids. In 2004, Congress amended the Act to prohibit making, selling, or possessing steroid precursors and provided funds for anti-steroid education.

Beginning in the late 1980s, the IOC instituted random drug testing for elite athletes. Officials expected athletes to inform them of their location and be prepared to submit a urine sample within 48 hours. If they refused, they would be treated as though they tested positive for banned drugs and would receive sanctions, which ranged from reprimands to permanent exclusion from sport. Even today, anabolic steroid use is a critical issue, as evidenced by the sanctions issued against the Russian Olympic team in the 2016 Rio de Janeiro and 2021 Tokyo Olympics for conducting a state-sponsored doping program.

Steroids and Professional Sports: In the United States, professional baseball and the National Football League introduced drug-testing programs in 2004 to stem the tide of drug misuse in sport. In December 2007, the Mitchell Report— commissioned by the Commissioner of Major League Baseball at the request of the U.S. Congress— concluded that drug use was widespread at all levels of the sport:

"For more than a decade, there has been widespread illegal use of anabolic steroids and other performance-enhancing substances by players in Major League Baseball, in violation of federal law and baseball policy. Club officials routinely have discussed the possibility of such substance use when evaluating players. Those who have illegally used these substances range from players whose major league careers were brief to potential members of the Baseball Hall of Fame. They include pitchers and position players, and their backgrounds are as diverse as those of all major league players."

A link to the full copy of the Mitchell Report is available in the references and is "must" reading for any sports student. (http://files.mlb.com/mitchtpt.pdf)

The Biological Passport: Initiated in 2008, it is WADA's latest effort to detect and discourage performance-enhancing drugs. The program established typical blood levels of various physiological markers. Changes in these markers would suggest illegal drug use, even when athletes passed drug tests.

Random drug tests, administered by WADA, were instituted in Olympic sports in 2004. Still, widespread steroid abuse persisted— most notably in an institutionalized drug program by the Russians at the Sochi Olympics. Systematic drug use in Russia has continued, resulting in further suspensions of Russian athletes in the 2021 Tokyo Olympics. Athletes still use steroids and play a cat and mouse game with drug testers to avoid detection.

Master's Sports: Older athletes, called masters, are not exempt from drug use. Many athletes have tested positive for anabolic steroids and other drugs since drug testing initiation in international competitions in 1995 and U.S. competitions in 2011. Drug testing is controversial in older adults because many drugs used medically to treat aging problems are on the banned substance list. Drug use by master's athletes is common in track and field, cycling, weightlifting, and CrossFit Games.

Typical Users: Today, the main steroid users are non-athlete recreationally active males and females in their 20s and 30s who want to look more muscular and athletic and middle-age and older adults for life-extension and quality of life. Testosterone and other anabolic steroids are legal in many countries worldwide and are readily available on the Internet, so recreational use of the drugs will continue for some time.

Summary

Anabolic steroids include testosterone or chemical modifications of testosterone. They have anabolic (tissue building) and androgenic (masculinizing) effects, so they are often called anabolic-androgenic steroids. Most governing bodies in amateur and professional sports ban anabolic steroids, but athletes and recreationally active people continue to use them, so it is important for coaches and personal trainers to understand them.

Testosterone was isolated and synthesized in the 1930s, and its applications have been controversial since then. Athletic applications began in the early 1950s in weightlifting by Russian athletes but spread rapidly to athletes in other sports and countries. By the 1970s, the German Democratic Republic (East Germany) and the Union of Soviet Socialist Republics (USSR) developed sophisticated state-sponsored steroid programs that was only revealed after the USSR breakup and the reunification of Germany. Systematic doping continued in Russia, leading to Russia's suspension from the Olympics in 2016 and 2021.

Doping control in sport gradually became more sophisticated with drug testing at the Grenoble Olympics in 1968, out-of-competition random drug testing in the 1980s, the formation of WADA in November, 1999, and the biological passport in 2002. The biological passport is an electronic record of baseline biological factors altered by doping such as hematocrit, hemoglobin, testosterone, and IGF-1.

Doping became an issue in professional sports due to scandals in baseball, American football, and soccer. Consequently, most sports instigated stringent anti-doping regulations and testing protocols, with severe consequences for failing tests.

Anabolic steroids became legal issues, with the U.S. Congress passing the Anabolic Steroid Control Acts of 1990 and 2004.

ANABOLIC STEROIDS

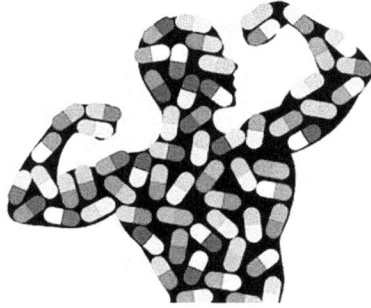

2

WHAT ARE STEROIDS AND HOW
DO THEY WORK?

S teroids are organic chemicals containing 17 carbon
atoms arranged in four-fused rings (Figure 2-1).
Steroids occur widely in nature in plants, animals,
yeasts, and molds. Even slight variations in chemical
structure affect their biological activity.

Cholesterol is the most abundant steroid in humans. It is a critical component of cell membranes, and
a precursor (chemical compound preceding another in
a metabolic pathway) of bile salts, sex hormones,
adrenal hormones, and vitamin D (Figure 2-2). Anabolic steroids (anabolic-androgenic steroids) are synthetic versions of the steroid hormone testosterone.

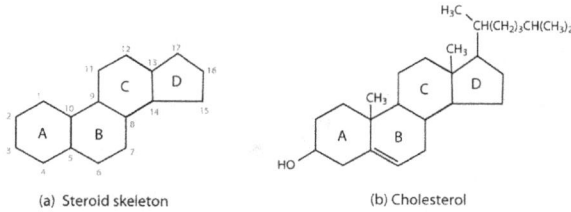

(a) Steroid skeleton   (b) Cholesterol

Figure 2-1: (a) The basic steroid skeleton contains 17 carbon atoms bound in four "fused" rings; b) cholesterol is the most common steroid in the body. It acts as a precursor for many other body chemicals. Figure 2-2 shows a simplified pathway for the conversion of cholesterol to testosterone. Source: Shutterstock.

Steroid Physiology: Steroid hormones have significant effects on human physiology and performance. *Hormones* are signaling chemicals produced by glands such as the testes and ovaries transported in the blood to distant organs and tissues to regulate physiology and behavior.

Hormones control many physiological functions, including the regulation of fats, carbohydrates, and proteins; fight-or-flight survival mechanisms (sympathetic activation during dangerous situations or getting "psyched" during athletic contests); programmed cell death, reproduction, growth and development (e.g., physical and emotional changes during childhood; menopause); immunity; and weight control.

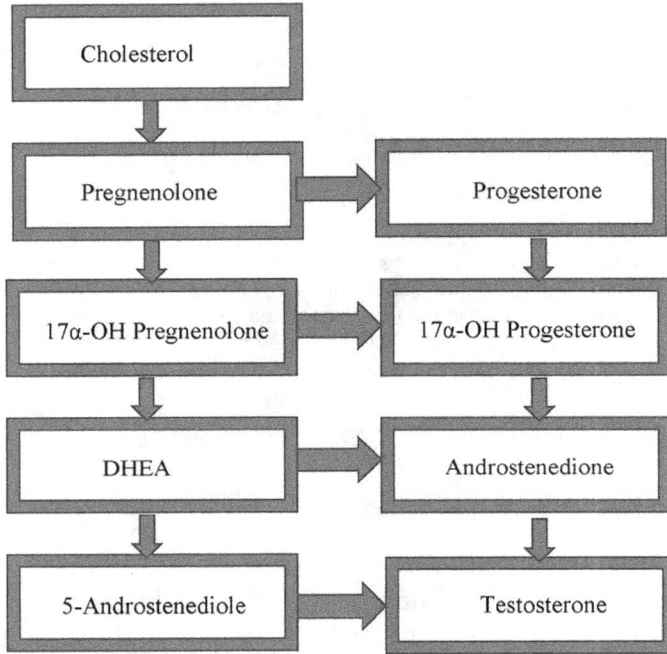

Figure 2-2: Simplified diagram of the conversion of cholesterol to testosterone. Notice that two substances— DHEA and androstenedione— are popular supplements (sometimes called "pro-hormones") taken to increase testosterone levels.

Athletes sometimes try to influence hormone balance by taking anabolic steroids or growth hormone. While this has temporary effects, the body reacts by producing fewer naturally occurring hormones (i.e., testosterone or growth hormone) that trigger challenges to hormone regulation and side effects (e.g., testicular atrophy or shrinkage). In the short run, these hormones increase strength, power, and muscle mass. They work best when accompanied by intense weight training, power training, and a higher protein diet.

. . .

Hormone Homeostasis: Hormones are essential parts of homeostasis: internal balance or equilibrium in body functions. Hormones are carefully regulated by other hormones, blood concentrations of glucose (sugar), the nervous system and thought processes, and environmental changes (e.g., heat, cold, altitude).

Steroid hormones work by binding specific receptors in target tissues that signal activation of gene activity and synthesize specific proteins (Figure 2-3). Steroid hormones can dissolve in fats, so they can cross membranes and enter the cell nuclei. In the nucleus, steroids influence genes to cause specific physiological effects such as promoting protein synthesis or the growth of sex organs. The DNA in the nucleus contains cell blueprints to construct proteins (see Figure 2-3 and 3-2). One of testosterone's important functions is to stimulate muscle protein production and increase muscle size and strength.

Not All Steroids are Anabolic: Corticosteroids are catabolic hormones (trigger atrophy) produced in the adrenal glands, often used in medicine to treat inflammation. The common phrase "on steroids" means that something is more significant or impressive than something else. The correct term should be "anabolic steroids" because the term could easily apply to corticosteroids and mean something smaller and less impressive.

Steroid Hormone Response

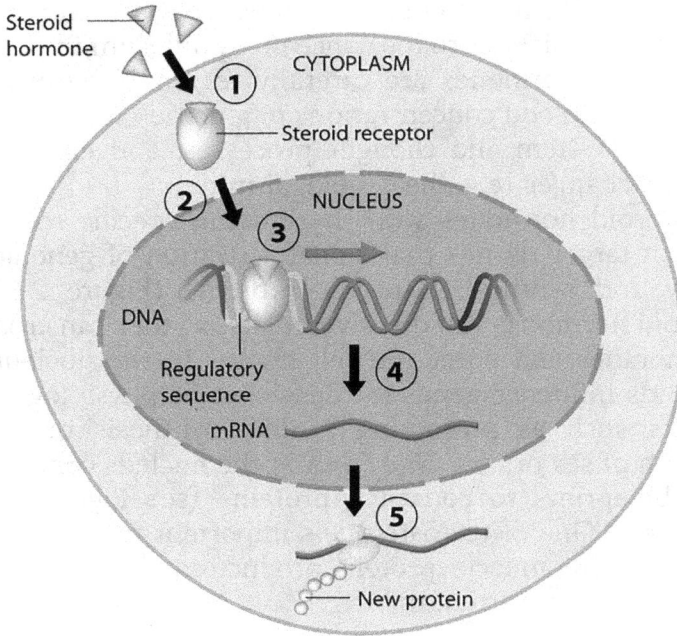

Figure 2-3: The steroid hormones testosterone and anabolic steroids work by entering the cell cytoplasm (1) and binding specific hormone receptors in the cells (2). The hormone-receptor complex enters the nucleus (3) and stimulates the genes to synthesize proteins (4,5). Source: Shutterstock.

Steroid Classifications

In animals, most steroids are hormones classified according to their binding chemicals in cells. These include:

1) **Sex steroids** (produced in the testes, ovaries, and adrenal glands):

- **Androgens** develop and maintain male characteristics by binding to androgen receptors, but they are present in males and females. Androgens can convert to estrogens. Testosterone is the principal androgen. Dehydroepiandrosterone (DHEA) and androstenedione are mainly produced in the adrenal glands and are less potent than testosterone. Androgens regulate testes formation, male pubertal development, sperm production, fat deposition, muscle mass, behavior (sex drive, aggression), and nerve formation in the brain's hippocampus (consolidates information in the brain).
- **Estrogens** develop and maintain female characteristics by binding to estrogen receptors. Estrogens include estradiol, estrone, and estriol, with estradiol most common (before menopause). Estrogens are most common in women but are essential in males for sperm maturation, sex drive, and body composition regulation. Estrogens help regulate metabolism, fat storage, female sexual characteristics, skin and blood vessel health, bone metabolism, liver protein synthesis, blood clotting, ovulation, sexual behavior, and mental health.
- **Progesterone** is involved in the menstrual cycle, pregnancy, skin health, and brain function.

2) **Corticosteroids:** produced in the adrenal glands regulate metabolism, immune function, blood volume, blood pressure, body water, and electrolytes.

- **Glucocorticoids** bind with the glucocorticoid receptor and are important regulators of immunity, inflammation, protein, and fat breakdown to promote carbohydrate metabolism, bone metabolism, and the fight or flight reaction to danger. Examples include cortisol, cortisone, prednisone, and dexamethasone. Medically, they are used to treat inflammation, altitude sickness, severe allergies, and autoimmune diseases.
- **Mineralocorticoids** also bind with specific receptors involved in electrolyte and water metabolism. Aldosterone is the principal mineralocorticoid.

3) **Vitamin D** refers to a subclass of steroids called secosteroids (type of steroid with a "broken" ring) that regulates calcium, magnesium, and phosphate critical in bone metabolism.

Testosterone and Anabolic Steroids in the Body

Testosterone is a steroid and the principal male hormone. The testicular Leydig cells produce most testosterone in males, while females produce testosterone in the ovaries and adrenal glands. After puberty, testosterone production is 15-20 times greater in males than females (Handelsman, et al., 2018).

Testosterone's Sexual Effects: Anabolic steroids include testosterone and synthetic drugs structurally like testosterone and have similar effects. Testosterone develops primary sexual characteristics such as the testes, penis, and prostate and secondary sexual characteristics male-pattern hair growth (face and underarm), deepening of the voice, linear growth, and muscle and bone growth. It promotes sperm and semen production in adults and is critical for sex drive in males and females.

Testosterone affects tissues throughout the body (Figure 2-4). Many anabolic steroid side effects stem from natural effects of the hormone unwanted in the recipient. Athletes are interested in increasing muscle strength, power, and size. The hormone also affects skin, bones, bone marrow, sex organs, and central nervous system. In addition to increasing muscle protein synthesis, testosterone affects tissues throughout the body (Figure 2-4). Effects on skin, bone, brain, bone marrow, and sex organs explain some of the drug's diverse side-effects.

Testosterone can increase oil secretion in the skin, bone density, red blood cell production, sex drive, sperm production, primary and secondary sexual characteristics, linear growth, and erectile function. A woman or child who takes anabolic steroids to increase strength might also experience voice changes, hair growth, closure of the bone growth centers, or clitoral hypertrophy. All effects are regular testosterone functions, except they are undesirable in the recipient.

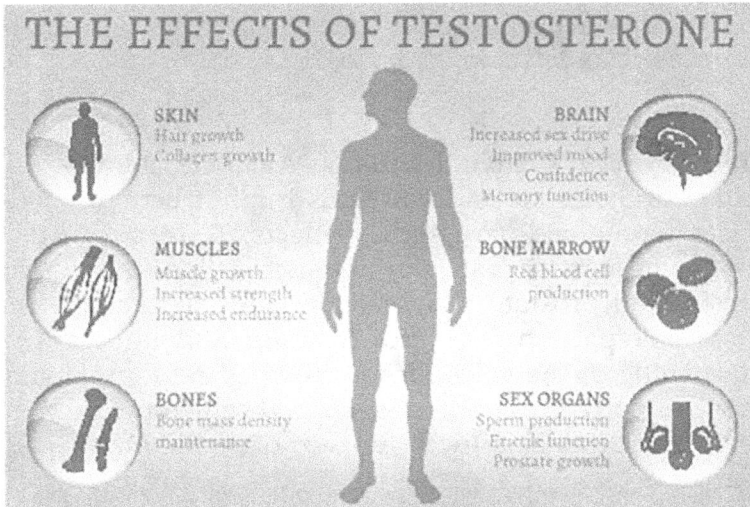

Figure 2-4: Testosterone affects a variety of tissues and organs. Source: Shutterstock.

Testosterone and Aging: Testosterone levels begin to deteriorate at about age 30— particularly the biologically active free testosterone (Figure 2-5). By age 50, free testosterone may be 50 percent of what it was at age 25. This decrease leads to decreased muscle mass and strength, abdominal obesity, poor sexual performance, cardiovascular disease, and depression (Bhasin, et al., 2021).

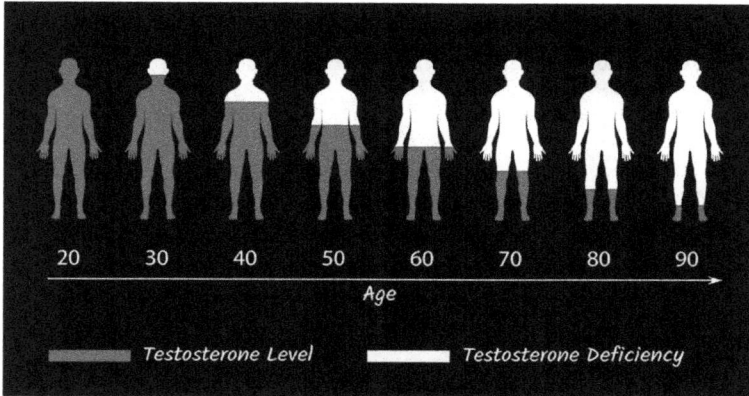

Figure 2-5: Decreases in testosterone with age in men. Some men have substantial decreases in testosterone by age 30-40 yr., which can contribute to heart disease, muscle weakness, loss of muscle and bone mass, depression, insulin resistance, and decreased longevity. The link between decreased testosterone levels and poor health has resulted in widespread testosterone supplementation in aging men. Source: Shutterstock.

Testosterone Replacement Therapy: Prescriptions for testosterone in middle-aged and older men have increased over 500 percent in the past ten years. Testosterone replacement therapy (TRT) causes impressive improvements in strength, physical and sexual performance, and well-being (Bhasin, et al., 1996). Some experts fear that the possible adverse effects of TRT on health may exceed the benefits. Physicians should monitor patients for sleep apnea, acne, gynecomastia (breast development), blood fat changes, increased red blood cell concentration, prostate enlargement, and testicular shrinkage. TRT is in its infancy. Until recently, hormone replacement was nearly standard in post-menopausal females until extensive clinical studies showed increased heart attack and stroke risk.

Scientists need to conduct similar trials in males before they can recommend TRT universally.

Summary

A steroid is an organic chemical containing 17 carbon atoms arranged in four-fused rings. They occur widely in nature in plants, animals, yeasts, and molds. Cholesterol, the most abundant steroid in humans, serves as a precursor for the steroid hormones testosterone, estrogens, and corticosteroids. Anabolic steroids include testosterone and synthetic drugs structurally like testosterone and have similar effects. Anabolic steroids increase muscle strength, power, and size, but they have biological effects on the heart, skin, bones, bone marrow, sex organs, and central nervous system. They bind to specific cell receptors, which influences protein synthesis controlled in the cell nuclei.

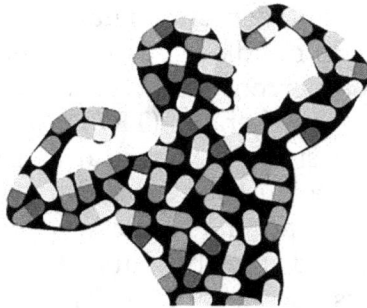

3

HOW ANABOLIC STEROIDS WORK IN THE BODY

A thletes mainly take anabolic steroids to increase muscle mass and strength, but they positively affect most human performance aspects. These elements include muscle capacity (e.g., muscle size, strength, power), motor control (e.g., skill development), recovery from training, training intensity, and psychological aggressiveness. Many personal trainers and strength coaches emphasize muscle function and neglect other critical factors determining success. They should understand these factors—even when their clients do not use anabolic steroids.

Anabolic Steroids Promote Muscle Protein Synthesis

Anabolic steroids promote muscle protein synthesis by influencing genes in the cell nuclei (Fig. 3-1). Protein synthesis is mainly controlled by the muscle cell nuclei containing genetic material called deoxyribonucleic acid (DNA).

THE GENE IS A UNIT OF HEREDITY

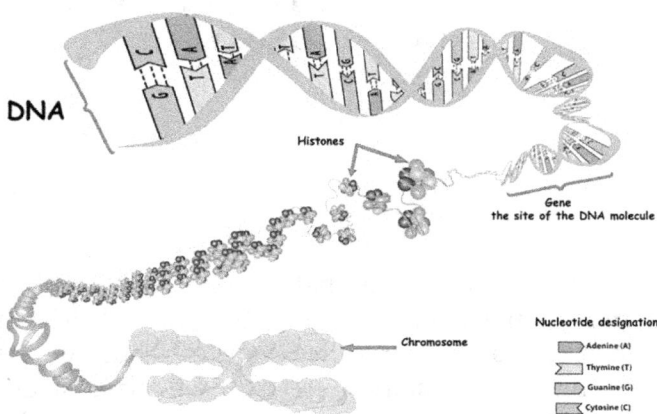

Figure 3-1: The general structure of genes. Chromosomes are long strands of DNA subdivided into genes. Genes are shorter strands of DNA containing precise codes represented by combinations of the nucleotides G, C, A, and T. The nucleotide uracil (U) substitutes for thiamine later in protein synthesis. Combinations of these nucleotides organize amino acids in precise order to make specific proteins. Source: Shutterstock.

Skeletal muscle cells have many nuclei, increasing further through training and stimulation by testosterone and other anabolic hormones. Muscle represents the body's most extensive protein-based tissue. Muscle proteins are constructed continuously and degraded to amino acids, proteins' essential building blocks. Muscle destruction appears metabolically wasteful, but it serves the vital function of tissue quality control, eliminating or repairing damaged tissues, and allowing muscles to operate at peak levels. Amino acids released during protein breakdown can be converted to glucose (blood sugar) through gluconeogenesis in the liver to fuel exercise, and help to maintain desirable circulating blood glucose levels.

Cell Nucleus: The cell nucleus contains 23 chromosome pairs— 22 chromosomes plus a sex chromosome pair— containing long DNA chains. DNA chemical codes serve as blueprints for all aspects of cell function. Smaller chromosome segments called genes have codes that carry out specific biochemical tasks such as making contractile proteins and regulating metabolism. These codes are sequences of nucleotides: guanine (G), cytosine(C), adenine (A), and thymine (T). The nucleotide uracil (U) substitutes for thiamine outside the nucleus.

Genes Control Phenotypes: The genes contain different nucleotide combinations that serve as codes to organize amino acids into specific proteins. Genes control phenotypes (characteristics) such as height, eye and hair color, or enzyme or hormone production. Slight variances in gene sequences called alleles or polymorphisms account for individual phenotype differences in strength, endurance, and body composition.

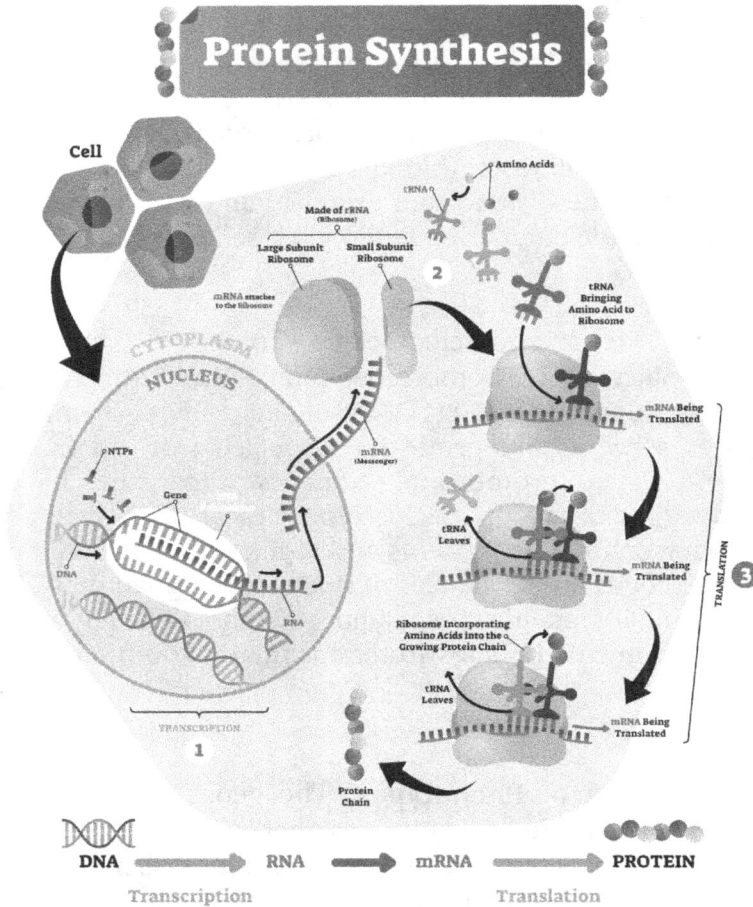

Figure 3-2: Basic mechanisms of protein synthesis. Source: Shutterstock.

Genes and Protein Synthesis: Figure 3-2 summarizes protein synthesis. Protein synthesis involves transcription and translation, which takes the codes for protein structure from the nucleus and arranges the amino acids in a precise order to make new proteins. The process begins with transcription— copying information from the DNA in specific genes to ribonucleic acid (RNA). The RNA blueprint called messenger RNA (mRNA) travels to cell structures outside the nucleus called ribosomes, small particles throughout the cytoplasm ("cell interior") that serve as protein-making factories. Each muscle cell contains roughly 10 million ribosomes.

The next step in protein synthesis is translation— the cell uses information from the mRNA to produce protein, which begins when an mRNA in the cytoplasm attaches to a ribosome. Nucleotides are subdivided into codons— three different nucleotides coded to line up with a specific amino acid. As each codon in the mRNA moves through the ribosome, the proper amino acid is brought into the ribosome by tRNA. In the ribosome, the amino acid transfers to building peptides (amino acid combinations) and proteins (long amino acids chains). This process continues until the ribosome reaches one of the three stop codons resulting in a complete polypeptide or protein.

Androgen Receptors and Protein Synthesis

Androgens (testosterone and other anabolic steroids)

bind to receptors in the cells, which triggers protein synthesis in the cell nuclei. Steroid hormones work

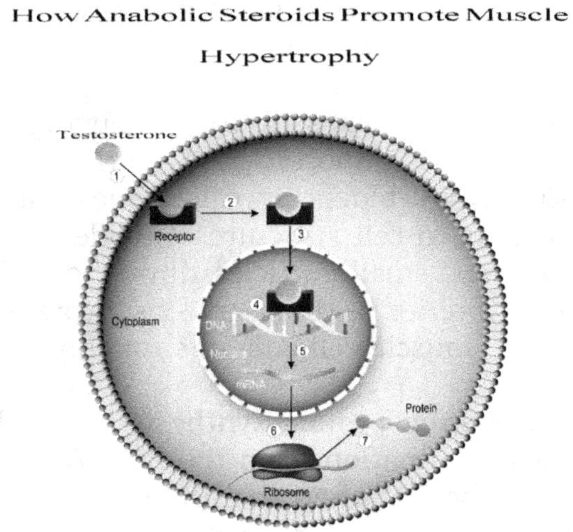
How Anabolic Steroids Promote Muscle Hypertrophy
Testosterone
Receptor
Cytoplasm
Protein
Ribosome

Figure 3-3: The influence of testosterone and the androgen receptor on protein synthesis. Source: Shutterstock.

by binding to receptor molecules to activate specific genes to synthesize proteins (Figure 3-3). Figure 3-3b shows a micrograph of an androgen receptor.

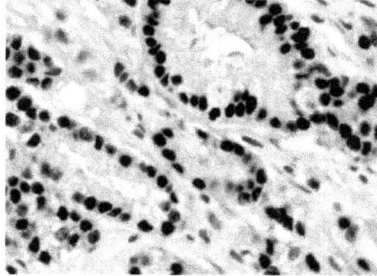

Figure 3-3b: Micrograph of an androgen receptor: The androgen receptor is activated by binding with testosterone or dihydrotestosterone and influences DNA to trigger gene activity such as promoting muscle hypertrophy, stimulating sex drive, or developing primary and secondary sexual characteristics. In females, the androgen receptor influences sexual function and psychological behavior. The receptor also affects nerve function, which helps explain why anabolic steroids improve performance in power sports. Source: Shutterstock.

This process works much like a lock and key. The key— the anabolic steroid— binds with a testosterone receptor— the lock, which begins a process to make new proteins. The result depends on the target cell. In muscle, steroids stimulate hypertrophy. In skin, they boost oil production and stimulate hair follicle growth, and so on. Anabolic steroids increase muscle growth factor (e.g., IGF-1) production, important for increasing muscle size.

Structural differences in synthetic anabolic steroids affect their binding affinities to the androgen receptors, influencing their anabolic (tissue building) and androgenic (sex-linked) effects. Slight structural differences are the rationale for steroid stacking— the simultaneous use of more than one type of anabolic steroid. Nandrolone and metenolone have a higher receptor binding affinity than testosterone, while stanozolol, methandienone, and fluoxymesterone have lower binding affinities (Bhasin, et al., 2021).

Muscle Hypertrophy: Large steroid doses promote muscle hypertrophy even without weight training (Bhasin et al., 1996). Combining steroids and high-intensity training magnifies the gains. Most research studies confirm that steroids work best in experienced weightlifters who use heavy weights and produce high muscle tension during exercise (Yu, et al., 2014). The effectiveness of anabolic steroids depends upon *unbound* receptor sites in muscle. Intense strength training increases the number of unbound receptor sites (Gustafsson, et al., 1984; Janne, et al., 1990; Vicencio, et al., 2014). More receptor sites make anabolic steroids more effective. Diets high in protein and calories can also increase anabolic steroids' effectiveness (Tamaki, et al. 2001; Rogozkin, 1979).

Anabolic Steroids Stimulate mTOR

While the nucleus directs most protein synthesis, a biochemical pathway in the cytoplasm (cell space outside the nucleus) called the mammalian target of rapamycin (mTOR) also regulates translation and repairs damaged tissues. Translation aligns amino acids on the ribosomes to produce new proteins. Anabolic steroids activate mTOR, which functions inside and outside the nucleus to promote protein synthesis (Jiang, 2010).

Factor Affecting mTOR

Exercise and Muscle Tension	Anabolic Steroids, Growth Factors, IGF-1, Insulin	Nutrients, branched chain amino acids, Calories

∨

mTOR Pathway in Cell cytoplasm

∨

Translation of Proteins on Ribosmes

∨

*Purpose: Cell Survival,
Cell Growth, Ion Channel Control, Cell Repair,
Nerve Cell Growth, and Repair*

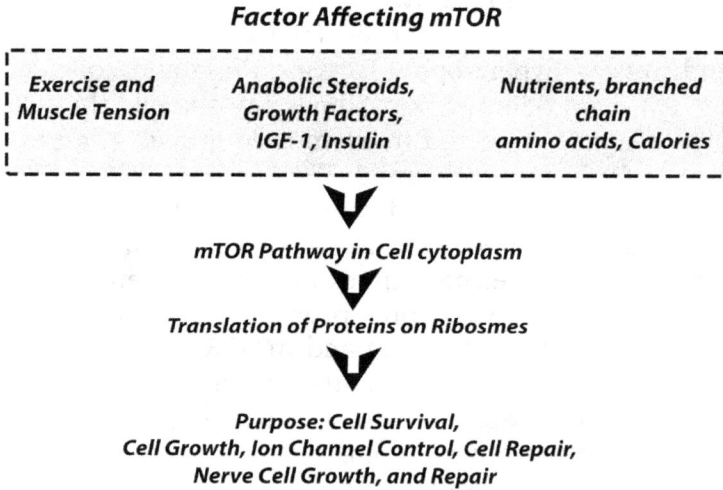

Figure 3-4: Factors affecting mTOR and their effects on protein synthesis.

Testosterone converts to dihydrotestosterone (DHT), which stimulates the mTOR pathway in the muscle cell to directly manufacture muscle proteins (Figure 3-4). In muscle cells, muscle tension, DHT, nutrients, insulin, and other muscle growth factors activates mTOR. This action is significantly faster than gene stimulation. DHT is a powerful testosterone metabolite synthesized in the prostate gland, testes, and hair follicles. DHT promotes amino acid uptake in fast and slow twitch muscle fibers and increases amino acid transporter activity. Testosterone is converted to DHT, which stimulates mTOR and promotes muscle hypertrophy.

· · ·

An Important Link: Two noteworthy studies support the link among testosterone (anabolic steroids), DHT, and muscle hypertrophy. Fanxing Zeng and colleagues (2017) from Beijing Sport University showed that DHT plus exercise triggered more muscle growth than exercise or DHT alone (Figure 3-5).

Basualto-Alarcon and co-workers (2013) from the University of Chile in Santiago conducted a molecular biology gene-altering "knockout" experiment demonstrating that testosterone promoted hypertrophy via androgen receptor binding and mTOR pathway stimulation. Knockout experiments measure the effect of blocking key steps in metabolism and measuring the effects on alternative factors.

They administered testosterone but blocked protein synthesis in the nucleus. The muscle fibers hypertrophied when given DHT, which showed that anabolic steroids also hypertrophy muscle (increase muscle size) via the mTOR pathway.

Exercise + DHT Increases Muscle Mass More Than Exercise and DHT Alone
Wet Muscle Mass (g)

Sedentary
1.95± 0.20

Sedentary + DHT
2.01±0.12

Exercise
1.99±0.09

Exercise + DHT
2.08±0.13

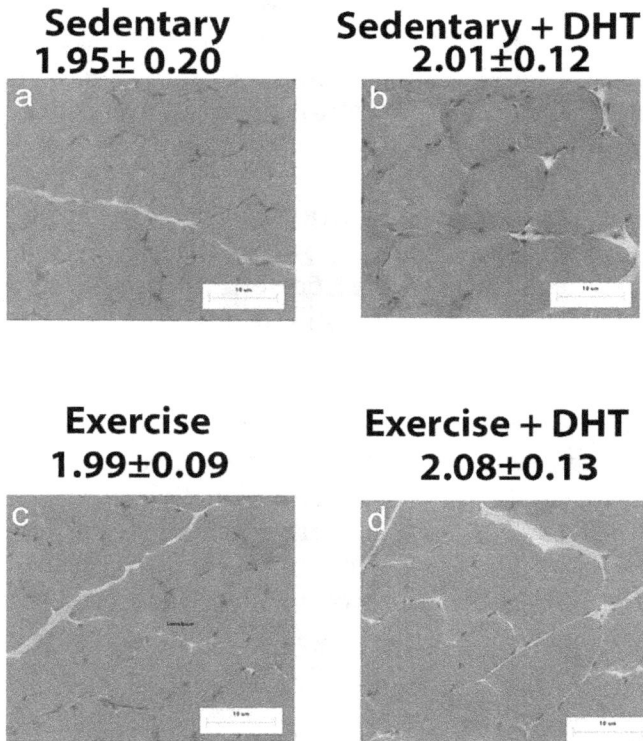

Figure 3-5: Source: Modified from Zeng, et al, 2017.

39

THOMAS D FAHEY & FRANK I KATCH

Factors Affecting Muscle Hypertrophy

Muscle protein synthesis and growth occur best when athletes consider all the elements for optimal adaptations to training. These include levels of anabolic hormones (e.g., testosterone, growth hormone, IGF-1, insulin), resistive exercise, the balance between anabolic and catabolic hormones, protein and increased total caloric intake, mTOR-triggering amino acid consumption (e.g., leucine), rest between workouts, and sleep.

Testosterone and growth hormone trigger the production of the muscle growth factor IGF-1. Testosterone and IGF-1 are powerful combinations to promote muscle hypertrophy. Testosterone and growth hormone work together to cause muscle growth. Muscle protein synthesis and growth are complicated and depend on intricate processes involving hormones, genes, and enzymes. Athletes are naïve to think that training, diet, supplements, or anabolic drug use by themselves will magically trigger muscle growth. The interaction of testosterone and growth hormone is essential to optimize protein synthesis and muscle growth.

Leucine and Other Branched-Chain Amino Acids (BCAA): BCAAs stimulate mTOR to promote muscle hypertrophy (Pedroso, 2015), which is essential information for drug-free athletes. Leucine is an amino acid that serves as a protein building block. It is also an important regulator in tissue repair, energy metabolism, and blood glucose control. Protein mixtures containing large amounts of leucine boost muscle hypertrophy.

Leucine regulates protein synthesis via mTOR. Stimulating mTOR with leucine regulates energy balance and food intake, which affects muscle mass and body composition. Protein supplements high in leucine (e.g., 5 g/day) influence protein synthesis in muscle, fat, liver, heart, kidneys, and pancreas. Leucine is a branched-chain amino acid (BCAA) that also includes isoleucine and valine. While leucine triggers protein synthesis by itself, it is more effective to promote muscle growth in the presence of other BCAAs.

Anabolic Steroids Increase Muscle Satellite Cells

The muscle cell's nucleus is the center of protein synthesis, but nuclei have difficulty servicing muscle cells as they grow larger. Fortunately, muscle cell nuclei increase in number as the cells grow. Skeletal muscle cells are elongated or tubular structures with nuclei on the outside part of the cells. As muscles hypertrophy (grow), they add nuclei to service the needs of the muscle cells. They do this through nuclear accretion, a cell process that balances muscle cell nuclei with cytoplasmic volume (Figures 3-6, 3-7, 3-8).

Satellite Cells: Part of muscle cell growth involves activating satellite cells—stem cells that contain only a single nucleus that can form new contractile tissue. These satellite cells furnish new nuclei as the muscle increases in size. When stimulated by testosterone or exercise, these new nuclei form myoblasts, and then myotubes, which are integrated into existing muscle fibers and increase their size.

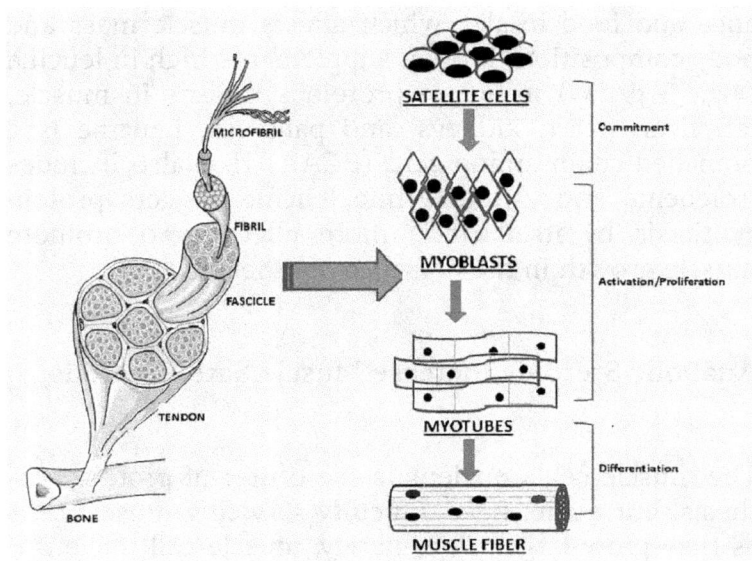

Figure 3-6: Muscles hypertrophy by integrating satellite cells into muscle cells. This process adds additional nuclei to cells, which further enhances their capacity for muscle hypertrophy and increasing muscle strength. Source: Shutterstock.

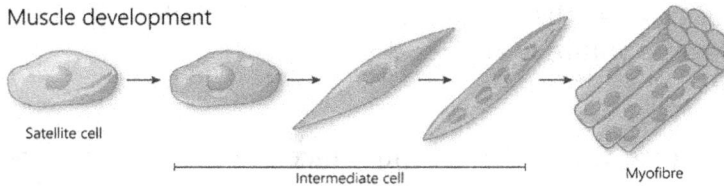

Figure 3-7: Integration of satellite cells into muscle. Source: Shutterstock.

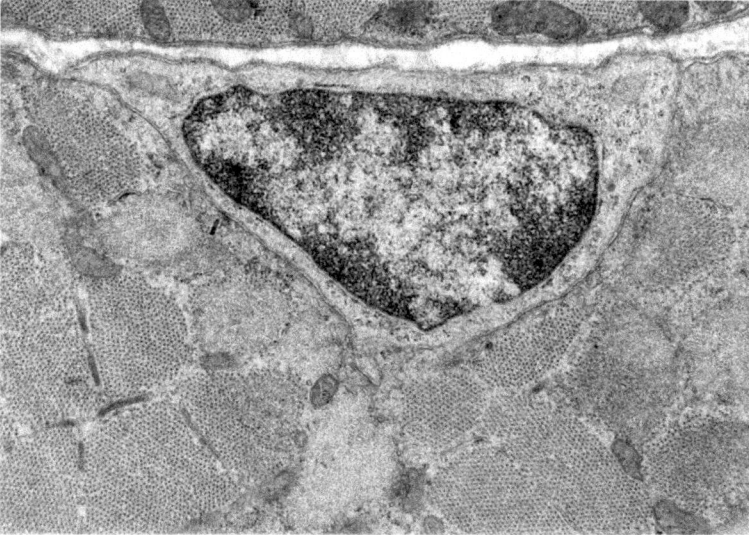

Figure 3-8: Micrograph of satellite cell. Source: Shutterstock.

Muscles hypertrophy in response to small injuries triggered by overload (e.g., weight training, sprinting, distance running). Satellite cells, stem cells that lie next to skeletal muscle fibers, are activated to help the fibers grow, repair, and regenerate Figure 3-9). The satellite cells are integrated into the muscle, forming new muscle cell nuclei. New satellite cells increase muscle size and enhance the fibers' capacity for protein synthesis. Factors affecting muscle hypertrophy include the anabolic hormones testosterone, growth hormone, insulin-like growth factor-1, and insulin; calories, protein, key amino acids (e.g., leucine), muscle overload, and rest intervals between workouts.

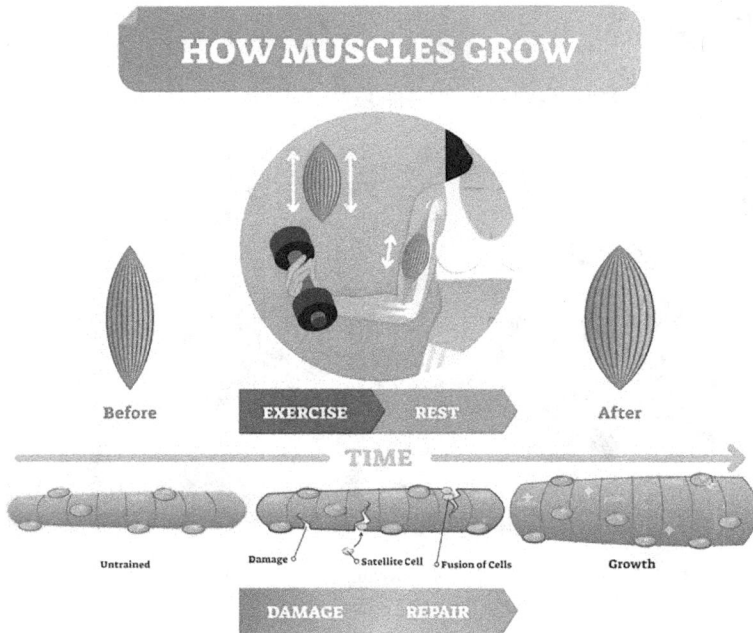

Figure 3-9: Muscle tension, particularly during eccentric (lengthening) contractions, trigger micro-injuries, stimulating satellite cell activation and muscle hypertrophy. Source: Shutterstock

Muscle growth factors can cause the satellite cells to combine with muscle cells stressed or damaged during training to assist in cell repair and adaptation. Anabolic steroids, combined with weight training, trigger muscle hypertrophy, increase satellite cells and muscle cell nuclei, and alter satellite cell structures. Factors associated with increased satellite cell activity include exercise stress, anabolic hormones such as testosterone, growth hormone, IGF-1, and linear growth. Satellite cells integrate into muscle following training-induced tissue damage, triggering muscle hypertrophy.

Muscle Memory: Anabolic steroids enhance cellular muscle memory that persists long after exposure to the drugs and intense training. Previous strength training —with or without anabolic steroids— makes it easier to regain strength or muscle mass when training resumes.

Anabolic Steroids Activate Satellite Cells

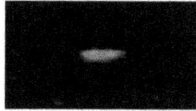

Sedentary/ Drug-Free

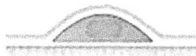

Trained/ Anabolic Steroids

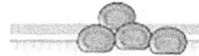

Inactive Satellite Cells

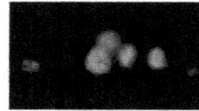

Activated Satellite Cells

Figure 3-10: Intense training and anabolic steroids activate dormant satellite cells that promote muscle hypertrophy, The activated satellite cells persist for years after active training or anabolic steroid consumption, which provides long-term advantages and makes it easier to regain strength and power after reconditioning. Source: Modified from Dumont, et al. , 2015.

Figure 3-10 shows how activated dormant satellite cells migrate to the cells' surface for integration into existing muscle fibers and increase active cell nuclei (Dumont et al., 2015). Satellite cells are in proximity to mature muscle fibers in a dormant state.

Upon activation by intense exercise or testosterone, satellite cells enter the muscle media and form new myofibers. When stimulated by testosterone or training, they form myoblasts, and then myotubes, which are integrated into existing muscle fibers, increasing their size.

Satellite Cell Benefits: Accumulating new satellite cells improves the capacity for protein synthesis and adding muscle—changes that might last a lifetime. For example, it may take three to five years for a young athlete to bench press 300 pounds, simultaneously building active satellite cells from the heavy training required to lift that much weight. He will lose strength when training stops.

But, he has a secret weapon when training resumes. Strength levels will regain more quickly by resuming training because the satellite cells will still remain operational! Instead of taking five years to bench press 300 pounds, the strength level might restore after only a few months. These effects are similar in males and females.

Egner, et al. (2013) induced large increases in muscle mass and muscle cell nuclei in mice using anabolic steroids and overload training. The drug was withdrawn, and muscle size reverted to pre-training levels, but the increase in muscle cell nuclei remained intact. Muscle size increased by 30 percent following retraining, compared to no change in control animals. Anabolic steroids have long-lasting effects on muscle tissue that could last a lifetime.

Many strength athletes and bodybuilders take anabolic steroids for short periods to boost muscle mass and cut fat. People using anabolic steroids for five to fifteen years are more muscular and less fat than equally trained people who did not use them (Yu, et al., 2014).

Swedish researchers (Yu, et al., 2014) compared long-time steroid users with equally trained nonusers using a sophisticated body composition measuring DEXA technique. Steroid users had over 20 pounds more muscle and nearly 5 pounds less fat than weight-trained non-steroid users or sedentary controls.

Steroid users also showed larger increases in lean leg mass, muscle fiber size, muscle cell nuclear density, and muscle capillary density. Anabolic steroids build strength, muscle mass, and give athletes an advantage even after they stop taking them.

Animal studies reported similar results. In mice, injecting steroids (testosterone propionate for 14 days) increased muscle cell nuclei by 66 percent and muscle fiber area by 77 percent (Egner, et al., 2013). The number of nuclei remained elevated even three months after steroid supplementation. Following a three-month layoff from training, muscle mass increased by 31 percent within six days, while control animals did not grow. With renewed training, muscle cell memory allows them to regain mass rapidly.

Steroids provide a long-term advantage, which might be a consideration when punishing athletes for doping violations. Mice only live for about two years, so it is difficult to generalize the results to humans.

. . .

Previous Anabolic Steroid Users

Previous anabolic steroid use gives users a profound advantage in sport. The Olympics at Rio de Janeiro set the record for the number of athletes competing with previously sanctioned for drug offenses. The older athletes won 35 of the 974 medals awarded. The number of athletes with positive drug results was undoubtedly underreported because of lax doping control procedures in many countries (Figure 3-11).

Approximately a third of the competing countries entered athletes banned for doping offenses. Russia entered six athletes who failed drug tests or implicated in the Olympic Committee's doping investigation of Russia.

The doping problem is not a matter of "forgive and forget." Suspensions for anabolic steroid violations range from two years to life. WADA reinstates many athletes following their first or second offense. This might not be enough.

Anabolic steroids' long-lasting effects persist many years after the athletes stop taking them, provided they continue to train hard. These drugs increase hormone receptor sites and muscle satellite cells that give an advantage for a lifetime.

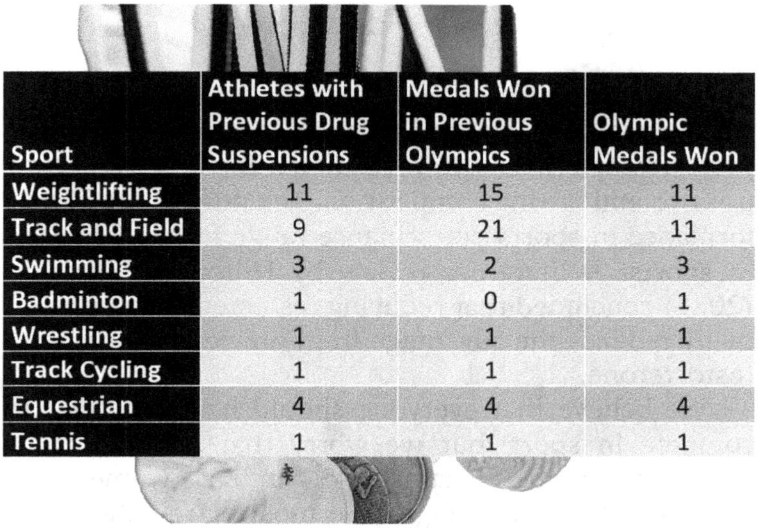

Sport	Athletes with Previous Drug Suspensions	Medals Won in Previous Olympics	Olympic Medals Won
Weightlifting	11	15	11
Track and Field	9	21	11
Swimming	3	2	3
Badminton	1	0	1
Wrestling	1	1	1
Track Cycling	1	1	1
Equestrian	4	4	4
Tennis	1	1	1

Figure 3-11 Reinstated athletes who previously received suspensions for anabolic steroid use performed exceptionally well at the Rio de Janeiro Olympics. Source: Produced from data published in The New York Times, Aug. 18, 2016.

Anabolic steroids plus intense weight training stimulate satellite cell formation. Satellite cells are integrated into muscle cells, making them bigger and stronger. They enhance the capacity for muscle protein synthesis. These effects remain after the person stops taking anabolic steroids.

Transexual Athletes: A related factor is the participation of trans women in women's competitions. Previous exposure of cells to testosterone— with or without anabolic steroids provides long-term increases in androgen receptor sites, myelin, and muscle satellite cells, even in athletes with suppressed testosterone levels.

The International Olympic Committee ruled that transgender women may compete as men if they suppress testosterone below 10 mol/L for at least 12 mo prior to and during competition. Sex differences in performance in sports performance range from 10 to 50% in sports. A literature review by Hilton & Lundberg (2021) concluded that reducing testosterone only minimally reduces the advantage from previous exposure to testosterone.

We believe that everyone should have the right to compete in sport, but we worry that allowing trans women to compete against CIS gendered women provides an unfair advantage. The most extreme example is Caitlyn Jenner. When she competed in Montreal's men's decathlon, Jenner ran the 400 meters in 47.51 seconds. Marita Koch from the German Democratic Republic (GDR— East Germany) holds the women's record at 47.60 seconds set in 1985. While Koch never tested positive for steroids, documents from coaching training diaries from the GDR implicate her. Jenner was a decathlete and not a 400-meter specialist. Proponents for full inclusion claim that trans-women are bullied in school, and preventing participation traumatizes them further.

Genetic Advantages in Sport: For the past 15 years, co-author Fahey collaborated in sports genetics studies with researchers from the University of Puerto Rico Medical School led by Dr. Miguel Rivera. These studies show that winning runners have genetic advantages over less successful athletes.

Finnish cross-country skier Eero Mäntyranta won two gold medals in cross-country skiing in the 1964 Winter Olympics. Later evidence showed he had a genetic mutation that greatly improved his oxygen carrying capacity. The famous exercise scientist Per Olaf Åstrand (deceased) once said, "If you want to be an Olympic gold medalist, choose your parents carefully." Trans athletes also have varied genes, so perhaps should not be singled out when the standards are not applied equally.

Anti-Catabolic Effects

Most athletes comment that steroids help them train harder and recover faster. They also have difficulty making progress or maintaining the gains when they stopped drug use. Anabolic steroids may have anti-catabolic effects, so the drugs may reduce post-exercise muscle breakdown and inflammation that accompanies intense exercise training. These effects include decreases in glucocorticoid receptor expression, glucocorticoid-induced muscle breakdown, and IGF-1 suppression prevention (Bhasin, et al., 2021). In this regard, IGF-1 is an important anabolic hormone.

Corticosteroids and Intense Training: During intense exercise, the adrenal glands release the glucocorticoid (GC) cortisol (C). C has beneficial actions during exercise: it degrades amino acids, helps maintain blood glucose (sugar) through gluconeogenesis in the liver; maintains normal vascular integrity and responsiveness; and protects the body from an overreaction of the immune system triggered by exercise-induced muscle damage (Duclos, et al., 2003).

Intense exercise is traumatic. It creates muscle damage, inflammation, and releases reactive oxygen species (He, et al. 2016), delaying recovery and slowing training gains. The hormonal profile ideally progresses from catabolic processes (breakdown) to anabolic processes (positive adaptation) during recovery. After intense exercise, corticosteroids remain elevated, slowing recovery, muscle hypertrophy, and strength and power (Duclos et al., 2003).

Anabolic steroids may partially block the effects of cortisol involved in tissue breakdown during and after exercise (Parr and Muller-Scholl, 2017). Anabolic steroids may prevent tissue destruction following intense workouts, which speeds recovery. Cortisol and related hormones, secreted by the adrenal cortex, also have receptor sites within skeletal muscle cells.

Anabolic steroids may block cortisol binding to its receptor sites, preventing muscle breakdown and enhancing recovery (Genazzani, et al., 2006; Rubinow, et al., 2005; Place, 2000; Isaacson, et al., 1993). While this is beneficial when athletes take the drugs, the effect backfires when they stop taking them. Hormonal adaptations occur in response to the abnormally high androgen levels present in the athlete's body. Increases occur in cortisol receptor sites and cortisol secretion from the adrenal cortex.

Chronic corticosteroid suppression is not beneficial. Extreme overtraining triggers corticosteroid insufficiency, with symptoms similar to Addison's disease (chronic fatigue, weakness, low blood pressure, weight loss) (Lehmann, et al., 1998). Anabolic steroids affect corticosteroid metabolism and training intensity, which might subject intensely training athletes taking anabolic steroids to severe overtraining.

Anabolic steroids interfere with the body's natural testosterone production. People who stop taking anabolic steroids have less testosterone than usual during the "off" periods. Cortisol's catabolic effects increase when the athlete stops taking the drugs, and they rapidly lose strength and muscle size.

Inflammation: Inflammation is the body's response to tissue and cell damage from injury, high blood pressure, intense exercise, air pollution, cigarette smoke, or poor metabolic health from abnormal blood lipids (fats) and poor blood glucose control. Acute inflammation is a short-term response to exercise and an important way the body improves physical fitness. For example, short-term inflammation triggers increased muscle protein synthesis that promotes muscle fitness and recovery from exercise. In contrast, chronic inflammation is a prolonged, abnormal process that causes tissue breakdown and diseases like atherosclerosis, glucocorticoid suppression, some cancers, and rheumatoid arthritis.

Exercise increases acute inflammation during and shortly after a workout, but it reduces chronic inflammation—if the training program is not too severe. For example, practicing endurance training three to five days weekly will reduce inflammation. Training excessively by running a marathon several times a month or doing strenuous cross-training workouts five to seven days per week, causes overtraining and chronic inflammation. We refer to this as the "Goldilocks effect":

training should not be too little or too much but just right.

The rebound effect of cortisol and its receptors present anabolic steroid-users with several serious problems:

1. Psychological addiction is more probable because they become dependent on the drugs because they lose strength and size rapidly when off steroids. To stave off deconditioning, athletes sometimes take the drugs for long periods to prevent falling behind.
2. Long-term administration increases the chance of severe side effects.
3. Cortisol suppresses the immune system, which makes steroid users more prone to diseases and colds and flu during the period immediately following steroid administration.

Many athletes combat a cortisol effect by never going off the drugs. Athletes cycle on and off steroids because they believe the receptors "down-regulate" to reduce drug sensitivity. Some people think that if the dosage is high enough, the receptors do not lose sensitivity and training gains will occur continuously. While it is difficult to prove this hypothesis, the incredible size of modern-day bodybuilders who purportedly stay on anabolic steroids continuously would support this position.

Metabolic Effects

Anabolic steroids have metabolic effects that help boost performance. They increase cell sensitivity to insulin and leptin, which enhances carbohydrate, fat, and protein metabolism. They increase glycogen synthesis and storage critical for intense exercise. They increase lactate transporters MCT1 and MCT4 to improve lactate clearance and its use as a fuel (Bhasin, et al., 2021).

Psychological Effects

Much is said about psychological side effects from anabolic steroids—"roid rage," psychosis, drug dependence, and paranoia. Some psychological effects might improve performance. Anabolic steroids increase aggressiveness and training intensity.

Steroid High and Aggressiveness: Some researchers believe steroids work by making athletes feel better and more aggressive. The improved sense of well-being and euphoria, and increased tolerance to stress, allows athletes to train harder.

The "steroid high," if it exists, helps experienced athletes more than novices because they know how to push themselves harder in practice and competition. Many studies show that anabolic steroids increase aggressiveness (Bronson, et al., 1996; Pagonis, et al., 2006), but no research has demonstrated this is responsible for improved performance or increased training intensity.

The balance between testosterone and corticosteroids partially controls dominance and aggressiveness on the playing field. High cortisol levels are linked to reduced competitiveness, dominance, and social defeat (Mehta, et al., 2010). Anabolic steroids suppress corticosteroids during exercise and recovery, which increases competitive aggressiveness, which might provide an advantage during competition and training. Increased aggression might cause greater performance intensity, but it is unclear if this is beneficial during competition. Reduced corticosteroids might give athletes the psychological capacity to train harder, which is beneficial—provided athletes avoid overuse injuries.

Most studies on the psychiatric or psychological effects of anabolic steroids examine the drugs' pathological effects. Increased aggressiveness might benefit athletes such as weightlifters or shot putters, yet interfere with performance in a football quarterback, golfer, or tennis player where judgment is more critical.

Neural Effects

The central nervous system comprises the brain and spinal cord. The body contains over 7 trillion nerves. They form nervous pathways that control movement. These carry instructions to the muscles to perform movements like swinging a golf club or running a complex football pass route.

Anabolic steroids might enhance neural control of movement. Motor control regulates movement by the nervous system and involves nerve tracts that activate muscles to perform the movement. External stimuli, such as performance anxiety when shooting a free throw in basketball, impacts reflex motor control. Harnessing motor control to train the nervous system is the secret of building powerful movements on the playing field.

Specificity and Neural Programming

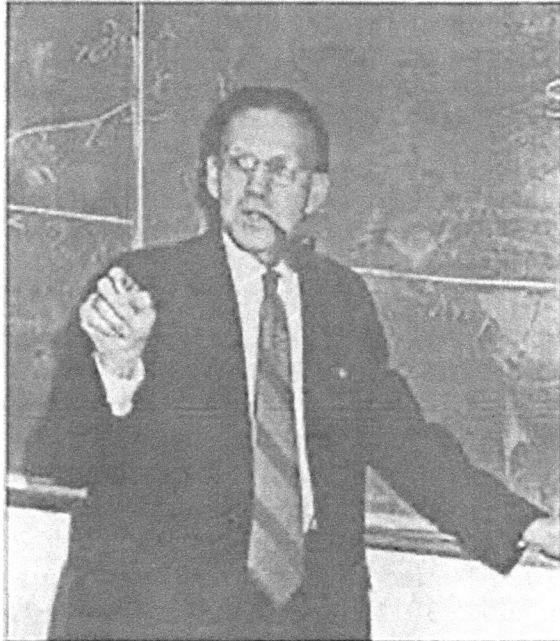

Figure 3-11: Franklin Henry, University of California, Berkeley

In 1960, Dr. Franklin Henry, from the University of

California, Berkeley (Figure 3-12), introduced the concept of motor programming and specificity as the basis to perform and improve skills. His work, called the "memory drum" theory of neuromotor reaction (Henry & Rogers, 1960), found that skilled movements such as the golf swing or throwing the discus are imprinted in the nervous system and "played back"— like a reflex — with repeated practice. Repeated practice on the driving range develops a "computer program" in the brain that can playback like a reflex on the course. The nonconscious motor pattern gets stronger with practice.

Sports skills are highly specific. The forehand in tennis, for example, is a different skill than hitting a baseball. Practicing one will not develop skill in the other. Performing skills slowly is not the same as performing them at full speed. Skilled movements represent precise motor pathway development.

Henry's theory was impossible to show experimentally— until recently. Advances in brain research showed that skill training (e.g., practicing the golf swing) builds and reinforces nerve tracts that control motor skills by laying down myelin along the nerve fibers (Figure 3-12). Myelin is a fatty substance that covers nerve cells and promotes nerve impulse speed. From the University of British Columbia in Vancouver, Canada, Boyd and colleagues showed that people improve skilled movements by increasing the myelin content of nerve tracts used to perform movements (Lakhani, et al., 2016).

Steroids' neural effects are under-appreciated and under-studied by scientists. Growth hormone has anabolic effects more significant than anabolic steroids, yet anabolic steroids remain the drugs of choice for power athletes. In the 1970s, several studies by Ariel (1972,

1973, 1974) showed that steroids enhanced neural activation. Steroids affect nerve cell's protein metabolism essential for nerve-cell survival, function, and nerve impulse transmission.

Neural Activation and Elite Sports Performance: Maximizing neural function is critical for sports performance. The motor unit, composed of a motor nerve and connecting muscle fibers, is the basic nervous structure that translates the intention to move and perform sports movements into muscle contractions that cause them (Figure 3-12). The nerve cell body— the axon— connects to the dendrite, which binds to individual muscle cells. Practice, training, and anabolic steroids enhance the myelin sheath to speed neural conduction.

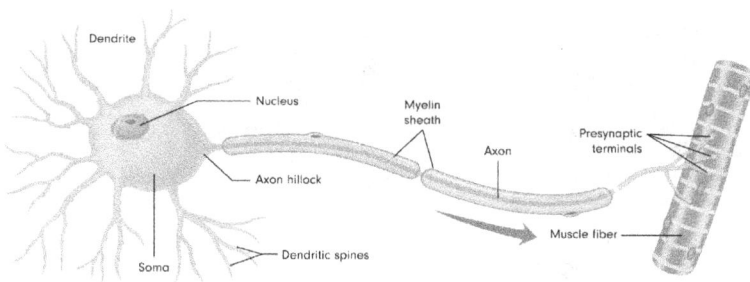

Figure 3-12: Motor nerve showing the myelin sheath, which promotes the neural conduction speed. Anabolic steroids promote myelin growth, which increases strength, power, and skill. These are long-term changes, which provide anabolic steroid users with extended advantages. Source: Shutterstock.

Anabolic steroids stimulate nerve growth in healthy

and injured subjects. Their most important effect is to increase the myelinated fiber diameter and myelin sheath thickness via oligodendrocytes (Figure 3-13). Anabolic steroids stimulate oligodendrocytes, which produce myelin— the covering of nerve cells that speed the rate of nerve impulses in the central and peripheral nervous systems.

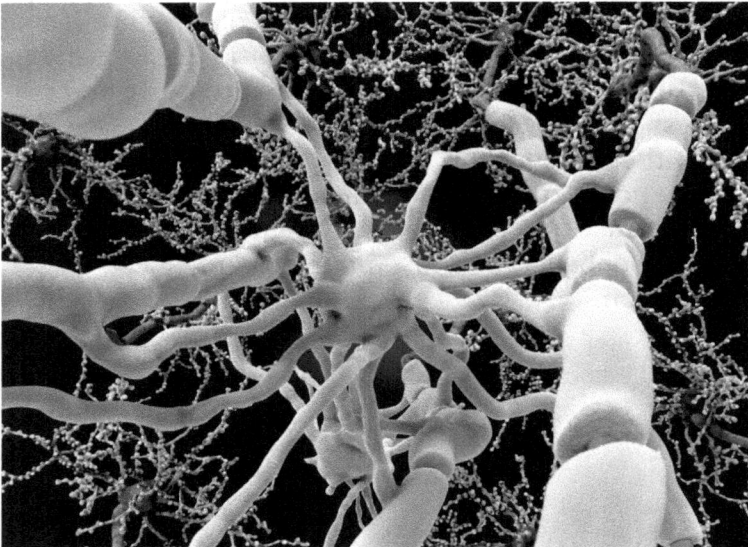

Figure 3-13: Testosterone and other anabolic steroids stimulate oligodendrocytes to produce myelin, which improves motor control, speed, and power. This effect is the most important reason steroids improve athletic performance. Source: Shutterstock.

Learning motor skills to throw a discus or perform a snatch involves progressively increasing myelin nerve coverings to allow faster and smoother performance. Anabolic steroids combined with intense strength training increase nerve cell myelination and motor control, which is an important reason that the drugs improve performance in high power sports (Neto, et al., 2017). Anabolic steroids are therapeutically powerful drugs that promote nerve healing following trauma. Training and anabolic steroids enhance myelin formation in specific nerve tracts, which improves power and sports performance.

Practice Makes Myelin: What evidence suggests that anabolic steroids influence neural performance? In a rat study, Neto, et al. (2017) concluded that an anabolic steroid (testosterone propionate) increased myelinated fiber diameter and myelin sheath thickness. Ghizoni and co-workers (2013), also using rats, showed that nandrolone promoted functional recovery from surgically induced nerve damage, while Cree, et al. (2017) showed that anabolic steroids promoted oligodendrocyte growth following hypoxic induced brain injury. The study by Ariel and Saville (1972) and more recent studies on myelin growth show anabolic steroids profoundly affect the nervous system, which accounts for the drugs' popularity with power athletes.

Selective Androgen Receptor Modulators (SARMs)

The next generation of anabolic steroids will be selective androgen receptor modulators (SARMs) targeting androgen receptors in specific muscle or bone tissues. SARMs are the Holy Grail of anabolic drugs because they build muscle without affecting other organs or tissues. These drugs will help speed healing following traumatic injuries and invariably help athletes improve performance. SARMs include Andarine (S4), Ligandrol (LGD-4033), Ostarine (enobosarm), RAD-140 (testolone, Figure 3-4), and Yk-11 (Bhasin, et al., 2021).

Function: Current anabolic steroids (including testosterone) bind and activate androgen receptors throughout the body, and their effects are not specific to any tissue. While they turn on protein synthesis in muscle, they also bind to androgen receptors in the prostate, sex organs, heart, liver, skin, and brain, which can cause unwanted effects in these tissues.

Figure 3-14: The SARM RAD-140 targets androgen receptors in muscle. Source: Shutterstock.

General receptor binding causes acne, prostate enlargement, thickening of the blood, and masculinization in women and children. SARMs target specific androgen sites in muscles and do not bind to receptors in other tissues, minimizing side effects and improving the drug's usefulness. The synthetic testosterone trenbolone has SARM-like effects because it is highly anabolic in skeletal muscle but has minimal side effects in other tissues.

Testosterone has an anabolic to androgenic ratio of 1:1, so anabolic effects that promote muscle hypertrophy are roughly equal to sex-linked effects such as male hair growth patterns and developing secondary sexual characteristics. The SARM RAD-140 (Figure 3-14) has a ratio of 90:1 (anabolic effects are 90 times

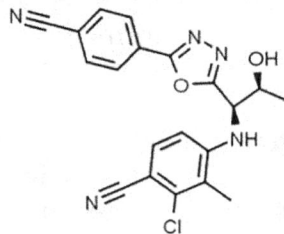

greater than androgenic effects). The World Anti-Doping Agency (WADA) bans the use of SARMs in sport.

Not Yet Approved: Endosarm (Figure 3-15) is a SARM developed by GTx, Inc. to treat muscle wasting in conditions such as cancer and

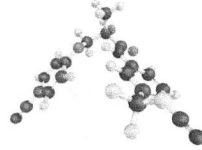

Figure 3-15: The molecular structure of Endosarm. Source: Shutterstock.

HIV, osteoporosis (loss of bone mass), and urinary incontinence (urine leaking) in women (https://www. gtxinc.com). It is undergoing phase II trials but is not approved by the Food and Drug Administration (FDA). Endosarm might increase the risk of heart attack, stroke, and liver damage. It increases lean mass, strength, power, and physical fitness (Dalton et al. 2011).

SARMs such as Endosarm are also banned by the World Anti-Doping Agency (WADA), even though the drug is not available clinically. WADA developed tests for all known SARMs. UFC fighter Sean O'Malley and Tennessee Titan offensive lineman Taylor Lewan tested positive for Endosarm in 2018 and 2019 from drugs purchased on the Internet.

Training and Muscle Hypertrophy

Anabolic steroids stimulate muscle hypertrophy—particularly when accompanied by intense training and sensible nutrition programs. They have anabolic (tissue building) and androgenic (sex-linked) effects. In boys, testosterone causes large increases in height, weight, and muscle mass during puberty and adolescence.

Anabolic and Androgenic Effects: The hormones have androgenic and anabolic effects. Androgenic effects are changes in primary and secondary sexual characteristics. These include penis and testes enlargement, voice changes, facial, underarm, and genital hair growth, and increased aggressiveness. Teenage boys' aggressive behavior is at least partly due to increased testosterone levels. Androgenic-anabolic effects include muscle, bone, and red blood cell growth and increased nerve conduction velocity.

Pharmaceutical companies make anabolic steroids to boost tissue-building properties (anabolic effects) and reduce effects on sexual tissues (androgenic effects). It is difficult to create a purely anabolic steroid —one with no sexual side effects because the androgenic effects are anabolic effects in sex-linked tissues. The effects of male hormones on accessory sex glands, genital hair growth, and skin oiliness are anabolic processes in those tissues. The steroids with the most powerful anabolic effects are also those with the most significant androgenic effects.

Females can expect considerable improvements in strength, power, speed, and muscle mass. For them, side effects reflect the hormone's normal action. Facial hair growth, increased libido, deepening of the voice, and enhanced aggressiveness are natural and desirable effects of androgen hormones in men. Such changes, however, may be unacceptable to females. The decision to take these drugs must balance the undesirable effects from increased muscle mass and power.

Summary

Athletes first used anabolic steroids in the early 1950s, and the practice has been controversial ever since. Anabolic steroids have short- and long-term effects on performance that give steroid users advantages over nonusers. Positive effects include:

- Stimulating protein synthesis by binding with androgen receptor sites on the cells and influencing the muscle cell nucleus to make more protein.
- Stimulating the mTOR pathway to make more muscle protein by a mechanism that does not involve the muscle cell nucleus.
- Promoting anti-catabolic effects, possibly involving cross-binding on corticosteroid receptor sites, which reduces corticosteroid uptake and speeds recovery and cellular adaptation processes.
- Increasing muscle satellite cells and muscle cell nuclei. Activated satellite cells persist long after discontinuing training.
- Increasing aggressiveness, which might promote training and competitive intensity.
- Increasing myelin production by the oligodendrocytes. Practice and anabolic steroids build faster and more powerful reflex motor pathways to improve performance.

4

ANABOLIC STEROIDS AND SPORTS

Anabolic steroids are synthetic variations of testosterone— a hormone produced in the male testes and the female ovaries. Testosterone is also generated indirectly from hormones produced in the adrenal glands. Athletes use anabolic steroids to gain weight, strength, power, speed, endurance, and aggressiveness. They are widely used in athletics, bodybuilding, weightlifting, and American football. Increasingly, males and females who do not play sports use steroids to improve physical appearance.

Steroids and Children: Even school-aged children use them. Studies of children world-wide found that four to eight percent of adolescents have tried the drugs, with one-quarter of them non-athletes (Buckley et al. 1988). Nicholls, et al. (2017), in a review of 52 studies involving nearly 200,000 young people age 10-21 years, concluded that almost 6 percent of boys and 5 percent of girls used anabolic steroids at least once and only half were athletes. The study noted that some children younger than ten had used the drugs. Use patterns remained steady in young athletes since the 1980s and an almost equal number of non-athletes as athletes used the drugs. Although the drugs can sometimes produce serious side effects, the lure of making rapid gains in strength, power, and muscle size makes these drugs irresistible to many athletes and active people.

Steroids and Bodybuilding: Anabolic steroids have profoundly affected bodybuilding, American football, weightlifting, baseball, and the throwing events in track and field. Steroid use is universal in elite bodybuilding.

Bodybuilding has changed dramatically during the past 120 years. Figure 4-1 shows champion bodybuilders Eugen Sandow (1901), Arnold Schwarzeneggar (1968), and Ronnie Coleman (2007). These athletes trained vigorously, yet the athletes differed greatly in body composition. We can assume that all had fat percentages below 10 percent, but Coleman outweighed Sandow by 120 pounds.

Anabolic steroids did not exist in 1900. Sandow was a serious athlete who made his living as a professional strongman and bodybuilder. Schwarzeneggar competed in the early days of anabolic steroid use. He was known for intense and dedicated training.

Steroid use was more widespread and sophisticated when Coleman competed, and athletes typically used scientifically-based nutrition programs and the anabolic drugs growth hormone and insulin. Modern athletes are much bigger and faster than before—champion bodybuilders of the past could not even qualify in current bodybuilding contests.

100 Years of Bodybuilding			
Name	Eugen Sandow	Arnold Schwarzenegger	Ronnie Coleman
Birth year	1867	1947	1964
Active years	1885-1922	1963-1980	1990-2007
Height (ft, in; cm)	5-9; 175	6-3; 191	5-11; 180
Weight (lb; kg)	190; 86.18	230; 104.33	310; 140.61
Arms (in: cm)	18; 45.72	22; 55.88	24; 60.96
Chest (in; cm)	48; 121.92	57; 144.78	58; 147.32
Waist (in; cm)	30; 76.2	30; 76.2	36; 91.44
Thighs (in; cm)	27; 68.58	28.5; 72.39	36; 91.44
Calves (in; cm)	18; 45.72	20; 50.8	22; 55.88

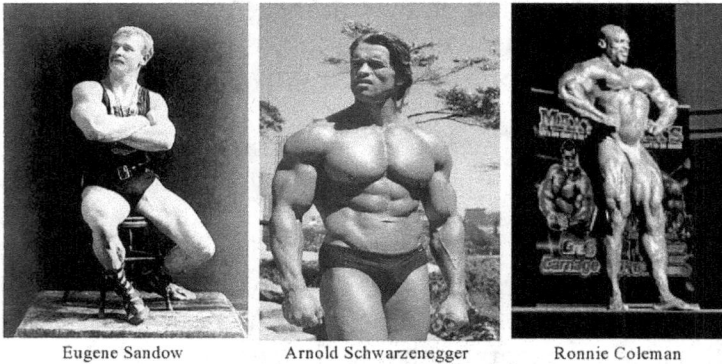

Eugene Sandow   Arnold Schwarzenegger   Ronnie Coleman

Figure 4-1: Changes in body composition in champion bodybuilders: Eugen Sandow (1901), Arnold Schwarzeneggar (1968), and Ronnie Coleman (2007). Source of photos: Wiki Commons.

1970s Discus Throwers and Shot-putters: Fahey, et al. (1979) studied elite strength athletes who competed in the 1970s. The sample included 30 elite strength athletes, including three world record holders, eight other world-class athletes, and 19 national class athletes. Average weights of discus throwers and shot-putters was 104.7 and 112.5 kg, which were comparable to professional football linemen in the 1970s. These athletes competed before anabolic steroid use was commonplace, and certainly before the high dose steroid regimens used by many athletes today.

American Football Players: In college and professional American football, 150-kg (330-lb) linemen are ordinary, while in the 1980s, NFL linemen rarely exceeded 285 pounds (Figure 4-2). Leading high school linemen average 270 pounds, and 300-pound athletes are now commonplace.

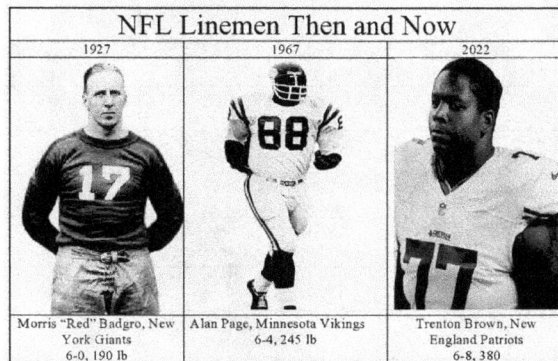

Figure 4-2: Changes in body composition of NFL Linemen since the 1920s: Moris Badro (1927), Alan Page (1967), and Trent Brown (2022). Source of photos: Wiki Commons.

Some of these athletes did not get that way through better training methods alone; they received help from taking anabolic steroids, growth hormone, and other supplements.

Table 4-1 shows notable linemen who played in the NFL between 1920 and 2020, college linemen competing in the NFL combine, and high school linemen competing in recruiting combines. Junior and senior high school linemen are as large as NFL linemen who played in the 1970s and 80s. Without casting dispersions on any athlete, elite football players' bodyweight requirements make it difficult to compete without these drugs.

Notable Linemen in the National Football League 1920-2020
NFL Combine 1999-2017
High School Recruiting Combines 2015-2016

Name	Position	Team	Years active	Height (ft-in	Weight (lb.)
George Halas	End	Decatur Staleys	1919-1929	6-0	182
Jim Otto	Center	Oakland Raiders	1960-1974	6-2	255
Anthony Muñoz	Offensive tackle	Cincinnati Bengals	1980-1993	6-6	278
Larry Allen	Guard	Dallas Cowboys	1994-2007	6-3	325
Marshall Yanda	Guard	Baltimore Ravens	2007-2019	6-4	305
La'el Collins	Offensive Tackle	Dallas Cowboys	2015-present	6-4	323
NFL Combine	Offensive Line	--	1999-2017	6-5	313
High School Combine	Offensive Line	--	2015-2016	6-1	268

Sources: Gillen, Z.M., et al. Res Q Exer Sport. 90:227, 2019, Wikipedia.

Table 4-1: Changes in body size among NFL linemen since 1919.

Research and the Real World: Surprisingly, the research literature is divided on anabolic steroids' ability to enhance physical performance. Yet, most athletes who consume these substances tout their beneficial effects. Many athletes feel they would not have been as successful without them.

There are several possible reasons for the large differences between experimental findings and empirical observations. An incredible mystique has arisen around these substances, providing fertile ground for the placebo effect. Also, anabolic steroid use in the "real world" is considerably different from that in rigidly controlled, double-blind laboratory research experiments.

In a double-blind study, neither the subject nor the experimenter know who takes the drug or placebo. Most studies did not use the same drug dosage used by athletes because institutional safeguards prohibit administrating high dosages of possibly dangerous substances to human subjects. Also, subjects in research experiments seldom resemble accomplished weight-trained athletes. Under these conditions, one must assess the results from research studies and clinical and empirical field observations to obtain a realistic profile of the use, effects on performance, and side effects of these substances.

Bodybuilders and power athletes have used anabolic steroids since the 1960s. It was not until the early 1970s that scientists studied their effects on body composition and athletic performance. Many studies showed that the drugs did not enhance performance. Scientists believed that most of the perceived gains were due more to psychological effects than the drugs' biological actions.

. . .

Dosage and Steroid Effectiveness: The discrepancy between empirical observations and the results from scientific studies raised the question, "How could anabolic steroids appear to be so effective in bodybuilders and power athletes but fail to show similar results in scientific studies?" Studies by Bhasin and coworkers (1996, 2001) and Storer, et al. (2008, 2017) answered the question. They found that steroid dosage was the key to the drugs' effectiveness.

In the first studies, they gave 600 mg/week of testosterone enanthate or a placebo for 10 weeks to subjects who were lifting weights or sedentary (not lifting weights). Unlike many previous studies, their research demonstrated steroids increased strength and muscle mass. Subjects who took large testosterone doses gained increased lean mass, strength, and muscle size without lifting weights. The experimental group improved 10 kg in the bench press and 15 kg in the back squat and made substantial gains in arm and thigh muscle size without lifting weights. These studies have been replicated in young and older men.

Modern bodybuilders and strength athletes sometimes take 20 to 30 times more testosterone than therapeutic doses used in the early studies. Larger doses in part account for the large increases in body size observed in modern bodybuilders and power athletes. A consensus statement from the American College of Sports Medicine (2021) concluded that anabolic steroids, when accompanied by a progressive training program, increase muscle strength, lean body mass, endurance, and power (Bhasin, et al., 2021).

· · ·

Table 4-2: Summary of Anabolic Steroid Actions and Effects on Athletic Performance:

- Anabolic steroids are synthetic male hormones resembling testosterone manufactured to enhance male hormones' anabolic properties while minimizing their androgenic properties.
- Anabolic steroids effectively increase protein synthesis rate in target cells, generating satellite cells in muscle, slowing protein breakdown during and after exercise, increasing neural transmission speed, and increasing aggressiveness and feelings of well-being. These effects help athletes improve faster and recover more rapidly from intense workouts.
- Anabolic steroids effectively increase strength, power, muscle size, and speed if the athlete is involved in an intense weight-training program.
- Anabolic steroids promote myelin production in nerve fibers, which speeds neural transmission and reinforces motor pathways. Combining precise skill training, anabolic steroids, and high-power training may improve high-power sports performance.
- Anabolic steroids do not improve maximal oxygen consumption. Still, they may improve performance in endurance events by increasing power output and allowing athletes to run, swim, ski, and cycle faster

and exercise at higher percentages of maximal oxygen consumption.

- Most studies have shown no effects of the drugs on body fat, although testosterone affects fat metabolism. Changes in food intake and physical activity in athletes may help to explain the discrepancies.
- Major differences exist between published research findings and popular conceptions among athletes about anabolic steroid effectiveness to improve athletic performance. These differences may be due to (1) the placebo effect, (2) low doses in research studies, (3) use of untrained test subjects, and (4) failure to document peaking techniques.

Subjects who lifted weights and took testosterone showed even more significant gains (Bhasin, et al., 2001). In 20 weeks, they increased nearly 22 kg in the bench press and 35 kg in the back squat and gained over 5 kg in lean tissue. The improvements made by subjects in this study were similar to those observed empirically in athletes taking anabolic steroids independently. They refuted older low dose studies showing anabolic steroids did not increase muscle mass or strength.

Strength Gains and Testosterone Levels: Other studies from Bhasin's group showed that gains in strength varied directly with blood testosterone levels —the higher the serum testosterone, the greater the gains in strength and muscle size — particularly in weight-trained subjects (Bhasin et al. 2001; Storer, et al., 2017). These studies showed that using low testosterone or anabolic steroids doses depressed testicular testosterone production.

The body controls testosterone levels through negative feedback between the hypothalamus, pituitary, and testes. When blood testosterone levels are low, the hypothalamus secretes gonadotropin-releasing hormone (GRH), which triggers luteinizing hormone (LH) and follicle-stimulating hormone (FSH) release from the pituitary. This stimulates the testes to produce testosterone. In athletes taking continuous high anabolic steroid doses, high testosterone levels overwhelms the normal testosterone control system, rendering the feedback mechanism moot. These athletes can expect serious side effects.

Why was there a failure to make any gains in muscle size and strength in studies that used low anabolic steroid or testosterone doses? Initially, the low-dose administration increased blood testosterone levels. This gave the training program a temporary boost. Then the body's hormone control system took over, which decreased testosterone control hormones (GRH, LH, FSH) and lowered blood testosterone back to normal. The reduction in testosterone production resulted in lower blood testosterone levels and established a lag time to restore natural balance.

Even without supplements, the capacity to gain strength depends on testosterone levels present in the blood. Normal blood testosterone in young men (18–40 yr) varies between 350 and 1200 ng/dL of blood. Large, rapid increases in strength or muscle mass depend on large blood testosterone concentrations. Bhasin and coworkers (1999) showed that taking 300 mg/week of testosterone was necessary to elevate blood testosterone above normal levels. Taking 600 mg/week increased blood testosterone to 2500 ng/dL of blood, which is more than double the normal range.

In the Bhasin et al. studies, 150 mg of testosterone weekly never increased blood testosterone above 500 ng/dL. Taking even standard therapeutic doses does not increase blood testosterone to levels needed to promote muscle hypertrophy and strength faster than normal. At least 300 mg would be required each week to exceed normal blood testosterone by even small amounts. Taking low doses shuts down normal testosterone production, so any concentration gains are quickly lost. Also, athletes may have side effects from the drugs, even at these relatively small doses.

Bodybuilders: Serious bodybuilders and power athletes who use steroids typically take at least 600–1000 mg/week of various forms of testosterone and anabolic steroids. They combine them with other anabolic supplements such as growth hormone, insulin-like growth factor (IGF-1), clenbuterol, and creatine monohydrate. They also take Nolvadex to prevent gynecomastia (growth of breast tissue), and human chorionic gonadotropin to boost normal testosterone production. These anabolic supplement programs probably account for the noticeable increases in size and strength in bodybuilders and other weight-trained athletes.

Studies before those of Bhasin and coworkers often found that anabolic steroids did not improve performance because they used low drug doses. Higher doses produce significant effects on muscle size and strength but also increase side effect risks.

Trained Athletes

Most changes in strength during the early part of the training are neural; that is, increased strength is mainly due to an improved ability to recruit motor units and establish basic motor (movement) patterns. However, anabolic steroids affect processes associated with protein synthesis in muscle. Studies lasting six weeks (typical study length) would largely reflect the neural changes and easily overlook the drug's cellular effects. The gains made by athletes in uncontrolled observations have been more impressive.

Studies on Trained Athletes: Studies are rare on the effects of anabolic steroids in accomplished training athletes For obvious reasons, athletes will rarely admit to taking banned substances, let alone allowing physical measurements.

Hartgens, et al. (1996, 2002, 2003) studied the effects of anabolic steroids in well-trained strength athletes. These were uncontrolled studies with few subjects, but they examined well-trained athletes using anabolic steroids under realistic conditions. Compared to control subjects, athletes gained body weight (4.4 kg), lean body mass (4.5 kg), and lost fat (1%). The changes persisted six weeks after the studies.

Little objective data exists on the anabolic steroid effects in elite athletes. Some training records have become available from elite athletes from the German Democratic Republic (i.e., East Germany). These athletes benefited substantially from the drugs, but the effects were impossible to substantiate. Since the Soviet Union and East Germany break-up, documents and testimony shed light on government-sponsored performance-enhancing drug use—particularly anabolic steroids. State-sponsored doping continued in Russia and resulted in significant sanctions against their athletes by the International Olympic Committee (see chapter 10).

World Records: Circumstantial evidence that steroids boost performance in elite athletes exists in abundance. Examining the world record progression in the men's shot put, discus, and hammer and the women's shot put and discus show unmistakable trends that reflect anabolic steroid use in these sports. The men's shot-put record progressed steadily from 15.54 meters in 1909 to 17.82 in 1950 and to 19.30 in 1960. Athletes first used steroids in the early 1960s. Shot-put records reflect this: 21.50 meters in 1965, 21.86 in 1976, 22.62 in 1985, and 23.12 in 1990. Progression in the world record stopped abruptly in 1990. After a 30 year hiatus, Ryan Crouser broke the world record at the 2021 U.S. Olympic Trials with a throw of 23.37 meters (76 ft 8 in).

The discus record progression was similar: 47.58 meters in 1912, 51.03 in 1930, 56.97 in 1949, 64.55 in 1964, 70.86 in 1976, and 74.08 in 1986. Again, there has been no progress in the discus world record since

1986. Similar trends exist in the men's hammer throw and women's discus and shot put. What can explain the abrupt halt in record progression in these sports?

Doping Control: Strict drug testing and the biological passport introduced in 2009 decreased anabolic steroid use in elite sport. Between the 1960s and 1990s, drug testing was unsystematic and typically administered at championships. After that, the World Anti-Doping Agency (WADA) introduced random drug tests in elite athletes. The athletic biological passport monitored selected biological markers that could directly or indirectly detect athletic doping. These trends do not prove that athletes used anabolic steroids. The trend was not evident in the women's hammer throw, which only recently became an official event in women's athletics, so performances reflect improved technique and increases in strength and power.

Female Athletes

Based on positive doping tests, anabolic steroid use in women athletes is relatively common, but data on anabolic steroid use in female athletes are rare. Historical data from the German Democratic Republic (GDR) and clinical observations provide information on these drug's effects on women.

Women Competing for the GDR: Reports from the GDR showed that anabolic steroid use was prevalent in speed and power events. Huang and Basaria (2017) estimated that anabolic steroid administration over four-years improved shot-put performance by 4.5-5 m, discus by 11 to 20 m, 400-m run by 4-5 sec, and the 1500-m run by 7-10 sec. Athletes took 10 to 100 times the therapeutic dosage of anabolic steroids.

Clinical studies of androgen treatment in non-athletic women show similar benefits (Dobbs, et al. 2002). Testosterone and estrogen increased upper and lower body muscle mass four to ten times more than estrogen alone in postmenopausal women. Greater improvements occurred in the bench press and loaded stair climbing (carrying weights). Women taking the highest dosage showed the largest changes in muscle mass and physical performance. These women were not athletes, but the changes were similar to those observed in world-class athletes from the GDR.

Hyperandrogenism: Women with hyperandrogenism (higher than normal testosterone levels) are more successful in women's sports. Bermon, et al. (2014) reported a higher prevalence of women with sexual development disorders and elevated androgens among successful female power and speed athletes. Congenitally higher androgen levels and anabolic steroids provide other advantages besides increased muscle mass and strength. Exposure to higher testosterone levels also triggers changes in muscle satellite cells, myelin, and androgen receptor concentrations, and provide long-term advantages.

· · ·

Non Athletic Women: Males sometimes lead females down the dark path of steroid use. The average male steroid user is 30 years old, physically active, employed, and never participated in organized sport. A new phenomenon is females in their late 20s who use anabolic steroids to improve body composition and sex drive.

Swedish researcher Borjesson (2016) interviewed eight non-athletic women who used anabolic steroids. Most women used two or more steroids concurrently for 58 weeks. Five women reported undesirable voice changes, clitoral enlargement, and body hair growth side effects. Seven of the eight had boyfriends who encouraged them to use the drugs.

Children

Politicians and sports administrators promote steroid bans in athletes to discourage their use by children. Only about 4-6 percent of high school students have ever used steroids, so the problem has been blown out of proportion.

Fahey, et al. (1979) measured blood testosterone levels before and after exercise in male children during different stages of pubertal development (Tanner pubertal stages 1-5). Male children do not reach adult levels of testosterone until stage 5, full sexual development. Anabolic steroids will have profound effects on performance, growth, and sexual development in less mature pubertal stages.

Steroids exhibit severe side effects in children. During adolescence, anabolic steroid exposure leads to virilization, accelerates bone growth and sexual development, promotes premature growth plate closure, alters nerve cell growth and brain serotonin levels, and increases aggressive behavior (Bhasin, et al., 2021). Many young people think anabolic steroids are harmless because they are readily available on the Internet. "They might be illegal, but they are not bad."

Epidemiology: Studies conducted over the last 30 years found that 4 to 6 percent of males and 1.5 to 3 percent of females have ever used anabolic steroids. Most school-aged steroid users are non-athletes who take the drugs to improve physical appearance and increase strength at the health club (see extensive reference list on "Steroid Use Epidemiology" in the reference section).

Steroid use is a problem among high school students, but it is less problematic than alcohol and recreational drug abuse. It is a minor problem compared to deteriorating athletic programs and overwhelming overweight and obesity among young people.

Drug Testing High School Athletes: We believe it is important to educate students about the health and legal risks of using performance-enhancing drugs, but we do not advocate throwing the baby out with the bathwater by directing precious resources to eradicate steroid use in school when there are more important needs for financial resources to support other educational programs.

Some states have expensive steroid drug-testing programs. Between 2007 and 2015, Texas had a drug testing program that cost $10 million but only netted 40 positive tests, so they abandoned the program because it was ineffective. A better use of the money should have been to fund professional, full-time coaches who could educate students about training, nutrition, and drug use.

Coaches who work with children should become knowledgeable about anabolic steroids and supplements but should never recommend them. Recommending anabolic steroids to children is unethical and could cause severe legal and professional consequences. Parents will sometimes ask about steroids, steroid sources, and advice about their use. Avoid these situations and vigorously defend drug-free sport.

Physical Performance in Middle-Aged and Older Adults

Based on the number of positive drug tests in master's sport, anabolic steroid use is as prevalent in master's sports as in open competition. High testosterone doses increase strength in middle-aged and older men by 35 percent. Studies in older adults used untrained subjects, so the effects would not be as dramatic as in athletes. Also, the high doses required to trigger these effects cause elevated hematocrit (percent cells in the blood) and hemoglobin levels, increasing the risk of blood clots.

Minimum anabolic hormone levels are necessary to increase muscle mass in older adults. Supplementing with testosterone and growth hormone is common in aging men. Sattler, et al. (2011), in a study of men age

65 to 90 years, showed that increasing total testosterone to 1046 ng/dL (200–400 ng/dL is normal in older men) was necessary to increase lean mass and enhance strength. The effects of testosterone were greater when the men also supplemented with growth hormone, but the incidence of elevated hematocrit increased with dose. The study showed that testosterone supplements in older adults increased muscle mass, strength, and movement capacity.

Sarcopenia: Sarcopenia (muscle loss) is common in aging adults but less prevalent in masters athletes. Testosterone supplements increase lean body mass by 1-3 kg. Testosterone stimulates muscle protein synthesis, decreases muscle protein degradation, improves amino acid utilization, and increases satellite cells and muscle cell nuclei. Storer, et al. (2008, 2016) studied older men taking testosterone supplements for three years. Compared to control subjects, testosterone replacement improved stair-climbing power, muscle mass, and power output capacity. These adaptations affect performance and health.

Muscle is critical for blood sugar (glucose) regulation because it is the main tissue using glucose as an energy source. Type 2 diabetes is common in older adults because lost muscle mass reduces the principle site of glucose use. Testosterone, particularly combined with resistive exercise, can reverse this trend by increasing or sustaining muscle mass.

Master's Athletes: These studies did not examine master's athletes (master's sports ban anabolic steroids). In 2005, a former master's world champion in the discus throw received a two-year suspension from competition for testing positive for anabolic steroids at the World Championships in San Sebastian, Spain. He took testosterone supplements to help treat type 2 diabetes and had applied for a medical exemption (Heo, et al., 2020). He never received the exemption and was vigorously pursued by doping control officials.

In 2011, the U.S. National champion in the shot-put receiving testosterone gel for health reasons failed a doping test for the same reason. Doping sanctions are common in master's sports because so many athletes take hormone supplements as anti-aging therapy.

Anabolic steroids have a profound effect on sports performance in older athletes. As discussed, testosterone supplements enhance the performance of motor neurons— particularly those recruited and overloaded during exercise. Steroids promote athletic performance by stimulating myelin production in specific motor pathways. These pathways are highly specific to sports movements.

Changes in sports performance are difficult to measure with conventional fitness tests. For example, testosterone may enhance power during a golf swing by enhancing the neural pathway through myelin production independent of changes in the squat, bench press, or grip strength.

In older adults, testosterone supplementation triggers 1-3 kg of fat loss in 12 to 16 weeks (Linderman, et al., 2020). These changes are modest compared to improvements in muscle mass and strength. Increased muscle mass boosts metabolic rate but has a small effect on fat mass. Changes in fat mass with anabolic steroids probably have minimal effects on performance in middle-aged and older competitive athletes.

2021 ACSM Consensus Statement (Bhasin, et al., 2021): A 2021 consensus statement from the American College of Sports Medicine (ACSM) concluded, "Androgen replacement therapy is approved for the medical treatment of several clinical diseases and abnormalities. The ACSM acknowledges the lawful and ethical use of AAS for clinical purposes and supports the physicians' ability to provide androgen therapy to patients when deemed medically necessary."

Summary

Anabolic steroids have influenced sport in the last half of the 20th century and beyond. In the previous 100 years, differences in body weight among champion bodybuilders and some American football players exceed 100 pounds. Anabolic steroids help athletes achieve these new requirements. The drugs have had a profound effect on performance, as demonstrated by changes in records before and after stringent doping control programs. There is little objective evidence on anabolic steroids' effects on performance in females, but training diaries from the GDR and performances in athletic contests in the years before effective drug testing suggest substantial effects.

Only about 4-6 percent of high school students have used anabolic steroids, so the problem has been overstated. We believe it is important to educate students about the health and legal risks of using perfor-mance-enhancing drugs, but we do not advocate drug testing athletes because the money is better spent hiring professional coaches and better funding athletic programs.

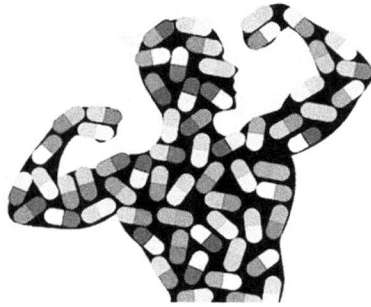

5

HOW ATHLETES AND RECREATIONALLY ACTIVE ADULTS USE STEROIDS

Non-athletes are the most significant abusers of performance-enhancing drugs. The Internet has made anabolic steroids, growth hormone, melanotan, weight-loss drugs, Botox, and dermal fillers available to anyone with negligible legal risk. Surveys of people who purchase steroids on the Internet show that steroid doses range from 250 to 3200 milligrams per week, while cycles averaged four to twelve weeks. Fifty-nine percent reported using over 1000 milligrams of testosterone weekly (Westerman, et al., 2016).

Athletes and non-athletes typically take various drugs and supplements, so isolating the effects of any substance in the "real-world" remains difficult. Drugs include human growth hormone, IGF-1, insulin, modafinil, ephedrine, amphetamines, and clenbuterol. Supplements include protein, individual amino acids (e.g., branched-chain amino acids such as leucine), caffeine, and creatine monohydrate.

Mode of Administration

People take steroids orally, intramuscularly (injected), and transdermally (gel or cream). They can also be taken buccally (absorbed under the tongue), intranasally, and as implanted pellets and patches.

The C17α-anabolic steroids are synthetic hormones are orally active and do not require intramuscular injection. Formulated oral anabolic steroids resist liver metabolism and have a high incidence of liver toxicity. Popular oral anabolic steroids include methandienone (Dianabol), oxandrolone (Anavar, Oxandrin), fluoxymesterone (Halotestin), oxymetholone (Anadrol), and stanozolol (Winstrol).

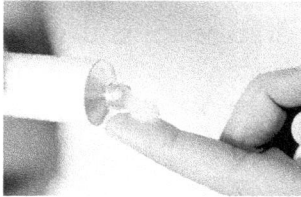

Figure 5-1: Testosterone cream. Source: Shutterstock.

Transdermal testosterone is popular with middle-aged and older adults to treat hypogonadism (low testosterone levels) (Figure 5-1). It has a short half-life and must be applied frequently. Examples include gels (Androgel and Testim), solutions (Axiron), and patches (Androderm).

Injectable anabolic steroids include testosterone oil solutions (e.g., testosterone cypionate, testosterone enanthate, testosterone undecanoate, nandrolone decanoate (Deca-Durabolin), Sustanon (combination of testosterone propionate, testosterone phenylpropianate, testosterone isocaproate, testosterone decanoate), and nandrolone phenylpropionate (Durabolin)). Testosterone propionate is no longer prescribed in the United States but is available on the Internet. Injectable steroids release slowly into the bloodstream.

Anabolic Steroids are Popular with Recreationally Active Non-Athletes

Athletes are not the primary users of anabolic steroids. Far more non-athletes 25–40-year-old males and females take these drugs to enhance physical appearance, body composition, and sex drive. An extensive survey by Cohen, et al. (2008) found that U.S. male steroid users were about 30 years old, highly educated, Caucasian, with full-time jobs and above-average salaries. They did not use the drugs in adolescence and were not motivated by athletic performance. The most popular anabolic steroids with non-athletes included single ester testosterone, Dianabol, Deca Durabolin, Winstrol, and Equipoise.

The typical steroid user is not an athlete, so their side effects substantially differ from strength athletes who train at much higher intensities. The news media portrays the typical steroid user as a rogue elite athlete who takes the drug to cheat the competition. The truth is far from that.

An anonymous survey of 231 male testosterone users by Westerman and colleagues from the Mayo Clinic in Rochester, Minnesota showed that in the United States, most are educated, employed, married, white, and economically well-off (Westerman, et al., 2016). Most have taken the drugs for over three years and take large doses greater than 800 milligrams a week (mainly testosterone). More than half bought their testosterone on the Internet and 28 percent from a physician. More than half spend $100 to $1000 a month on performance-enhancing drugs. Seventy-five percent had routine lab tests performed, and most took more than one performance-enhancing drug. Surprisingly, only 57 percent had played high school sports. Over 80 percent took testosterone or other anabolic steroids to increase muscle mass and decrease fat.

Most side effects are mild in recreational users and include acne, gynecomastia (breast growth), and stretch marks. Steroid users typically used three or more other drugs or supplements. Using performance-enhancing drugs is linked to cocaine use, training years, and training frequency. Most users get their information about steroid use patterns from the Internet or other users.

Anabolic Steroids Sources

While physicians can prescribe testosterone for legitimate medical reasons (e.g., hypogonadism in aging adults, low libido), strict regulations prohibit physician prescriptions for athletes to improve performance and recreationally active people to improve appearance.

The Internet is the number one source of black market anabolic steroids and growth hormone in the United States and has created the world's largest drugstore! Numerous websites provide detailed information about anabolic drugs and their side effects and sometimes maintain lists of fraudulent operators designed to direct business to their own companies. The United States Food and Drug Administration (FDA) admits that offshore steroid Internet sites are virtually immune from prosecution for illegal or unsafe practices.

Several FDA and European health organizations studies reported that about 50% of drugs purchased on the Internet are counterfeit and sometimes contain toxic substances that can cause illness or death (McBride, et al., 2018). Typical problems with Internet steroids include products without active ingredients, incorrect quantities of active ingredients, wrong ingredients, fake packaging, copies of original products, products containing impurities and contaminants, and outdated drugs purchased from other companies. People risk getting ripped off, arrested, or sick when they buy anabolic medications on the Internet.

Italian researchers surveyed 10 websites selling anabolic drugs online (Cardaro, et al., 2011). Fifty percent of the websites originated in the United States, and 30 percent originated in Europe. Nandrolone, methandrostenolone, and testosterone were the most common anabolic steroids offered for sale. Other typical performance–enhancing drugs included clenbuterol, growth hormone, IGF-1, thyroid hormones, erythropoietin (EPO), and insulin. Recommended doses on the websites were typically much higher than the therapeutic prescription drug counterparts, which could harm public health. The researchers did not report on the reliability or product quality offered on the sites.

Legislation to Control Anabolic Steroid Use and Distribution

The 1990 and 2004 Anabolic Control Acts: The United States Congress has tried to limit steroid use by athletes and non-athletes. The Anabolic Control Acts of 1990 and 2004 identified anabolic steroids as a separate drug class and classified several dozen anabolic steroids as controlled substances.

The 2004 legislation banned the sale of steroid precursors (e.g., androstenedione) and increased penalties for making, selling, or prescribing anabolic steroids for recreational purposes. This legislation made it nearly impossible for people to obtain anabolic steroids from physicians for non-medical reasons. People mainly buy drugs on the Internet or from countries without restrictions.

The "War on Drugs" is usually associated with marijuana, cocaine, heroin, and methamphetamine. Operation Pangaea III led by Interpol (International criminal police organization with 194 member countries) pursued counterfeit medications sold online. Counterfeiters can make a fortune from a small investment.

Counterfeit drugs often contain contaminants that can cause extreme illness or death, and many contain none of the active ingredients listed on their labels. Counterfeit medications include drugs for preventing heart attacks and treating hepatitis and HIV infections. Scientists have developed sophisticated methods to determine the content and source of counterfeit medicines. Unfortunately, the high cost of drugs literally drives people to the black market.

Popular Anabolic Steroids and Their Clearance Rates

Testosterone and related hormones are produced naturally in the testes, ovaries, and adrenal glands. Figure 5-2 shows endogenous (naturally occurring) and exogenous anabolic steroid (drugs) sources. Synthetic anabolic steroids change the basic testosterone molecule. They stay in the system longer, alter the androgenic vs. anabolic effects, and minimize side effects.

Synthetic drugs stay in the system longer than physiologically-produced testosterone. Athletes who use these drugs try to estimate clearance rates to avoid detection. The blood testosterone half-life is 10 to 100 min. The testosterone esters testosterone cypionate and testosterone enanthate have 8-day half-lives, but clearance rates are longer in old versus young men (Coviello, et al., 2006). The anabolic steroid Dianabol (methandrostenolone) has a half-life of about 5 hr.

Athletes Beware: Clearance rates for various anabolic steroids are available on the Internet. Athletes subject to doping control who take anabolic steroids should be wary of this information because it is not based on scientific studies. Also, people vary in the rate they clear testosterone. Genetics and age account for most individual differences in testosterone clearance rates. In some people, injected testosterone was undetectable after three days, while it persisted for several weeks in others. Measuring anabolic steroid metabolites has extended detection to 3-weeks or more (Schanzer, et al., 2006).

Nandrolone Decanoate (Deca-Durabolin) is detectable for at least 9-months in some people according to a study from Sweden's Karolinska Institute, (Garevik et al., 2016). Subjects received a single 150 mg dose of nandrolone decanoate. They monitored urine for nandrolone and two of its metabolites (19-norandrosterone and 19-noretiocholanolone) for nine months.

Popular Anabolic Steroids

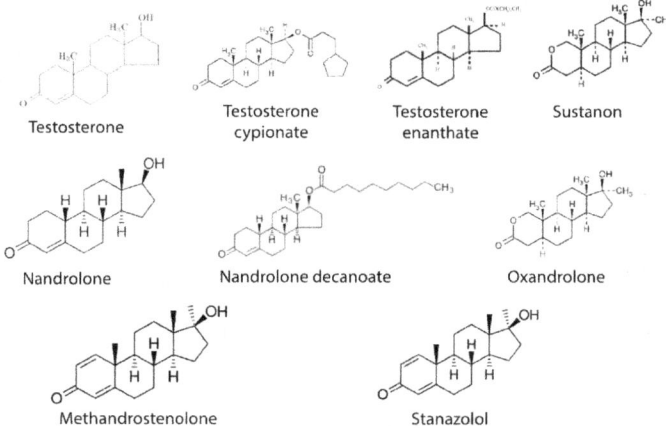

Figure 5-2: Chemical structures of commonly used anabolic steroids. Source: Modified from Shutterstock.

Nandrolone is a notorious drug among athletes because of drug suspensions in athletes using it. These included Olympic medal winners and elite athletes Linford Christie (sprinter), Merlene Ottey (sprinter), Ben Plucknett (thrower), and Dieter Baumann (distance runner). Large differences in clearance rates existed in these athletes, with some athletes testing clean in 30 days and others detectable after nine months.

Dosage, length of use, body fat level, and genetic-linked clearance rates determine how long the drug remains detectable.Steroid clearance rate tables on the Internet are not based on actual data!

Testosterone Gels, Creams, and Oral Anabolic Steroids: These are undetectable in blood or urine within hours or days. Changes in factors measured as part of the *athletic passport* can persist for weeks. These include red blood cells (hematocrit and hemoglobin), growth hormone, IGF-I, testosterone and its metabolites, liver enzymes, and blood lipids. One of us reported data on high-density lipoproteins (HDL) changes in world-class athletes during repeated anabolic steroid cycles (Peterson and Fahey, 1985). HDL decreased when the athletes took the drugs but increased when they went off the drugs. The changes in HDL took at least a week during the dosing cycles.

Stacking and Cycling: Many steroid users use several drugs simultaneously, hoping to increase their effects and vary the doses for each drug during different cycling periods. Table 5-1 shows the anabolic steroid dosing schedule from a world-class power athlete from the 1980s obtained from his training diary.

Table 5-1			
Anabolic Steroid Therapy Program of a World Class Athlete with Weight Training			
week	Injectable Steroid	Oral Steroid Journal	Training Program
1-2	250 mg of Sustanon every 5 days	8 mg Winstrol	Heavy weight training: high volume, medium intensity
3-4	250 mg of Sustanon every 5 days	10 mg Winstrol 10 mg Dianabol	Heavy weight training: high volume, medium intensity
5	250 mg of Sustanon every 5 days	10 mg Winstrol 20 mg Dianabol	Heavy weight training: high volume, medium intensity
6	250 mg of Sustanon every 5 days	Progressive dose decrease	Low volume, lowintensity; Rest week
7-8	No injectables	Non-oral	Low volume; high intensity
9	No injectables	10 mg Dianabol	Low volume, high intensity; Heavy lifting once
10	200 mg testosterone enanthate every 5 days	15 mg Dianabol	Low volume, high intensity; lift heavy objects once during the week
11	200 mg testosterone	20 mg Dianabol	Training with low volume and low intensity weights.

Table 5-1: Steroid and weight training program of a world-class power athlete. Source: Brooks, et al. *Exercise Physiology: Human Bioenergetics and its Applications*. New York: Amazon, 2020. 5th. Edition.

The athlete took the highly androgenic drugs Delatestryl (testosterone enanthate) and testosterone propionate close to competition because their molecular structures are more comparable to testosterone with a greater effect on aggressiveness. A closer look at the athlete's cycling and stacking program show coordination with the training program.

The steroid dosage increased gradually during the first five weeks, and corresponded to a load weight training cycle involving high volume and high resistance training. The athlete stopped taking the drugs for three weeks and then took highly androgenic drugs during the remainder of the training cycle before a competition.

The pre-competition drugs maximized aggressiveness. Training used peak set training emphasizing low repetitions and high weight, followed by several day's rest before competition. Modern leading bodybuilder's drug regimens use considerably higher doses.

Testosterone Shut-Down: Athletes cycle anabolic steroids to avoid a shutdown of natural production in the hormone. Typical anabolic steroid cycles last six weeks. A negative feedback mechanism involving testosterone levels and hormones released by the hypothalamus and pituitary glands in the brain (hypothalamic releasing factor, luteinizing hormone, follicle stimulating hormone) control testosterone production. Figure 5-3 shows the hormone controls to produce testosterone.

Male Hypothalamic-Pituitary-Gonadal Axis

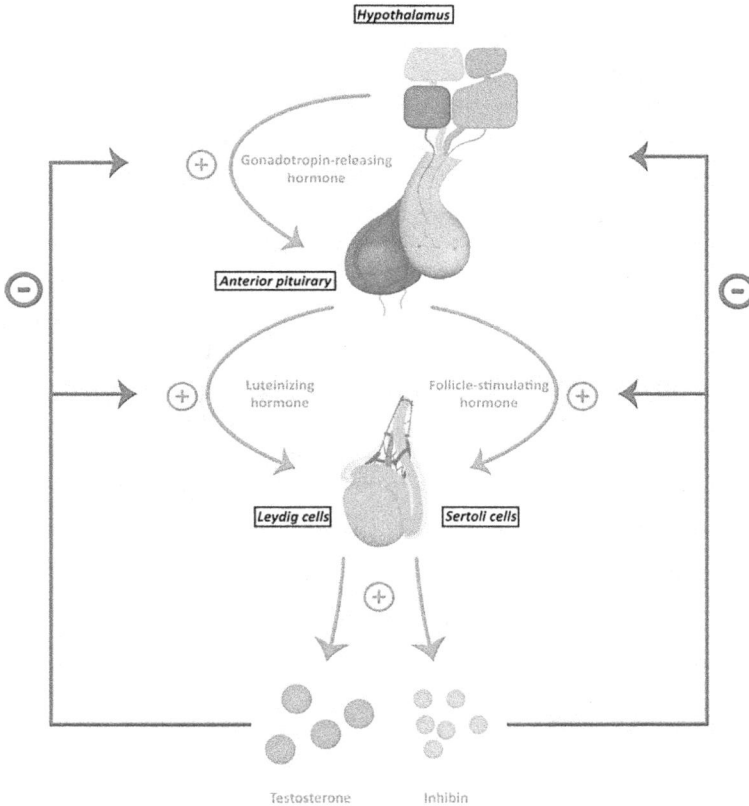

Figure 5-3: The hypothalamic-pituitary-gonadal axis controls testosterone production. Increases in testosterone (or testosterone-like drugs) suppress controlling hormones in the hypothalamus and pituitary, which reduces testosterone production. Source: Shutterstock.

Tightly Regulated: The hypothalamic-pituitary-gonadal axis tightly regulates the natural testosterone production in the testes. The body interprets anabolic steroids as an excess in testosterone. The perception of excess testosterone triggers a decrease in controlling hormones in the hypothalamus and pituitary, which in turn decreases natural testosterone production.

Athletes cycle anabolic steroids to "restart" natural testosterone production. Some athletes take higher doses and never go off the drugs. Higher doses and longer administration lead to more side effects.

A closer look at the athlete's cycling and stacking program show coordination with the training program. The steroid dosage increased gradually during the first five weeks, and corresponded to a load weight training cycle involving high volume and high resistance training. Load cycles employed high sets, moderate repetitions, pushing athletes to the max (e.g., bench press, 5 x 5, 350-400 lb). The athlete stopped taking the drugs for three weeks and then took highly androgenic drugs during the remainder of the training cycle before a competition.

Peak cycle weight training during the competitive season involved training 1-2 times per week using near maximum weight for 3-5 sets and low repetitions (e.g., bench press: one workout per week, 3-5 sets, 1-2 reps, 425-500 lb). Athletes employed no more than four lifts in their competitive workouts. Lifts might include bench press, squats, cleans or snatches, and deadlifts. The pre-competition drugs maximized aggressiveness. Training emphasized low repetitions and high weight, followed by several day's rest before competition. They performed all lifts explosively.

Contrary to power athletes in American football

and the throwing events in the 70s and 80s, leading bodybuilders use considerably higher doses of anabolic drugs and emphasize failure training in their workouts. The combination of intense training programs, high doses of anabolic drugs, and effective nutrition and supplement programs account for the incredible size of modern bodybuilders.

Testosterone is Bound or Unbound: Some testosterone binds to sex hormone-binding globulin, which severely decreases its biological availability. Bhasin and co-workers (2017) showed that bound testosterone increases during low-dose testosterone supplementation, yet this decrease shuts down normal testosterone production, and the remaining testosterone becomes less effective. Athletes taking steroid doses surrender their capacity to achieve substantial training gains. They quickly lose prior gains and deplete natural testosterone levels.

Summary

The 1990 and 2004 Anabolic Steroid Control Acts make it illegal for physicians to prescribe anabolic steroids to improve athletic performance. Some athletes still take the drugs despite stringent drug testing in Olympic and professional sport. The average user is a 30-year old recreationally active male or female non-athlete trying to improve body composition or a middle-age or older adult attempting to improve quality of life or longevity.

Athletes and recreationally active adults purchase steroids on the Internet or in countries where they are legal, while testosterone is widely prescribed. Oral anabolic steroids are formulated to prolong their metabolism in the liver. They exhibit a high incidence of liver toxicity, so testosterone gels and injections are commonly prescribed alternatives.

Drugs vary in their detection rate, but information published on the Internet are not based on objective data. The hypothalamic-pituitary-gonadal axis regulates natural testosterone production. Anabolic steroids suppress natural testosterone levels, so steroid users often "stack" different steroids (taking two or more drugs together) and cycle on and off the drugs to maximize their effectiveness and minimize their side effects.

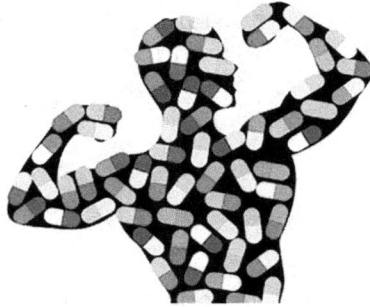

6

HEALTH EFFECTS OF ANABOLIC STEROIDS: INTERACTION WITH INTENSE TRAINING

People are upset and confused about steroid use in sports. The media sensationalizes notorious cases of purported steroid use. Examples include Oakland Raider football great Lyle Alzedo (died from brain cancer at age 38), New York Yankee home run hitter Jose Canseco, and pro wrestler Chris Benoit (murder-suicide). Dramatic TV coverage makes it difficult to objectively assess the effects, health risks, and ethics of anabolic steroid use.

We have created 12 general categories for the reported anabolic steroid side effects.

1. Urogenital and Sexual

- Reduced fertility
- Depressed spermatogenesis
- Lowered testosterone production
- Reduced gonadotropin hormone production (LH, FSH)
- Increased urine volume
- Increased or decreased libido (sex drive)

- Sore nipples
- Testicular atrophy (shrinkage)
- Impotence (erection problems)
- Priapism (persistent erections)
- Gynecomastia (enlargement of male breast tissue)
- Spontaneous erections (random erections)

2. Heart Disease and Stroke

- Elevated blood pressure
- Dyslipidemia (increased LDL, cholesterol, triglycerides; decreased HDL, Apo-A1)
- Blood clots
- Myocardial infarction (heart attack)
- Increased stroke risk (blood clots and arteriosclerosis)
- Elevated blood glucose (blood sugar)
- Cardiac enlargement
- Arrhythmias (abnormal rhythm on the electrocardiogram)
- Cardiomyopathy (disease of the heart muscle)
- Left heart enlargement
- Sudden cardiac death

3. Children

- Premature epiphyses closure in children (bone growth centers)
- Short stature
- Precocious puberty (early onset puberty)
- Delayed puberty
- Masculinization (adult male sexual

characteristics)
- Voice changes

4. Vascular Disorders

- Increased thrombosis risk (blood clots); platelet aggregation, protein coagulation
- Elevated hematocrit (percent cells in the blood)
- Elevated hemoglobin (transports oxygen and carbon dioxide)
- Edema (swelling)
- Epistaxis (nose bleeds)
- Dizziness

5. Women

- Amenorrhea (abnormal absence of menstruation)
- Reversible infertility
- Irreversible voice changes
- Clitoral enlargement
- Abnormal hair growth
- Hair loss
- Altered sex drive
- Breast atrophy
- Painful menstruation
- Uterine atrophy

6. Cancer

- Testicular cancer
- Wilms' tumor (kidney)
- Prostate hypertrophy

- Prostate cancer

7. Skin

- Acne vulgaris (skin disease, mainly on the face, back, and chest)
- Acne conglobate (severe acne form)
- Seborrhea (excessive discharge from sebaceous glands)
- Stretch marks (from enlarged muscles)
- Abnormal hair growth
- Increased apocrine sweat gland activity (oil secreting glands found in under arms, groin, and feet)
- Increased sebaceous gland secretion (oily skin)
- Hair loss and baldness

8. Psychological and Brain

- Increased aggressiveness
- Increased nervous tension, mood swings, depression
- Muscle dysmorphia (excessive desire for muscularity)
- Psychosis (abnormal thinking and perceptions)
- Violent or criminal behavior
- Suicide
- Dependence
- Nerve cell apoptosis (nerve cell death)
- Substance abuse (gateway drug)

9. Musculoskeletal

- Muscle cramps and spasms
- Increased soft tissue injury risk (strains and sprains)
- Overtraining injuries
- Rhabdomyolysis (muscle cell destruction)
- Muscle hypertrophy (enlargement)

10. Metabolic

- Elevated creatine kinase (CK)
- Elevated lactate dehydrogenase (LDH)
- Altered electrolyte balance
- GI distress (stomach and intestinal problems, diarrhea)
- Disturbed thyroid function
- Depressed immune function
- Glucose intolerance (poor blood sugar control)
- Insulin resistance (poor blood sugar control)

11. Liver Side Effects

- Elevated levels in critical liver enzymes
- Increased bromsulphalein (BSP) retention
- Hepatocellular carcinoma (liver cancer)
- Peliosis hepatis (blood-filled cysts in the liver)
- Cholestasis (blockage of bile ducts in the liver)
- Jaundice (yellowing of the skin from liver disease)
- Hepatoxicity (toxic liver disease)
- Altered liver function tests (LDH, ALP, AST, ALT)

12. Kidney

- Nephropathy (kidney disease)
- Kidney failure
- Cancer

Note: Many of the side effects have been reported in clinical observations but not demonstrated in well-controlled experimental studies.

Unfortunately, anabolic steroids are so politicized that most people do not care about the truth. As usual, discussions about steroids and doping received considerable media attention at the Olympic Games in Tokyo, Rio de Janeiro, London, and Beijing.

Poor Advice: For years, physicians told athletes that steroids do not work and cause catastrophic side effects. In reality, anabolic steroids improve performance —particularly in high doses. While steroids sometimes show undesirable side effects, they are usually minor unless the user takes high doses. Steroids—along with progress in training, technique, and sports nutrition— are partially responsible for improved performance in baseball, track and field, swimming, weightlifting, and bodybuilding, and contact sports athletes' increased size.

Paradoxically, low testosterone levels may cause premature death, cardiovascular disease, sarcopenia (muscle loss), osteoporosis (bone loss), decreased sexual performance, and psychological depression in middle-aged and older men (Bhasin, et al., 2018). This has promoted "anti-aging" programs by supplementing with testosterone and growth hormone. Side effects are less in these groups because they take doses lower than younger athletes and recreationally active participants.

Anabolic Steroids, Intense Training, and Side-Effects

Athletes train more intensely than the average recreational sports enthusiast. Elite power athletes on steroids typically bench press over 400 pounds, squat nearly 600 pounds, and deadlift over 600 pounds, and they often do this for many years (Fahey, 2002). Sprinters and jumpers also exercise at high power outputs for many years, resulting in eventual muscle and joint deterioration.

Heavy training loads cause tissue overload, rotator cuff tears, joint deterioration, and enlarged hearts. These changes resulted from intense long-term training that would not have been possible without prolonged anabolic steroid use. While tissue deterioration may be due to heavy training loads rather than steroids, athletes would not be capable of developing such high tissue stress levels without the drugs.

In the 1970s, Fahey performed echocardiograms on elite strength athletes, all of whom used anabolic steroids. Interventricular septum diameter (wall separating the left and right ventricles) was directly proportional to maximum squat weight. The strongest athlete squatted 900 lb (409 kg). Out of a sample of 15 athletes, three died of cardiac arrest or myocardial infarction in their 50s and 60s (unpublished observations).

· · ·

Overtraining: Prolonged, intense training programs are sometimes linked to an overtraining condition causing severe damage to muscles and myositis (muscle inflammation (Figure 6-1).

Rhabdomyolysis (Rhabdo) is muscle destruction triggered by trauma or excessive training that results in the muscle contents emptying into the bloodstream, which can cause intense pain, weakness, vomiting, confusion, kidney failure, cardiac arrhythmias, dark-colored urine, and ultimately death. Kidney failure stems from releasing the muscle breakdown products myoglobin and creatine kinase.

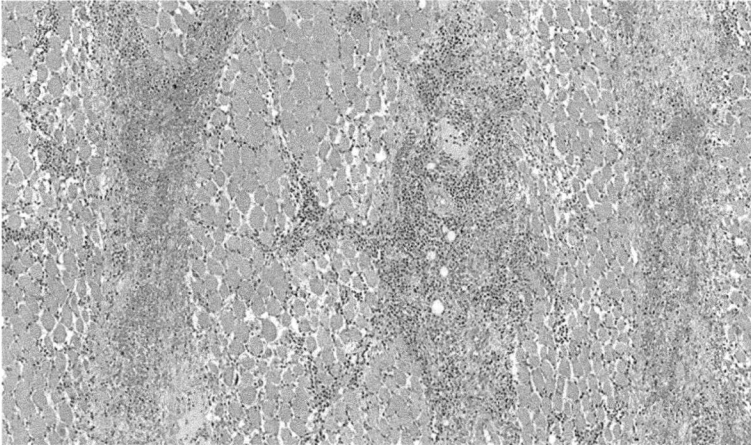

Figure 6-1: Micrograph of myositis in muscle tissue. Rhabdomyolysis is an extreme form of myositis resulting in muscle tissue destruction. Anabolic steroid users may be more susceptible to muscle inflammation because they can train harder and more intensely. Source: Shutterstock.

Rhabdo often results from severe trauma caused by auto accidents or falls, electrical injury, heatstroke, lack of blood flow, snake bite, and prolonged immobilization. Increasingly, rhabdo results from overtraining in "boot camp-style" or bodybuilding training programs that consistently push muscles to failure.

Muscle overexertion can destroy individual muscle cells. Anabolic steroids might contribute to training-induced rhabdo by allowing athletes to train even more intensely. Several clinical observations reported rhabdo in intensely training athletes taking anabolic steroids (Farkash, et al. 2009; Hageloch, et al. 1988; Braseth, et al., 2001; Pertusi, et al. 2001). The observations could be due to higher physical capacity, greater motivation, and a property of anabolic steroid use that allows athletes to train harder.

Anabolic Steroids and Soft Tissue

Tendon Rupture: Anabolic steroids increase tendon rupture risk. Reports of anabolic steroid side effects routinely cite an increased musculoskeletal rupture risk. While this information has been known for over 40 years, there is little evidence to support it. Sedentary rats developed stiffer tendons following anabolic steroid treatment (nandrolone decanoate; Marqueti, et al., 2012). Jump trained animals showed increased capacity to store elastic energy (Marqueti, et al., 2014). If these results can be applied to humans, it would support the claim that anabolic steroid use increases tendon rupture risk. However, rats are not humans, particularly sedentary rats!

Anabolic steroids and heavy weight training accelerate muscle protein synthesis more than weight training alone. The combination does not affect tendon size in the same way. In athletes involved in long-term heavy weight training, tendons were 15 percent larger in non-steroid users than steroid users. Steroids increased muscle fiber angles (pennation angle), which made the muscles more dense. Denser muscles and smaller tendons could increase tendon injury risk in steroid users.

The observation that steroids increase tendon injuries might be a chicken or egg argument. Steroids increase strength, particularly in serious strength-trained athletes. Is it the steroids or the increased strength that cause soft tissue injuries? Those who bench press 200 pounds are less susceptible to tendon injury than those who bench 400 pounds because they simply do not train as hard or as long. The extreme loads experienced by elite strength-trained athletes put extraordinary stresses and joint torques that push muscles, tendons, ligaments, and joint surfaces (chondrocytes) to the breaking point.

Side Effects and Dosage

High Doses Effective: Anabolic steroids are most effective at higher doses, but side effects also increase with dosage. It was not until the early 1970s that scientists studied the effects of anabolic steroids on muscle mass, strength, and athletic performance. Many of these studies, including Fahey's doctoral dissertation (Fahey & Brown, 1973), showed that the drugs did not improve performance or change body composition. Scientists believed that the placebo effect caused the most gains. Placebos work because they are effective by the power of suggestion.

In 1977, mainstream scientists and the American College of *Sports Medicine*—strongly condemned anabolic steroid use (ACSM, 1977). The ACSM considered that any gains in muscle mass, strength, or endurance were small and not worth the potentially deadly health risks. In the gym, many males made substantial gains with minimal side effects. Serious strength athletes knew that most sports scientists and physicians were misinformed about anabolic steroids.

A 2021 ACSM consensus statement admitted that steroids improve athletic performance and body composition but condemned their use (Bhasin, et al., 2021). However, they endorsed hormone replacement therapy in aging, hypogonadal men.

Low Doses Ineffective: Low testosterone or anabolic steroid doses have negligible effects on performance or body composition. Initially, supplementation increases blood testosterone levels, which gives the training program a temporary boost. However, the body's hormone control system quickly kicks in, which decreases testosterone level control hormones (GRH, LH, FSH) and reduces blood testosterone to either normal or below. Difficulties arise when athletes stop taking testosterone supplements. They have lower than normal blood testosterone levels, and it takes time to restore normal androgen control. Athletes sometimes combat diminishing returns by increasing dosage. Unfortunately, this strategy increases undesirable side effects.

. . .

Health Risks Accelerate with Higher Anabolic Steroid Doses

Normal blood testosterone levels in young men 18-40 yr vary between 350-1200 ng/dL (12-42 nmol/l). Even without supplements, the ability to gain strength depends on how much testosterone is in the blood (Storer, et al., 2003). To increase gains in strength or muscle mass, athletes must increase blood testosterone above normal levels. Bhasin and co-workers (1999) showed that it took 300 mg or more of testosterone per week to increase blood testosterone above normal levels. Taking 600 mg per week increased blood testosterone to 2500 ng/dL, which is more than double the highest level in the normal range.

Taking 150 mg testosterone per week never increased blood testosterone above 500 ng/dL. Taking even standard doses (200 mg for most types of testosterone) does not increase blood testosterone to levels needed to build muscle and strength faster than normal. Athletes need at least 300 mg a week to exceed normal blood testosterone by even a little. Low doses shut down normal testosterone production, so they quickly lose any gains when they cycle off the drugs.

Typically, serious bodybuilders and strength athletes who use steroids take stacks of at least 600-2000 mg per week of various forms of testosterone and anabolic steroids. They combine steroids with other anabolic supplements such as growth hormone, IGF-1, clenbuterol, creatine monohydrate, and Nolvadex to prevent gynecomastia, and human chorionic gonadotropin (hCG) to boost normal testosterone production. These anabolic supplement programs account for the incredible increase in size and strength in bodybuilders and other weight-trained athletes.

Side Effects Increase with Dosage: Large doses decrease HDL cholesterol and APO-A1, which may protect against heart disease. Only time will tell if athletes who take high dose testosterone supplements suffer more cardiovascular complications and heart attacks.

Prostate problems are a big fear in the medical community because prostate cancer is the second leading cancer-related cause of death in men. Little evidence shows testosterone supplements cause prostate gland enlargement in middle-age and older men (Morentaler, 2021). Prostate-specific antigen (PSA) values remain normal during normal dose testosterone administration. PSA is a blood test used to predict prostate enlargement and cancer. Little data exists, however, on the effects of extremely high doses of anabolic steroids on PSA or prostate health.

Another anabolic steroid risk is "roid rage." Most objective studies show that "roid rage" is mostly a myth and at occurs in susceptible people, particularly in high doses. About 10% or more bodybuilders who take over 600 mg testosterone weekly can expect severe and possibly dangerous psychological side-effects.

What Research Confirms about Dosage and Anabolic Steroid Effectiveness

Doses below 300 mg per week will not raise testosterone levels above normal, except for a brief time after the injection (Bhasin, et al. 1996). The body decreases its natural testosterone production, which reduces blood testosterone levels to normal or even below normal levels.

The risk of side effects increases at higher doses. The steroid (oral or injectable, oil or water-based, gel or cream) also influences the nature and seriousness of these side effects. Serious bodybuilders and strength-trained athletes who use steroids typically also use drugs to prevent gynecomastia and testicular atrophy. High oral anabolic steroids doses can be toxic to the liver. Oral drugs stay in the system longer, which then can negatively affect liver function.

Dose and Positive Drug Tests: High testosterone doses increase the chances of testing positive during a drug test. The test measures the ratio between testosterone to epitestosterone— a natural testosterone breakdown product. High doses will elevate the ratio above allowable levels. Taking low doses to escape detection provides few benefits because testosterone levels will drop to normal or below.

Steroids tempt almost every bodybuilder or strength athlete. Research studies have confirmed that long-term effectiveness requires high testosterone doses, but high doses cause more side effects. Effective, inexpensive, legal supplements (creatine monohydrate, caffeine, whey protein, and leucine) may work almost as well or better than taking low testosterone doses or testosterone-like anabolic steroids. Excessive amounts of testosterone— 300 mg/week or more— will increase muscle mass and strength in most athletes— even without weight training but will invariably precipitate negative side effects.

Are Athletes Guinea Pigs for Large Dose Steroid Research?

The long-term effects of anabolic steroid use in athletes remain unknown. In the 1970s in the United States, a typical steroid dose for serious bodybuilders was 200 mg Deca Durabolin each week, stacked with 25-50 mg Dianabol a day, with perhaps 20 mg Anavar added.

Today, many athletes greatly exceed these levels. Some athletes take over 3000 mg testosterone a week stacked with growth hormone, insulin, clenbuterol, and a host of nutritional supplements. Any substance —even water—used in excess will cause side effects. Modern strength-trained athletes who take large doses of these drugs will undoubtedly have potentially lethal side effects.

Will high steroid doses cause premature death, heart attack, and cancer? We will not know until scientists conduct large-scale epidemiological studies. With over 17 million anabolic steroid users in America and millions more worldwide, scientists have a large population to study!

Anabolic Steroids and Longevity

Athletes—in particular bodybuilders, throwers, weightlifters, and football players—have consumed anabolic steroids since the 1950s. Physicians predicted increased mortality and morbidity for these athletes, but no large-scale epidemiological evidence has ever supported those claims.

Widespread steroid use in athletics started in the 1960s. Many athletes who competed in the 1960s and 70s and used anabolic steroids have now crossed into middle and older age. Yet, there is little evidence they have a higher incidence of premature death or cardiovascular morbidity than non-athletes who never took steroids.

Most athletes do not care much about atrophied testicles, acne, or low sperm counts but do care about prematurely dying in 10-20 years. Athletes have been using steroids for over 60 years, but there has been no apparent epidemic of premature deaths in aging bodybuilders, throwers, American football players, weightlifters, or gym members.

Health Consequences: Several studies with few subjects investigated the long-term health consequences of steroid use in serious athletes. Parssinen and colleagues (2002) examined death rates in 62 male powerlifters who competed between 1977 and 1982 compared to an age-matched control population of over 1000 men. They assumed a high rate of anabolic steroid use in the powerlifters.

They reported 12.9% of the powerlifters died compared to only 3.1% in the control population. Powerlifters died from suicide (3 athletes), myocardial infarction (3 athletes), liver failure (1 athlete), and non-Hodgkin's lymphoma (1 athlete). The authors stated that these findings add to the growing evidence of an association between anabolic steroid abuse and early death and support the belief that measures to decrease steroid abuse in competitive and amateur athletes are justified.

While the researchers may be correct—steroid users may not live as long as non-users—this evidence was unfortunately based on selective evidence. First, they examined the deaths in only 8 athletes, three of whom died by suicide. Researchers must examine longevity in many more athletes to arrive at a consensus conclusion.

The lifestyle of former powerlifters may have a lot to do with their longevity. Studies in older athletes show that life-long exercise habits, diet, and health habits are critical for long life (Lee, et al., 1995, 1997). Powerlifters may die young because they become physically inactive later in life and avoid aerobic exercise. They may have other habits—excessive alcohol or drug consumption, poor diet, or cigarette consumption—that contribute to early death.

Finally, shorter, lighter men may live longer than those who are taller and heavier (Samaras and Storms, 1992). Powerlifters may simply die earlier because they have excessively greater muscle mass than the average person. The Aerobics Center Longevity study found that physical fitness rather than body mass index was a more important life-span predictor than body size variables (Lee, et al., 2011).

Horowitz, et al., (2019) examined the longevity of 644 men sanctioned for not submitting to a doping test compared to 5450 age-matched controls. These men were presumed anabolic steroid users, with death rates three times higher than non-users. Hospital visits and minor side effects (erectile dysfunction and gynecomastia) were higher in the anabolic steroid users.

Prescriptions Soar: In 2016, physicians wrote over 4 million testosterone prescriptions for middle-aged and older men. While most were non-athletes, it provides a large subject pool to assess the effects of anabolic steroids on longevity.

A large population study by Comhaire (2016) showed that testosterone replacement therapy increased survival rate by 10 percent in five years in men suffering from low testosterone levels. They took lower doses than young athletes taking anabolic steroids, but the information is useful for keeping the problem in perspective.

Improved Life Quality: Studies led by Bhasin et al. (1999, 2018) showed that testosterone replacement therapy might play a role in improving the quality of life in older adults. Middle-aged men given high testosterone doses (600 mg weekly) increased muscle mass, strength, and decreased abdominal fat. They showed no heart disease signs, elevated blood pressure, prostate enlargement, or severe changes in blood lipids (fats). It is unclear whether these benefits outweighed the possible risks.

Animal Studies: Animal studies showed mixed results on steroids and longevity. Bronson, et al. (1997) gave mice anabolic steroids for six months at doses either five times or 20 times their normal circulating testosterone levels. Fifty-two percent of the mice on the high dose died prematurely compared with 35% of the mice given the low dose, and only 12% of the control mice given no steroids. Steroid-using mice that died showed severe heart and liver damage. Conversely, hamsters given nandrolone decanoate lived longer than control animals (Davis et al., 1997). Other studies cast doubt on steroids' long-term health risks (Dickerman et al., 1997; Fineschi, et al., 2001). Scientists do not know whether long-term anabolic steroid use leads to premature death.

Consequences of Low Testosterone Levels (<300 ng/dL): Low testosterone levels in middle-aged and older men increase heart disease risk, muscle loss, depression, poor sexual performance, and longevity (Bhasin, et al., 2018). Several studies showed that testosterone therapy promotes good health and possibly lifespan, but these results may not aptly extrapolate to young athletes taking high drug doses. Aging athletes are reluctant to discuss steroid use during their athletic careers, so it will be challenging to definitively assess the risk of long-term steroid use on health and longevity.

Can Testosterone Replacement Therapy Increase Lifespan? Limited data show that anabolic steroids favorably affect cell structures that extend the lifespan (Yeap, et al., 2016). The gene telomere structure form the ends of the DNA strands and hold them together. The telomeres shorten over time, reducing their effectiveness and increasing the risk of bone marrow failure, liver cirrhosis, pulmonary fibrosis, cancer, and death. Danazol prevented telomere shortening in those with telomere diseases according to a 2016 study from the National Heart, Lung, and Blood Institute (Townsley, et al., 2016). These results might not apply to people with normal telomeres. If they do, anabolic steroids, at least in therapeutic doses, might increase longevity.

Testosterone levels vary widely in men over 50 (300-800 ng/dL). Is normal optimal? Most aging men want a vigorous lifestyle that increased testosterone can provide. Also, the biologically active free testosterone decreases steadily with age, even though testosterone levels might remain unchanged. *Optimal health and vitality are more important than the absence of disease.*

Summary

Anabolic steroids have many well-documented side effects, but the research is so politicized that it is sometimes difficult to draw accurate conclusions. Side effects are widespread; they include disorders affecting the liver, kidneys, urogenital system, skin, psyche, metabolism, and soft tissue.

Some steroid side-effects are due to their effects on strength. Steroid users sometimes developed strength levels that would be impossible to achieve without the drugs. The capacity for high intensity workouts increases the risk for cardiac hypertrophy and heart failure, rhabdomyolysis, and severe joint damage to knees, hips, and spine and premature death. High doses are linked to severe psychological problems.

Paradoxically, low testosterone levels in middle and

older age are linked to myocardial infarction, stroke, depression, sarcopenia, and osteoporosis. Testosterone replacement therapy may improve quality of life and longevity in aging men with medically diagnosed low testosterone levels.

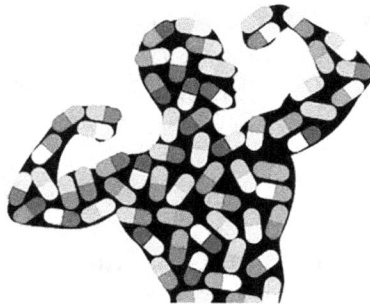

7

ANABOLIC STEROIDS AND SYSTEMIC DISEASE: HEART, CIRCULATION, CANCER, LIVER, KIDNEYS

Health experts cite premature death and heart attack as the primary reasons for avoiding anabolic steroids. Circumstantial evidence rather than experimental research accounts for most of these opinions. Case studies involving steroid users have documented strokes, heart attacks, sudden death, testicular and prostate cancer, heart enlargement, abnormal blood chemistry, and increased blood pressure.

Cardiovascular side effects often occur in athletes using several drugs simultaneously. Athletes take much higher steroid doses than they did 20 years ago, increasing side effect risks. Cardiovascular risks are rare in athletes taking average anabolic steroid doses but increase dramatically at higher levels. Higher doses cause large increases in hematocrit (blood thickness), which increase heart attack and stroke risk.

Low Testosterone Levels Increase Coronary Artery Disease Risk: The effects of recreational use of anabolic steroids on cardiovascular health are unknown. Go to almost any locker room worldwide and you will see warning signs against using anabolic steroids and testosterone. The signs warn—in bold letters—that steroids promote atherosclerosis and heart attack.

Coronary Artery Disease Mechanisms: Figure 7-1 shows the mechanism of myocardial infarction (heart attack) and stroke from arterial disease. Both conditions cause poor blood flow to the heart or brain resulting in cell death. The figure shows the physiological progression that leads to a heart attack or stroke:

1. Endothelial dysfunction, disruption in the cells lining the arteries
2. Fatty-streak formation, the deposition of fatty material in the endothelial cells
3. Plaque formation, which narrows the artery
4. Plaque rupture and blood clot, which blocks blood flow to part of the heart or brain

High-dose anabolic steroid use may promote each stage in blood vessel disease (D'Ascenzo, et al., 2007). Conversely, low-dose hormone replacement enhances endothelial function in hypogonadal men (Bhasin, et al., 2021).

ARTERY DISEASE
ATHEROSCLEROSIS
BLOOD CLOT

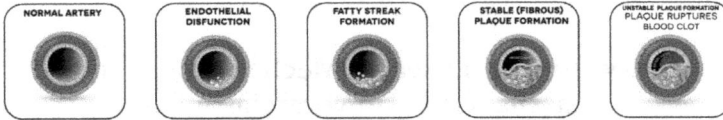

| NORMAL ARTERY | ENDOTHELIAL DISFUNCTION | FATTY STREAK FORMATION | STABLE (FIBROUS) PLAQUE FORMATION | UNSTABLE PLAQUE FORMATION PLAQUE RUPTURES BLOOD CLOT |

STROKE

HEART ATTACK

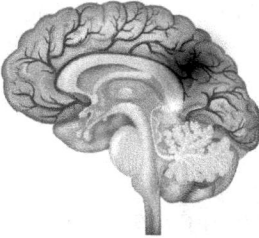

**BLOOD CLOT BLOCKS
BLOOD FLOW TO THE BRAIN**

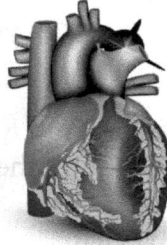

**BLOOD CLOT BLOCKS
BLOOD FLOW TO THE HEART MUSCLE**

Figure 7-1: Coronary artery disease. Source: Shutterstock.

A literature evaluation reveals that not only is testosterone not linked to atherosclerosis, but it may promote the health of the cells lining the blood vessels—the endothelium—to prevent disease. Men with higher testosterone levels have less abdominal fat, better functioning endothelial cells, and better blood glucose control—showing that having at least average testosterone levels is heart-healthy. Low free testosterone levels may be a risk factor for atherosclerosis (Philips, et al., 1994). In middle-age and older adults with low testosterone levels (<300 ng/dL), hormone supplements could protect against the disease (Bhasin, et al., 2018; Bhasin, et al., 2021).

What about the high dose testosterone and anabolic steroids used by some bodybuilders? That may be another story. Some studies suggest that abnormally elevated testosterone levels (or testosterone-like drugs) may promote changes in cardiac structure and insulin resistance. These conditions may lead to high blood pressure, endothelial disruption, abnormal blood lipids, and abnormalities with blood clotting (Barbosa, et al., 2018; Rasmussen, et al., 2018). There is little evidence about the long-term effects of high testosterone doses on the heart and blood vessels.

Large steroid doses build skeletal muscle, even absent exercise (Bhasin, et al., 1996). The heart is a muscle and will grow in response to heavy weightlifting and anabolic hormones. Heart damage is the most significant long-term risk with heavy steroid use, but the evidence for heart damage is not clear. Bodybuilders and power athletes often have enlarged hearts—even when they do not take steroids (Santos, et al., 2014). While high steroid doses decrease HDL, the drugs have no effects or even reduce LDL and triglycerides—blood lipids that promote heart disease. Also, steroids increase the antioxidant superoxide dismutase activity that protects against heart disease (Delgato, et al., 2010).

Steroids and Inflamatory Markers: High anabolic steroid doses disrupt endothelial cell metabolism on the arteries' inner lining (D'Ascenzo, et al. 2007). Elevated testosterone levels and anabolic steroids may increase blood markers signifying inflammation, which can cause a variety of degenerative diseases, trigger DNA damage, and suppress the immune system. Blood vessel inflammation triggers abnormal fluid movement, interferes with cellular repair, promotes blood vessel fibrosis, and promotes blood clot formation. Recall that Figure 7-1 showed blood vessel disease progression that leads to blocked blood flow to the brain or heart.

Steroids and HDL: Steroids decrease HDL levels. HDL is a negative risk factor for heart disease—high HDL levels reduce the heart disease risk. The decrease in HDL cholesterol levels in steroid users might not promote heart disease. It might reflect an accelerated cholesterol transport rate.

HDL levels decrease dramatically when athletes take steroids and revert to normal when they stop taking the drug (Figure 7-2). A normal value for young men is 45 mg/dL. Steroid users often have levels less than 20 mg/dL—anything under 35 mg/dL suggests increased coronary artery disease risk. Despite years of steroid use, no definitive study has observed an increased death rate from heart disease in aging bodybuilders and other weight-trained athletes.

Figure 7-2 shows the effects of anabolic steroid cycles on HDL in elite strength athletes. Peterson and Fahey (1985) discovered this effect by accident. The researchers noted that some people tested in their lab had wildly fluctuating HDL levels. Further investigation showed they were elite strength athletes. They recruited them for a study that tracked HDL levels during steroid cycles. HDL values plunged when they were taking steroids and normalized when they stopped taking the drugs.

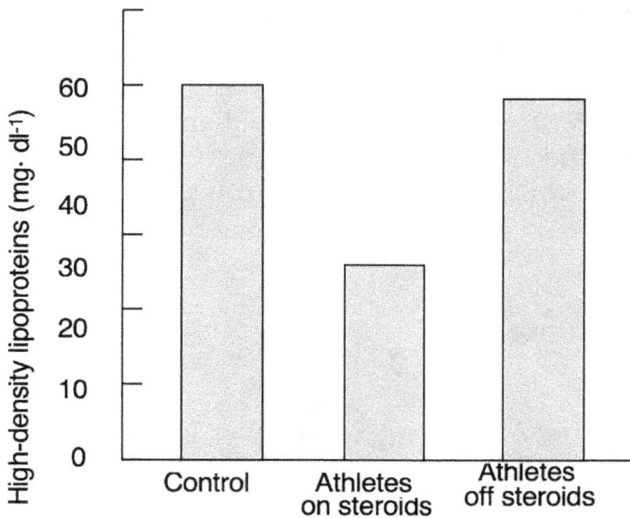

Figure 7-2 HDL during steroid cycles in elite athletes. Source: Peterson and Fahey, 1985.

Anabolic steroids disturb cholesterol metabolism, but the mechanisms remain elusive. Swedish researchers found that injecting 500 milligrams of testosterone enanthate increased HMG-CoA reductase enzyme, which increased cholesterol by 15% (Garevik, et al., 2012). Testosterone also decreases HDL cholesterol, probably by speeding its breakdown. The study showed that even a single anabolic steroid dose could interfere with cholesterol metabolism. The long-term effects of anabolic steroids on cholesterol metabolism remain unresolved.

Elite power athletes who use steroids also use other drugs and often follow diets linked to developing coronary artery disease. In the 1980s, one of us (Fahey) studied an elite anabolic steroid-using power athlete who consumed 30 eggs daily. His cholesterol was 300 mg/dL and his HDL was 12 mg/dL (Peterson and Fahey, 1986). He is now 73 years old and still apparently healthy and relatively physically active. Each athlete is unique, which makes disease processes difficult to study.

Heart Failure

Athletes who take high doses of anabolic steroids sometimes show increases in heart size, particularly in the interventricular septum— the wall separating the left and right ventricles (Figure 7-3). Increased heart wall size is probably due more to lifting heavy weights than the steroids themselves. However, the extreme increases in strength might not have been possible without the drugs, so steroids play a role in cardiac enlargement–at least indirectly.

Several heart studies in anabolic steroid users showed increases in heart mass, left ventricular hypertrophy, heart cell abnormalities, and disruptions in impulse conduction in the heart (i.e., abnormal electrocardiogram) (Sullivan, et al. 1998; Welder, et al. 1993; Far, et al., 2012; Polito, et al., 2017, White, et al., 2018). Anabolic steroids allow athletes to train harder, which increases the load on the heart and blood vessels.

Left Ventricular Hypertrophy: This condition occurs in elite strength athletes by increasing the left ventricle's heart wall size (Figure 7-3). This powerful heart chamber pumps blood to the general circulation. Factors that load the heart include heart rate, preload, afterload, and heart muscle contractility (Bruanwald, E, 1976). Heart rate increases during exercise and increases the energy demand of the heart. Preload is the stress of blood returning to the heart and "stretching" the heart wall and becomes significant during endurance running. Afterload is the resistance the heart gets from attempting to push blood into the circulation.

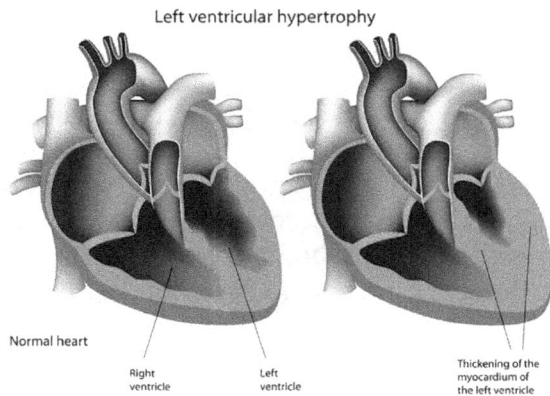

Figure 7-3: Cardiac hypertrophy is common in elite weight-trained athletes. Steroids allow athletes to lift more weight, which increases afterload stress on the heart. Source: Shutterstock.

Intense Weight Training: The leg and arm muscles contract at maximal levels and restrict blood flow from the heart, causing the heart to enlarge. Larger hearts take more energy to contract, which can then lead to heart failure as the athlete ages. During heavy squats in elite strength athletes, blood pressure can reach 480/350 mm Hg, demonstrating the extreme afterload stress in powerlifting (MacDougall, et al., 1985).

Lifting heavy weights loads the heart, which increases heart wall size and reduces the left ventricular chamber size (Figure 7-3). The left ventricle deteriorates as the athlete deconditions and ages, increasing heart failure risk.

Impaired Heart Function: Few data exist demonstrating chronic intense strength training effects on decreased heart function in anabolic steroid users. Heart enlargement is a common side effect of anabolic steroid use. Researchers from Uppsala University in Sweden (Far, et al., 2012) conducted autopsies on 87 men who tested positive for anabolic steroids and 173 aged–matched deceased men who had not taken the drugs. Deceased steroid users had the largest hearts. Increased heart size also was linked to body weight, height, age, and death from trauma.

What can we infer from these results? Anabolic steroids allow people to lift heavier weights, which increases the load on the heart and triggers cardiac enlargement. Did steroids or heavy lifting increase heart wall size? Perhaps people would be less capable of lifting heavy weights if they had not taken steroids.

Weight training causes a pressure load on the heart. Intense muscle contractions during squats or bench presses cause resistance in blood vessels, so the heart must work harder to push blood into the circulation. Steroid users are usually stronger than nonusers, so they experience greater heart pressure loads during exercise.

A Massachusetts General Hospital study showed that long-time steroid users had weaker hearts (Baggish, et al., 2010). The normal heart can pump 55 to 70 % of the blood delivered to it during each beat—a measure called the ejection fraction. Eighty-three percent of long-time steroid users had abnormally low ejection fractions at less than 55%. The steroid users took over 600 mg testosterone a week for at least nine years. The researchers speculated that decreased heart function in these athletes could eventually lead to heart failure.

Some athletes who died from heart attacks and heart failure were steroid users. Animal studies reported that large steroid doses damage heart muscle (Hassan, et al., 2009; Karhunen, et al., 1988; Melchert et al., 1992; Seara, et al., 2019). No large population study has demonstrated an increased death rate among former or current anabolic steroid users, so it is premature to say that steroids *cause* heart problems.

Strength-trained athletes who used steroids should know the warning signs that can lead to heart problems. These signs include hypertension, abnormal blood lipids (high cholesterol, LDL, triglycerides and low HDL), shortness of breath, chest pain, and abnormal blood chemistry (e.g., elevated creatine kinase, lactate dehydrogenase, C-reactive protein).

· · ·

Sudden Death: This is rare in young people but common in middle-aged and older people. Sudden death is the first symptom of cardiovascular disease in 33 percent of people. Italian researchers (Montisci, et al., 2011) reported four cases of cardiac–related sudden death in former anabolic steroid users. All the men showed evidence of left ventricular enlargement, and some showed heart cell abnormalities. No study has shown a cause-and-effect relationship between steroid use and sudden death. Steroids allow people to lift heavier weights than usual, adding excessive stress to the heart.

Fahey and Swanson (2008) developed a model for predicting sudden death from daily physical activity levels based on data from the Physicians Health Study. With the assumption that the relative sudden death frequency during exercise is linearly related to the proportion of time spent exercising, the analysis rendered a "U-shaped" curve between the relative sudden death risk and the weekly volume of moderate intensity exercise. The model predicted that men 40 to 80 years should exercise 30 minutes a day (6 METS intensity) six days a week to receive the benefits of exercise and minimize the risk of sudden death.

The Harvard Alumni studies directed by Ralph Paffenbarger showed that current physical activity patterns were more important for predicting cardiac morbidity and mortality than collegiate athletic experience (Lee, et al., 1997). Runacres, et al. (2021), in a study of 165,000 elite athletes, found that endurance and mixed/team athletes had a lower incidence of cardiovascular disease and cancer compared to the general population, while power athletes showed no risk reduction. Former power athletes (including former steroid users) must do the requisite amount of aerobic exercise to optimize health and longevity.

Arrhythmias

We can infer from some evidence that consuming high anabolic steroid doses triggers electrical instability in the heart, which may increase the risk of heart–related sudden death. While several case studies have reported isolated sudden death incidents in steroid-using athletes, this has not been demonstrated in any large-scale study.

A British study reported an increased incidence of instability in the electrocardiogram after exercise in athletes who used anabolic steroids compared to nonusers (Sculthorpe, et al., 2016). Post-exercise electrical instability in the heart increased the risk of heart–related sudden death. More research is needed before the science can conclude that anabolic steroids increase sudden death risk.

Figure 7-4 shows a normal electrocardiogram. Each element (P, QRS, T) precedes contractions in the heart's atria and ventricles. Figure 7-5 shows ventricular tachycardia (rapid heart rate) and ventricular fibrillation, both often leading to cardiac arrest and sudden death.

Normal Sinus Rhythm

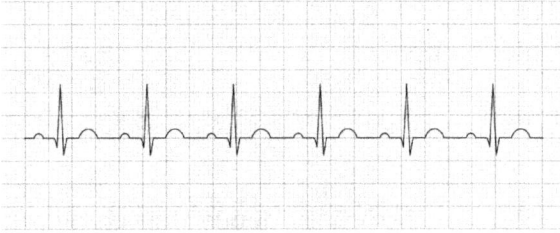

Figure 7-4: The normal electrocardiogram.
Source: Shutterstock

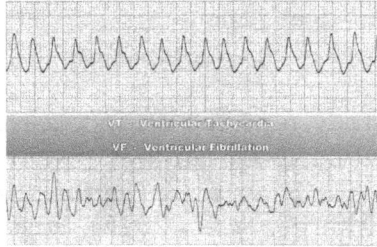

Figure 7-5: Dangerous arrhythmias: ventricular
tachycardia (upper); ventricular fibrillation (lower).
Source: Shutterstock.

Several researchers reported an increased atrial and ventricular tachycardia and fibrillation risk in long-time steroid users (Carbone, et al. 2017; D'Andrea, et al. 2018; Schollert, et al. 1993; Sullivan, et al. 1999). The atrial arrhythmias increase the risk of stroke (the atria are the heart's top chambers). These studies were clinical observations involving only a few athletes. They showed that long-term use of anabolic steroids is linked with heart abnormalities. These abnormalities include enlargement of the left ventricle, increased diastolic blood pressure (lower blood pressure number), arterial stiffness, and disturbances between the heart's electrical and contractile functions.

The researchers reported increases in atrial fibrillation (linked to fainting and stroke), chest pain, congestive heart failure, blood clotting, and palpitations. They also reported an increased incidence in cardiac arrhythmias in the atria of trained bodybuilders. They noted that bodybuilders did not appear to be more susceptible to other heart rhythm abnormalities.

Cardiomyopathy

Cardiomyopathy is a heart muscle disease that compromises the heart's capacity to contract and pump blood. The principal disease types include hypertrophic, dilated, and restrictive. Hypertrophic cardiomyopathy disease is inherited and the principal cause of heart-related sudden death in people under age 35. Anabolic steroids may cause dilated cardiomyopathy and heart failure in long-time steroid drug users (Garner, et al., 2018; Han, et al., 2015; Sullivan, et al., 1998). Steroids plus weight training initially increase heart wall-size due to pressure loading. Larger hearts take more energy to contract. This gradually weakens the heart muscle so the walls become thinner, resulting in a large, weak heart and chronic hypertension.

Blood

Testosterone and anabolic steroids stimulate red blood cell production by increasing erythropoietin, and erythroid progenitor cells, (Bhasin, et al., 2021). Increased hematocrit (percent cells in the blood) and hemoglobin are significant testosterone replacement therapy and anabolic steroid side effects. These changes increase the risk of dangerous blood clots, heart attack, and stroke (Yang, et al., 2018).

In males, increased hemoglobin levels associate with greater blood heme iron levels to increase coronary artery disease risk and sudden cardiac death (Kaluza, et al., 2014). University of Florida researchers (Beggs, et al., 2014) found that testosterone altered iron metabolism and stimulated red blood cell production independently from dihydrotestosterone. They measured blood changes during testosterone supplementation with and without concurrently administering finasteride—a drug that blocks dihydrotestosterone formation and used to treat male pattern baldness. Men experiencing increases in hematocrit and hemoglobin during testosterone therapy should donate blood regularly or stop taking the drugs!

Anabolic Steroids and Cancer

Cancer is a disease linked to genetic coding errors in DNA that trigger rapid cell growth that can travel to many different cells and tissues. The most common cancers affect the lungs, prostate, colon, rectum, skin, and breasts. Anabolic steroids increase cell growth rate, but there is little evidence they cause or promote cancerous growth.

Unfortunately, young people sometimes die from cancer. Because one cancer patient also took anabolic steroids in the past does not mean that steroids caused the problem. When the famous Oakland Raider pro football player Lyle Alzedo died of brain cancer at age 38 (1949-1992; active pro player 1971-1985), many people blamed anabolic steroids— even without evidence. Alzedo died from brain lymphoma, which is not associated with elevated testosterone levels.

High doses of anabolic steroids increase growth factor IGF-1, which might promote cancers of the colon, pancreas, and prostate. Oral anabolic steroids can be toxic to the liver and may trigger liver tumors. As with heart disease, indirect evidence implicates high dose steroid abuse with increased cancer risk. Any substance that triggers high tissue growth rates might also increase cancer cell growth, but no large population studies link anabolic steroid use with cancer.

Prostate Cancer: Prostate cancer is the leading cause of cancer death in men (Figure 7-6). Testosterone promotes the normal prostate growth and repair. A common treatment is to suppress testosterone metabolism by reducing production in the testes, blocking testosterone binding throughout the body, and blocking testosterone production from adrenal androgens (DHEA and androstenedione). However, several researchers reported that testosterone supplements did not increase prostate cancer risk (Debruyne, et al., 2017; Eisenberg, et al. 2015).

Prostate Cancer

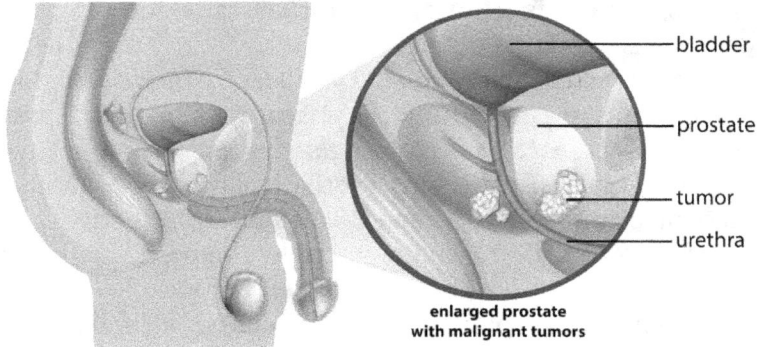

enlarged prostate
with malignant tumors

Figure 7-6 Supplemental testosterone's role to promote prostate cancer is highly controversial. Source: Shutterstock.

Testosterone supplements for aging men are highly controversial because it could increase prostate cancer risk. A British study of 1365 men reported that testosterone replacement therapy for up to 20 yr showed no increase in prostate cancer incidence (Eisenberg, et al., 2015). Prostate cancer rate was one case per 212 years of treatment and comparable to the average population. Testosterone treatment was not related to changes in prostate-specific antigen (PSA). Men taking testosterone supplements and receiving regular annual prostate exams had a lower prostate cancer risk than men not receiving treatment.

Athletes take anabolic steroids to promote muscle tissue growth. Cells throughout the body contain androgen receptors that have widespread anabolic effects. As mentioned previously, and with scarce data if any, some researchers have warned about the possibility that anabolic steroids *could* promote cancer.

. . .

DNA Damage: Several studies found evidence of DNA damage and cell death in anabolic steroid users. Damage to DNA can theoretically serve as a link between anabolic steroids and increased cancer risk. Abbasnezhad, et al. (2021) reported that anabolic steroid use in bodybuilders caused DNA damage and decreased telomere length in blood lymphocytes. Recall that many athletes have been using these drugs for over 50 years, and no study has shown an increased cancer risk in former steroid users.

Testicular Cancer: High-dose anabolic steroid use might increase testicular cancer risk. Cancer involves runaway cell growth in specific tissues that can migrate to other body areas. Ordinarily, genes limit tissue growth rates, but their controlling mechanisms fail to work in cancer cells. Spanish researchers presented evidence that anabolic steroids and tissue growth factor IGF-1 triggered testicular cancer growth in rats with a genetic susceptibility to the disease (Garcia, et al., 2012). If these results apply to humans, anabolic drugs may promote cancer growth in men who already have testicular cancer.

Growth hormone, EPO, and anabolic steroids promote tissue growth. Scientists have speculated that athletes taking these drugs might be more susceptible to cancer or cancer cell growth, particularly in high dosages. A literature review by Italian scientists concluded insufficient evidence links these drugs to cancer (Salerno, et al., 2018). Athletes typically combine powerful drugs, making it difficult to assess the health risks of specific agents. Most studies showing a link between these drugs and cancer are anecdotal case studies that do not show they triggered the disease. However, anabolic drugs can promote cancer cell growth, but more research is required to determine the risks.

Testosterone and anabolic steroids trigger rapid growth rates that could promote cancer cell growth. The genes carefully regulate cell growth, which have mechanisms for dealing with unintended mutant gene coding errors. Ultraviolet light, obesity, environmental toxins, and physical inactivity influence genetic coding, so it is conceivable that anabolic steroids *could* affect these processes.

Anabolic Steroids and Liver Disease

The liver is a vital metabolic organ involved with processing fats, carbohydrates, and proteins, hormone secretion, detoxification, bile production, cholesterol synthesis, processing vitamins, and enzyme synthesis. Figure 7-7 summarizes these effects.

Chemically altered oral anabolic steroids stay in the system longer than other anabolic steroid forms. C-17 alkylated androgenic steroids may cause liver injury, including cholestasis (blocked bile ducts), peliosis hepatis (blood filled cysts), nodular regenerative hyperplasia (high blood pressure in liver blood vessels), hepatic adenomas (hormone induced liver tumors), and hepatocellular carcinoma (liver cancer) (Lovisetto, et al., 1979, She, et al., 1994).

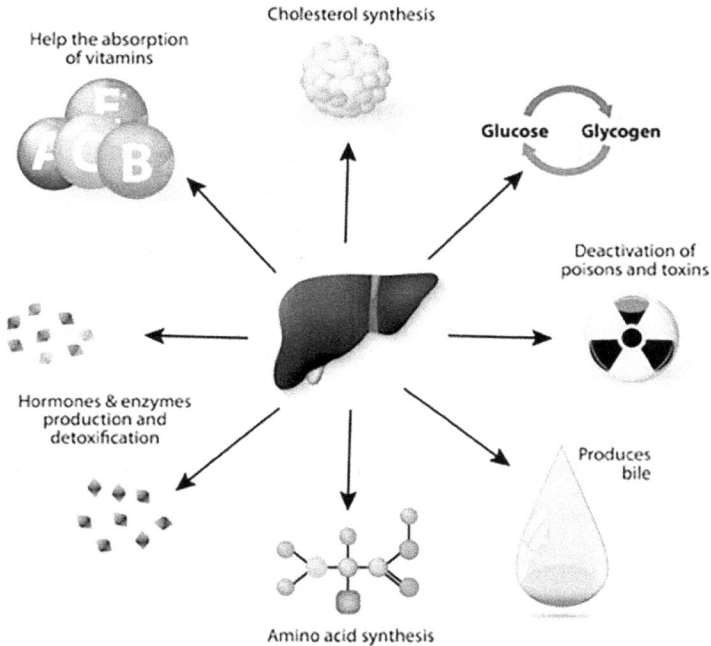

Figure 7-7: Summary of Liver Function. Source Shutterstock

Several clinical observations presented cases of liver damage in bodybuilders and other strength athletes who used steroids, and required hospitalization. Many cases also experienced kidney damage, although there were no deaths. The bottom line: athletes who take steroids should avoid oral anabolic steroids. These drugs are widely available in Latin America and Asia. They increase the risk in unsophisticated users of developing liver toxicity.

. . .

Blood Chemistry: Intense training can alter blood chemistry in users and nonusers of anabolic steroids. The steroid users might have trained harder than the nonusers, which would explain any minor differences in blood chemistry between the two groups. Many "clean" athletes who train hard will have elevated values of common liver function tests such as aspartate transaminase (AST), alkaline phosphatase (ALP), gamma-glutamyltransferase (GGT), albumen, total protein, and L-lactate dehydrogenase. Anabolic steroid use can also elevate these enzymes. Athletes who take anabolic steroids should monitor these blood constituents.

Anabolic steroid users have a slightly lower risk for contracting hepatitis B and C. In a study of 63 men, Australian researchers found that 9.5% of steroid users had hepatitis C antibodies, and 12% had hepatitis B antibodies (Aitken et al., 2002), significantly lower than the general population. Risk factors for hepatitis C included past heroin use, imprisonment, tattoos, and hepatitis B virus exposure. While steroid users had a lower risk of hepatitis than other men in the study, 12% exhibited antibodies to the disease.

Fatty Liver Disease (FLD): FLD involves fat accumulation in the liver. Causal factors include obesity, type 2 diabetes, hepatitis C, and alcohol consumption (Figure 7-8). It is a risk factor for liver fibrosis, liver cancer, cirrhosis, and esophageal pathologies. FLD affects 90% of alcoholics, 30% of people in Western countries, 10% of children, and 10% of Asians. It is common in unfit men and older adults. Environmental poisons and drugs can cause liver damage and FLD.

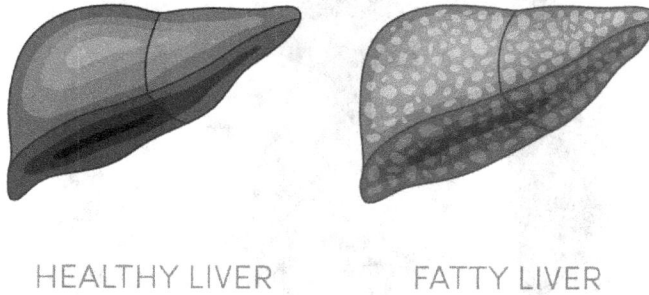

HEALTHY LIVER   FATTY LIVER

Figure 7-8: Fatty liver disease is excessive fat accumulation in the liver that may eventually lead to liver cancer and liver failure. Some reports link anabolic steroids to fatty liver disease.

Brazilian scientists compared markers of liver metabolism in 95 bodybuilders who used steroids with 85 nonusers (Nogueira, et al. 2014). They noted blood chemistry abnormalities in 12.6% of steroid users but only 2.4% of nonusers. None of the athletes in the study showed any adverse symptoms. They suggested that steroid use could be a risk factor for fatty liver disease.

Anabolic Steroids and Kidney Disease

The kidneys are bean-shaped organs about 4.3 inches long, located against the upper abdomen's back (Figure 7-9a). These vital organs control body fluids, blood pressure, waste product elimination, acid-base balance, and drug metabolism and excretion (Figure 7-9b).

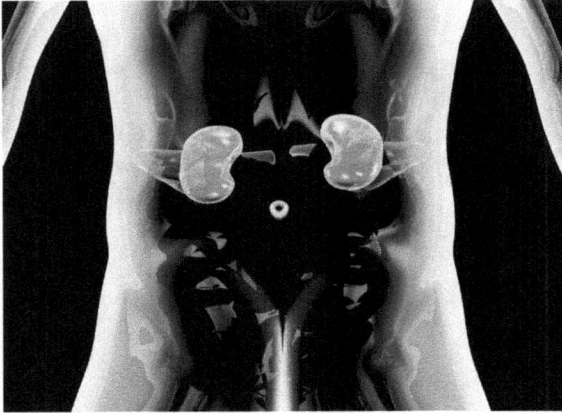

Figure 7-9a: Kidneys' location in the abdomen.
Source: Shutterstock.

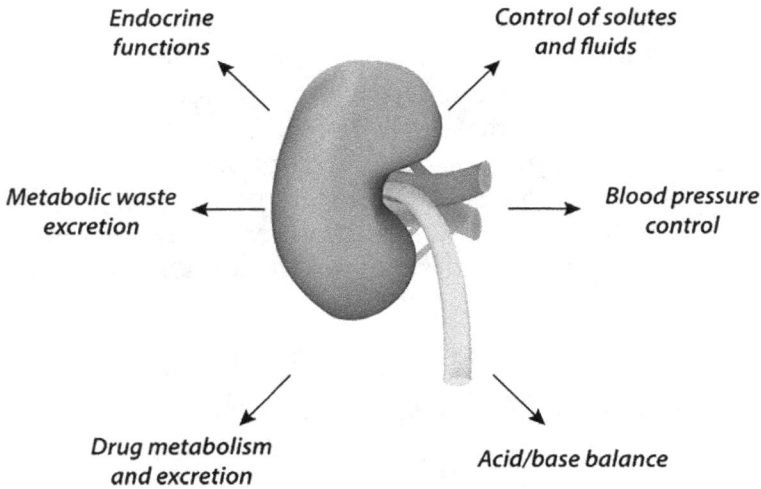

Figure 7-9b: Summary of kidney function. Source:
Shutterstock.

Kidney disease involves damage to the kidney in one of two types—inflammatory (nephritic) and non-inflammatory (nephrotic). Chronic kidney disease results in a gradual deterioration in kidney function leading to kidney failure requiring dialysis or kidney transplant. Roughly 13 percent of Americans have chronic kidney disease with the disease becoming more prevalent with age, particularly past age 50. The environmental toxin lead can cause kidney pathology.

In most people, kidney disease develops due to hypertension, type 2 diabetes, and the non-steroidal anti-inflammatory drugs (NSAIDs) aspirin and ibuprofen. Intensely training athletes often overuse NSAIDs, which can lead to kidney disease and stomach ulcers. Steroids allow people to train harder, which increases overtraining soft tissue injury risk and pain.

Intense weight training triggers acute increases in blood pressure. Blood pressure—measured directly inside the arteries—has reached as high as 480/350 mm Hg during heavy squats (resting blood pressure is typically 120/80 mm Hg). Blood pressure usually returns to normal after an intense weight training session, but repeated resistance training causes increased arterial stiffness, which can lead to chronic hypertension. Changes in arterial stiffness are minimal in middle-aged people who lift weights or in young people who lift light weights.

High blood pressure is sometimes called the silent killer because there are few obvious symptoms, but nevertheless can lead to coronary artery disease, heart failure, stroke, erectile dysfunction, and kidney disease. Chronic anabolic steroid use promotes increased blood pressure. Users often develop incredible strength levels that can add a significant load on the heart.

Blood Vessel Stiffness: Blood vessel stiffness is an important mechanism for developing high blood pressure and loading the kidneys. In a study on rats, Brazilian scientists found that long-term treatment with nandrolone decanoate caused increased resistance in the blood vessels supplying the gut, important for blood pressure regulation (Caliman, et al. 2017). We do not know if these results apply to humans.

Anabolic steroids make it possible to lift heavy weights, particularly in the squat, deadlift, and bench press. Fahey studied heart wall sizes in elite throwing athletes who were some of the strongest men in the world. For example, one athlete had a max squat of 900 pounds and several bench pressed over 600 pounds. Heart wall changes—a marker of pressure overload during training—were greatest in athletes with the highest squats (Fahey: unpublished observations, 1984). These athletes took anabolic steroids.

Lifting heavy loads triggers explosive increases in blood pressure. Trained athletes who lift heavy weights because they take steroids can expect increased blood pressure and an increased kidney disease risk. Clinical observations suggest that kidney problems reverse when the athletes stop taking the drugs.

The link between anabolic steroids, hypertension, and kidney damage is less evident in mid-level strength athletes. Testosterone and anabolic steroids caused kidney damage in some studies, but these findings were inconsistent and thus remain controversial.

Dietary Salt: Dietary salt influences the effects of testosterone on blood pressure. In a study on salt–loaded rats, Liu and Ely (2011) reported that 8 weeks of testosterone supplementation increased blood pressure more than in rats that were not salt-loaded.

If these results apply to humans, athletes who take testosterone and anabolic steroids should reduce dietary salt intake. Intense weight training causes arterial stiffness. Unfortunately, most Americans consume relatively high salt diets. Combining the effects of testosterone, high salt diets, and weight training could trigger long-term cardiovascular problems.

Combined Drug Effects: Determining the effects of individual drugs in athletes can be difficult because most take more than one drug and supplement simultaneously. Some of the drugs can interact and cause unpredictable side effects.

Schafer, et al. (2011) reported the case of a bodybuilder who injected oil-based testosterone and erythropoietin simultaneously (EPO is a blood-boosting drug). The athlete developed abnormally high calcium levels, which triggered multiple organ failure including severe kidney and liver injury. The athlete also trained intensely, so his condition could have been related to rhabdomyolysis, which involves destroying muscle cells and emptying the muscle contents into the bloodstream. It is difficult to determine whether multiple drug use or intense training caused the athlete's adverse condition.

Nandrolone decanoate, a popular drug with some bodybuilders, might be harmful to the kidneys. Nandrolone decanoate may cause kidney problems—according to a study on rabbits led by Greek researchers (Tsitsimpikou, et al., 2016). Long-term drug use led to structural and functional changes in the kidneys, including increases in blood urea, creatinine, SGOT (AST), and SGPT (ALT). The tissues became inflamed and fibrotic, and kidney cell telomerase activity increased.

The telomeres form the ends of the chromosomes and cell death (apoptosis) occurs when the telomeres unravel. Kidney cells also showed evidence of severe oxidative damage. If these results apply to humans, then long-term use of nandrolone could disrupt kidney function.

Summary

Case studies of steroid users document strokes, heart attacks, sudden death, testicular and prostate cancer, heart enlargement, abnormal blood chemistry, and increased blood pressure leading to hypertension. Cardiovascular side effects often occur in athletes using several drugs simultaneously. Athletes take much higher steroid doses than they did 20 years ago, which increases side effect risks. Cardiovascular risks are rare in athletes taking regular doses but increase dramatically at higher doses. Steroids stimulate extreme strength levels that generate higher than normal pressures in the circulation. Intense training loads increase ventricular afterload, arterial stiffness, and hypertension. Little research ties anabolic steroids to cancer, but clinical observations link steroids to prostate and testicular cancer.

Oral anabolic steroids increase liver damage and perhaps liver cancer risks, but injectable steroids are seldom implicated. High doses link to kidney damage. Intense training can alter blood chemistry values, which might be mistaken for the steroids' pathological effects.

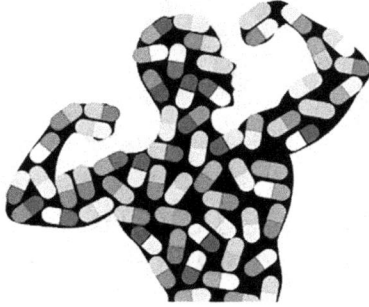

8

SEXUAL AND PSYCHOLOGICAL
EFFECTS OF ANABOLIC STEROIDS

Testosterone and the synthetic anabolic steroids increase muscle mass and affect cells throughout the body. Testosterone, like all hormones, is tightly regulated by a negative feedback loop involving other hormones—an increase in one hormone shuts down another hormone, which reduces the first hormone's production (Refer to Chapter 5, Figure 5-3). Injecting large doses of anabolic steroids disrupts normal regulatory functions and ultimately decreases natural testosterone production.

Sexual side effects represent anabolic steroids' most common negative consequence. They include testicular suppression, testicular atrophy, decreased sperm count, impaired semen quality, premature sperm cell death, abnormal cellular changes in the testes, and abnormal genetic changes in sperm cells. Prolonged anabolic steroid use depresses testicular function and fertility and can be intractable in long-time users . Infertility is common in young adults who use anabolic steroids, while hCG therapy usually restores normal testicular function.

With testosterone and anabolic steroids, it is not an easy task to separate politics from legitimate data. A literature review from the Münster University in Germany is an excellent example (Nieschlag and Vorona, 2015). They estimated that 6.4 % of males and 1.6 % of females worldwide have used anabolic steroids. The researchers gleaned most effects from single-subject clinical observations that could have been attributed to other factors. Sexual side effects linked to steroid use included testicular tumors, prostate enlargement and cancer, infertility, hair growth, hair loss, clitoral growth, deepening of women's voices, and increased breast cancer risk in both sexes. While these risks are real, the true incidence and risks remain unknown.

As one doping expert from Europe said, "We expect the most stringent evidence to support positive effects of these drugs but accept the most trivial anecdotes to prove side effects" (Brooks, et al., 2020). Testosterone and anabolic steroid use is widespread in athletes trying to improve performance, active people trying to improve appearance, and older people trying to slow the aging process. Researchers need accurate data from scientists rather than political posturing and political correctness from health experts.

Long-Term Effects: Anabolic steroid use has an adverse long-term effect on gonadal function by suppressing natural testosterone production. Hormones function on a feedback system that regulates production based on circulating levels. When one takes testosterone or other anabolic steroid drugs, the hormone regulators reduce naturally produced testosterone. When one stops taking the drugs, the feedback system gradually adjusts and restores the hormone balance to normal.

Harvard researchers reported that former steroid users had smaller testicular volumes and lowered circulating blood testosterone levels, even though they had not taken the drugs in 3 to 26 months (Kanayama, et al., 2015). Former users also showed reduced libido, greater incidence of depression, and erectile dysfunction compared to an athletic control group who never took steroids. Two men in the study failed to restore regular sex drive or erectile function even when given testosterone therapy.

Infertility: Anabolic steroids promote infertility. Millions of men in the United States take testosterone or other anabolic steroids. About fifty percent have taken the drugs for three or more years, and most take supra-physiological doses that increase blood testosterone above normal levels. Most studies of sexual function in men show that anabolic steroid use impairs fertility (Bhasin, et al., 2021).

Testosterone supplements cause a decrease in testosterone-controlling hormones LH and FSH, which promote a rebound testosterone decrease. These changes also reduce sperm production in the testes. Gradually, steroids cause testicular atrophy. The best treatment for testosterone-induced infertility is when users stop taking the drugs.

Females

During the Cold War (from 1947-1991), athletes from the Soviet Union, German Democratic Republic, and other Eastern Bloc countries used steroids systematically—sometimes without their knowledge or consent (Huang & Basaria, 2018). Clinical evaluation showed that females developed physiological changes consistent with testosterone's effects in males. These included abnormal hair growth (e.g., facial and back hair), acne, widening of the upper torso, deepening voice, male pattern balding, clitoral hypertrophy, and breast atrophy. Anabolic steroid use linked to irregular and painful menstruation (i.e., oligomenorrhea, amenorrhea, and dysmenorrhea) and infertility. The drugs also caused accelerated muscle hypertrophy, depression, and mood instability—all known testosterone side effects. Anecdotal information from former athletes from East Germany showed that many of these sexual side effects became life-long problems that adversely impacted their personal and family lives.

Children

Children taking anabolic steroids first experience accelerated maturation, followed by premature closure of the epiphyseal growth centers in the long bones. Anabolic steroid use in early adolescence can stunt growth. Varney (1999) suspected that some young female gymnasts have taken anabolic steroids specifically to stunt growth because small stature is an advantage in women's gymnastics.

Anabolic steroid use by adolescent athletes may predispose them to increased musculoskeletal injury risks. Studies in rats found that soft-tissue tensile strength diminishes in animals given anabolic steroids, perhaps from rebound increase in corticosteroid hormones with consistent drug use. Corticosteroids' catabolic effect results in tissue breakdown. This catabolic rebound effect may make young athletes' tendons and ligaments more injury prone. Anabolic steroids also may show such effects in adults.

Gynecomastia

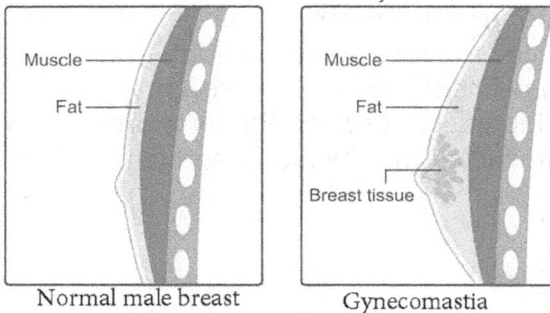

Muscle
Fat
Normal male breast

Muscle
Fat
Breast tissue
Gynecomastia

Figure 8-1: Gynecomastia is common in anabolic steroid users when testosterone converts to estrogen by aromatization. Source: Shutterstock.

Developing female–like breast tissue in men, called gynecomastia, can occur with excessive anabolic steroid use (Figure 8-1). Gynecomastia is a sexual side effect because it occurs due to testosterone and estrogen interaction. A portion of testosterone converts to estrogen by aromatization to promote breast tissue growth. In aromatization, aromatase catalyzes the conversion of testosterone into estradiol.

Some athletes take tamoxifen or raloxifene to prevent estrogen increases and reduce gynecomastia risk, yet some cases require surgery. The incidence of gynecomastia often increases with age because of changes in relative testosterone and estrogen levels. Gynecomastia usually gets better with time. Clinical observations of gynecomastia in anabolic steroid users include studies by De Luis, et al. 2001; Friedl, et al., 1989; Orlandi, et al., 2010; and Babigian, et al., 2001.

Many bodybuilders take aromatase inhibitors (e.g., Arimidex) to prevent converting testosterone to estrogen. Excessive estrogen triggers gynecomastia. Recent studies showed that suppression of estrogen promotes body fat deposition. Gibb, et al. (2016, 2019) from the British Heart Foundation Center for Cardiovascular Science at the University of Edinburgh in Scotland, found that aromatase inhibitor use promoted insulin resistance. They measured blood glucose disposal rates and fat formation following aromatase inhibitor administration. The studies showed estrogen is an important regulator of blood glucose in men—just as other studies show that estrogen helps to control fat mass.

Psychological Effects

Many bodybuilders and power athletes thrive when taking anabolic steroids because it activates brain reward centers. The pleasure is a lot more than they get from lifting 50 lb more in the bench press or sprinting 100-m faster. Athletes report a general feeling of well-being from taking the drugs besides the pleasure they get from improved performance. A study on rats given ready access to cannabinoids in the lab by Struik and colleagues (2016), found two week nandrolone decanoate administration increased the drug seeking behavior in the animals. Nandrolone triggers pleasure-seeking behavior in the brain.

"Roid Rage:" The media portrays steroid users as crazy people who often fly off the handle. According to them, steroid users are violent, irrational, and unstable. Psychiatric studies from Harvard University showed that while "roid rage" is real, it affects only a minority of steroid users (Pope, et al., 1988, 1996; Choi, et al. 1994).

Swedish researchers from the Forensic Psychiatric Clinic in Goteborg administered a mental health questionnaire to 683 athletes who competed between 1960 and 1979 in wrestling, weightlifting, powerlifting, and throwing events (Lindqvist-Bagg, et al., 2019). Twenty percent of the athletes admitted using anabolic steroids. They were more likely to seek help for psychological problems and had turned to illicit drugs. These results might reflect the people who use steroids rather than the effects of the drugs themselves.

Males

The psychological side effects of anabolic steroids—the so-called "roid rage"—have become an urban legend. The psychiatric literature shows that clinical cases of steroid-induced psychosis are rare but do occur. The media immediately linked the 2007 murder-suicide of pro wrestler Chris Benoit to steroid use. Benoit killed his wife and son before hanging himself. It is impossible to say what role steroids played in the tragedy.

Young people—even athletes—sometimes develop mental illness. That does not mean steroids caused the illness. For example, men with schizophrenia usually develop the disease in their late teens to early 20s. These are the peak years for dedicated sports participation. Schizophrenia symptoms could easily be mistaken for anabolic steroid side effects. No definitive study links steroid use to mental illness, but they increase aggressiveness and the risk of psychotic episodes in some people.

In many men, anabolic steroid use is symptomatic of poor body image. Before 1980, trained athletes used anabolic steroids to improve performance and body composition. The popularity of intense CrossFit sports and ultra-cut movie actors has placed unrealistic expectations on non-athletic men, which many have difficulty achieving.

The modern male's obsession with body image has led to previously rare depression and muscle dimorphism (obsessed with muscle mass). While eating disorders are rare in men, surprisingly about 5% of millennials resort to anabolic steroids, plastic surgery, and facial makeup to make them feel better about themselves.

The modern emphasis on gender equity has caused many modern young males to question their masculinity (Griffith, 2018). Most females have no trouble talking about their insecurities, but most males hide them. Feelings of physical inadequacy are new psychological challenges for modern people, and anabolic steroid use is symptomatic.

Violent Crime: Several European studies linked anabolic steroid use to violent crime. A popular perception about steroid users is that they are subject to irrational, violent rages. Most psychiatric studies show that while "roid rage" is mostly an urban legend, about 10% of steroid users have severe psychological side effects. A Swedish study from the University of Uppsala reported that anabolic steroid users were 65% more likely to commit violent crimes than non-users (Klotz, et al., 2010). The data says more about steroid users than steroids per se because violent crime rates were equal in present and former users. *Correlational studies do not prove steroids trigger violent crime, only that steroids and crime are related.*

Females

Actor and fitness guru Jane Fonda caused a stir when she revealed that she took testosterone to maintain muscle mass and sex drive. Women produce testosterone just like men, but the concentration is very low.

. . .

Personality: Indian researchers reported that females with higher testosterone levels were more opinionated (Tajima-Pozo, et al., 2015). They measured their performance before and after testosterone therapy. The group decision-making capacity decreased after receiving the hormone. Higher testosterone levels have been linked to anti-social behavior, aggressiveness, and reduced ability to trust.

Additional studies have reported contrasting results: Swiss researchers showed that testosterone promoted cooperative behavior (Eisenegger, et al. 2010, 2011). Females received either testosterone or a placebo they believed was testosterone and measured fair bargaining behavior. A single testosterone dose increased fair bargaining behavior, reduced bargaining conflicts, and smoothed social interactions. Females who took the placebo but thought they were receiving testosterone behaved more unfairly and stubbornly. Testosterone promoted socialization. Testosterone supplements increased sex drive and promoted more aggressive behaviors.

Sexuality: Anabolic steroids promote sex drive and sexuality in females, but they vary in their behavioral responsiveness to the drugs. Some effects might be due to increasing bioavailable estrogen. They may be secondary to their direct effects on mood.

The relationship between anabolic steroids and sexuality might be confused with other psychological mechanisms related to growth and sympathetic nervous system stimulation. In fact, females respond to lower anabolic steroid levels than males. Doses that do not affect males might trigger substantial changes in psychological and sexual responses in females.

Anabolic Steroid Addiction

Addiction to anabolic steroids could be widespread and a minor reason why some people seek substance abuse treatment. General anabolic steroid use did not become common until the 1980s. Former steroid users are now middle-aged and might be experiencing cardiovascular and reproductive side effects.

An on-going debate is whether steroids are addictive or just convenient to take. Steroids make it easier to train and improve performance in power events. They promote increases in strength, power, and muscle mass, so they are attractive to athletes and physically active adults—regardless of the potential health consequences, either short or longer term.

Anabolic steroids affect the central nervous system by stimulating the brain's mesolimbic reward system. Most mental health professionals have observed a 30% dependence rate at their clinics among steroid users. Most anabolic steroid users also take growth hormone, insulin, clenbuterol, IGF-1, stimulants, and opiates, so separating anabolic steroids' true addictive effects is difficult.

Steroids also stimulate the oligodendrocytes in the brain to produce myelin—the covering of nerve cells that speed the rate of nerve impulses in the central and peripheral nervous systems. Increased nerve cell myelination may be an essential reason that anabolic steroids improve performance in high power sports. Such effects on the brain make it easy to see why athletes have difficulty abandoning the drugs.

Anabolic steroids do not cause physical dependence like heroin or methamphetamines, but they might cause psychological dependence. An Internet survey by scientists from Touro University College of Pharmacy (Ip, et al., 2016) showed that over 23% met psychological dependence criteria, which included a history of illicit drug and alcohol abuse, sexual or physical abuse, and various psychiatric conditions. Steroid dependent individuals used higher doses for a longer duration and were more likely to suffer from depression. Nevertheless, the results might not apply to all anabolic steroid users.

Kicking the Steroid Habit: Many athletes and fitness enthusiasts take anabolic steroids for over 10 or 20 years. Some experts think that steroids are addictive and that athletes might need help to "kick the habit."

A Harvard University clinical study concluded that treatment depends on the addiction (Kanayama, et al., 2009). Some athletes who take steroids suffer from muscle dysmorphia and become addicted to steroids because of the effects on appearance. They might benefit from psychological counseling and properly prescribed drugs by a physician to treat depression. Others suffer from gonadal suppression from prolonged steroid use. They might benefit from human chorionic gonadotropin or clomiphene that restore normal reproductive hormone function and also minimize existing gynecomastia. *There is no documented widespread anabolic steroid addiction problem.*

Proper treatment can help people suffering from anabolic steroid addiction or psychological dependence. Steroids have a hedonic effect, so athletes get pleasure from the drugs' effects (i.e., satisfaction from lifting big weights in front of friends). They might benefit from naltrexone used to treat dependence on street drugs. SAMHSA's National Helpline is a free, confidential, 24/7, 365-day-a-year treatment referral and information service (in English and Spanish) for individuals and families facing mental and/or substance use disorders (https://www.samhsa.gov/find-help/national-helpline; **1-800-662-HELP** (4357)).

Anabolic Steroids as Gateway Drugs

Anabolic steroids are banned substances (legally and in sports) because athletic and law enforcement experts consider them gateway drugs for more dangerous substances. Anabolic steroid use is linked to alcohol, illicit drugs, and the legally performance-enhancing creatine monohydrate (Kanayama, et al., 2018).

The links between steroids, cigarette smoking, and marijuana are less clear. Often, steroid users want to maximize performance and health, so they avoid cigarette smoking with its obvious destructive effects on the body. *There is little evidence that steroids act as a gateway drug to more dangerous substances.*

Anabolic Steroids and the Brain

According to the Norwegian Doping Control Laboratory, long-term anabolic steroid use reduces brain volume and cortical thickness (the combined thickness of the cerebral cortex layers), (Bjornebekk, et al., 2017). The researchers performed structural magnetic resonance imaging scans in 82 current or former steroid users and 68 non-using weightlifters. Steroid users exhibited smaller brain mass, particularly in gray matter, cerebral cortex, and putamen (the outermost part of the basal ganglia). There were no differences in intelligence quotient (IQ), anxiety or depression, attention span, or behavioral problems (i.e., criminal behavior), despite structural changes. Anabolic steroid use is often associated with psychological disturbances related to structural changes in the brain.

Anabolic steroids can influence complex human behaviors such as negotiations and motivation. Swedish researchers (Kopsida, et al., 2016) found that testosterone altered performance in a behavior game called "The Ultimate Game." Players respond to reasonable, unreasonable, and neutral proposals involving money. Rational players will respond to valid offers that bring rewards. Male and female players accepted unreasonable offers more often after applying testosterone gel to their skin. Brain scans showed that testosterone activated the brain's amygdala involved in emotional reactions. The results suggest that testosterone participates in emotional responses during human interactions.

High-intensity exercise moderates the effects of steroids on the brain. Anabolic steroids trigger increases in oxidative stress in the brain. Free radicals produced naturally during metabolism are highly reactive chemicals that damage cell membranes and DNA and suppress the immune system. Oxidative damage in the brain may promote Parkinson's disease, Alzheimer's disease, multiple sclerosis, and Lou Gehrig's disease. *Intense exercise plays an important role in reducing the effects of free radicals on the brain.*

Sleep Apnea

Sleep is a critical part of mental and psychological health. Anabolic steroids disturb sleep and can induce sleep apnea. Sleep apnea is a dangerous disorder involving a collapsed airway during sleep, causing snoring, gasping, and interrupted sleep (Figure 8-2).

Sleep apnea promotes cardiac arrhythmias, heart attack, diabetes, auto accidents, and obesity. Large neck and body size, common in anabolic steroid users, is linked to sleep apnea. The condition is common in overweight, middle-aged men who are also more likely to take testosterone supplements. High testosterone doses (e.g., 1000 mg) made sleep apnea symptoms worse (Killick, et al., 2013). Testosterone reduced oxygen saturation during sleep and increased nighttime airway obstruction frequency. The severity of sleep apnea symptoms is unrelated to initial blood testosterone levels. Sleep apnea is a potential risk in people taking anabolic steroids and testosterone supplements.

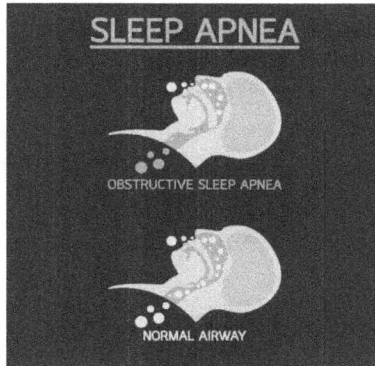

Figure 8-2: Anabolic steroids increase obstructive sleep apnea risk— a severe condition that saps energy levels and can lead to potentially fatal cardiac arrythmias. Source: Shutterstock.

Summary

Anabolic steroids have sexual and muscle-building effects, which is why many experts call them *anabolic-androgenic steroids*. They influence primary and secondary sexual characteristics. In females, they decrease fertility and alter menses and have masculinizing effects such as abnormal hair growth, voice changes, extreme muscularity, increased sex drive, and premature closure of the epiphyses (bone growth centers). In males, they alter fertility and libido and promote gynecomastia, male-pattern baldness, aggressiveness, premature maturation, and decreased testicular volume.

Anabolic steroids can have severe psychological side effects. Some users experience "roid rage," psychotic behavior, and dependence, but most media reports overstate steroids' psychological effects. They cause mood changes in many users, and some studies have linked steroids to criminal and violent behavior. The psychological effects are highly variable. *Steroid use can cause sleep apnea— probably due to increased body size and neck circumference triggered by the drugs rather than any property of the drugs themselves.*

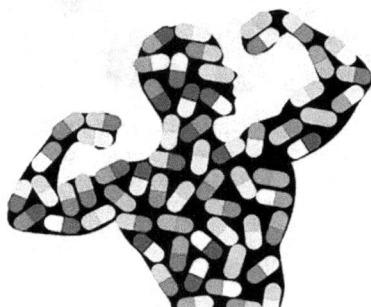

9
_____

MEDICAL USES FOR TESTOSTERONE AND ANABOLIC STEROIDS

Physicians widely use testosterone and other anabolic steroids to treat cachexia (weakness and tissue wasting) from AIDs, cancer, and chronic kidney disease (Laurent et al., 2019). Anabolic drugs decreased death rates and disabilities in these patients. These drugs increase body weight, lean body mass, muscle strength, and quality of life (Bhasin, et al., 2021). The drugs are safe if taken in moderate doses. Anabolic drugs are valuable for preventing muscle wasting (atrophy) with aging. Bad publicity linked to anabolic steroid and growth hormone use in athletes and political pressure related to the 1990 and 2004 Anabolic Steroid Control Acts make physicians reluctant to prescribe these drugs to their patients (Morgentaler, 2015).

Between 20 and 50% of middle-aged and older men have testosterone deficiency. Many of these men get testosterone replacement therapy, but is it safe? Researchers from the Mayo Clinic, in a meta-analysis of 51 studies, concluded that testosterone supplements increase hematocrit and hemoglobin, which thickens the blood (Fernández-Balsells, et al., 2010) and decreases HDL cholesterol. Testosterone therapy did not result in premature death, prostate disease, urological problems, heart attack, stroke, or increased cardiovascular disease risk factors. Men might reduce the risk of hemoconcentration (thick blood) by using testosterone creams or gels or donating blood. Injections cause spikes in testosterone that can stimulate red blood cell production. Nevertheless, testosterone therapy can benefit many aging men.

Should Hormone Supplements Be A Normal Part of Anti-Aging Therapy?

The United States' life expectancy for males and females has increased from about 47 in 1900 to 77.8 in 2020 (National Center for Health Statistics, 2021). Life expectancy at birth for men was 75.1 yr in 2020, representing a decline of 1.2 yr from 76.3 yr in 2019— primarily due to the COVID-19 epidemic. Hopefully, the suppressing effect of the COVID epidemic represents only a temporary pause in increasing lifespan in modern humans.

It is only natural that people want to enjoy these extra years and prevent disability. Decreases in testosterone and DHEA are related to decreased bone and muscle mass, diminished vitality, poor sexual performance, and psychological depression (Linderman et al., 2020).

In a literature review, Swiss scientists concluded that hormone replacement therapy is an underutilized medical technique for preventing aging effects (Samaras, et al., 2014). They recognized the potential side effects of hormone therapy and stated that it was inappropriate to use hormone supplements as a general anti-aging strategy. Hormone therapy is appropriate when physicians identify hormone deficiencies that might be remedied by treatment.

Not all studies were positive. Vigen and co-workers (2013) studied 1223 patients on testosterone therapy and recovering from coronary angiography and 7486 similar patients not taking testosterone. After five years, the risk of death, heart attack, and stroke increased in the patients taking testosterone. This study had a chilling effect on testosterone prescriptions in aging men. Critics of the study observed that Vigen, et al. misinterpreted their data. The number of adverse events divided by the number of patients was lower by half in the testosterone-treated group than the untreated group—10.1% vs. 21.2% (Morgentaler, 2015).

Most studies show that testosterone therapy is safe and effective. A large international study involving medical centers in 23 countries found that testosterone replacement therapy improved libido (sex drive), reduced erectile dysfunction, and enhanced quality of life in middle-aged men (Zitzmann, et al., 2012). Over 89% of patients were satisfied with the treatment. Side-effects were mild to moderate and included increased hematocrit, increased PSA (prostate enlargement marker), and pain at the injection site. The study found no cases of prostate cancer. Testosterone replacement therapy is a safe and effective treatment for aging men with low testosterone levels (< 300 ng/dL).

Testosterone therapy's application has been limited because of steroid scandals in baseball, cycling, track and field, and football. Scary tales promoted by the media and some medical community segments link testosterone to deadly heart attacks, cancer, liver disease, and psychotic behavior. Many physicians are reluctant to prescribe testosterone to their patients.

Before age 60, males have more heart attacks than females. Many scientists reasoned that since males have much higher testosterone levels than females, the hormone must cause heart attacks. New research shows the opposite. Low testosterone levels (T) increase heart disease and type 2 diabetes risk and decrease the risk in muscle and bone mass loss, prostate cancer, and depression (Linderman et al., 2020). Low T impairs metabolic health, promotes obesity, and decreases sexual performance. It is a serious public health issue that robs men of their energy levels and quality of life.

Boden, et al. (2020), in a study of 2118 men, found that aging men with low testosterone levels increased their risk of heart attack, stroke, metabolic syndrome, and sudden death compared to men with normal levels. Low testosterone levels in middle-aged and older males pose a significant premature death risk.

Harvard University urologist Abraham Morgentaler, is a vocal proponent of testosterone therapy in aging men. He hopes to change public perception about the dangers of low T and the beneficial effects of testosterone therapy (Morgentaler, 2015). He touted his 30 years of research and clinical experience to present a convincing argument for actively treating men with low testosterone levels. He believes that testosterone therapy can increase energy levels, libido, and outlook on life and decrease erectile dysfunction risk.

Testosterone, Sexual Performance, and Lifestyle

Testosterone levels decline in men after about age 35. The age-related decrease in testosterone is sometimes called andropause ("male menopause"), linked to muscle atrophy, psychological depression, declining sexual performance, and reduced interest in sex. Research supports the claims that testosterone improves sexual prowess, muscle mass, and self-image in hypogonadal aging men (Bhasin, et al., 2021).

Testosterone has important effects on sex drive and sexual performance. The hormone contributes to sperm cell production and semen volume, sex drive, and the capacity for erections. Low T decreases sex drive and makes it more difficult to get and maintain erections. Sexual problems related to low T levels can begin as early as the mid-20s.

Many experts say there is no "male menopause" because testosterone levels remain within typical values in most men — even in older age. Biologically available testosterone levels clearly decline during middle- and old age. In adolescents, minor changes in testosterone result in substantial changes in physical performance and sex drive (Fahey, et al. 1979). Middle-age men often experience a 50% decline in the biologically active free testosterone between ages 30-60 (Cabral, et al., 2014). They can expect reductions in sexual and physical capacities—even though total testosterone remains within normal limits.

Adequate differs from optimal. Treating men with low T levels should boost sexual performance, prevent degenerative diseases, and improve quality of life (Bhasin, et al., 2021).

Only about 8% of men with low T levels (total testosterone less than 400 ng/dL; free testosterone less than 15 pg/mL) are ever diagnosed, and even fewer seek or receive treatment (Morgentaler, et al., 2019). Their physicians often tell them to accept declining sex drive and energy levels, lost strength, depression, and fatigue as a part of natural aging.

Low T is a highly treatable medical condition. T therapy can turn the lights back on and make men feel better, improve relationships, boost mental and physical health, and may even prolong life. Physicians routinely treat sore joints, poor blood sugar regulation, and high blood pressure but ignore muscle atrophy, impotence, and middle-age male depression. Eyesight declines with age, but doctors do not tell their patients to accept it and not wear glasses. They should deal with testosterone deficiencies as they would diabetes, thyroid disease, or any other medical condition requiring intervention strategies.

Many physicians will not prescribe testosterone to aging men because they fear it might promote prostate cancer—the second leading cancer-related cause of death in men. Studies from Harvard University showed that low T levels increase prostate cancer risk (Morgentaler and Caliber, 2019). T therapy only promoted the disease in castrated men. The researchers noted that no study found any difference in cancer outcomes for men with T concentrations of 200, 500, or 800 ng/dL.

Physicians should suspect low testosterone levels if their male patients have decreased sex drive, erection problems, chronic fatigue, depression, increased abdominal fat, and muscle mass and strength loss. Consider this strategies for men with these symptoms:

- **Get a thorough physical examination** that includes measurements of total and free testosterone. Men with total testosterone less than 400 ng/dL or free testosterone less than 15 pg/mL might benefit from testosterone therapy. Other necessary baseline tests include luteinizing hormone (LH), prolactin, hematocrit, hemoglobin, prostate-specific antigen (PSA), and bone density.
- *T therapy is for men with low testosterone levels and should not be used in high doses to increase athletic performance.*
- **Lose weight.** Excess body fat lowers testosterone by increasing steroid hormone binding globulin (which reduces the biologically active free testosterone) and increases testosterone conversion to estrogen by aromatization. Increased estrogen levels in overweight men cause breast development (gynecomastia).
- **Monitor blood chemistry:** Any drug can cause side effects, and the ideal drug dose varies with the individual. As part of the treatment, the physician will monitor total and free testosterone, hematocrit, hemoglobin, PSA, HDL, and blood pressure, and carefully monitor sperm count and motility in those wishing to conceive.

Testosterone Supplements: Which Work Best?

Options for T therapy include injections, patches, gels, compounded testosterone creams, buccal tablets (under the tongue), pills, and testosterone-boosting drugs. Each has benefits and limitations. Considerations include:

- **Intramuscular Injections.** These are best for creating higher circulating testosterone levels but cause large "peaks and valleys" in hormone concentrations (high T levels after injection and low T levels before the next injection). They require home injections or expensive office visits. Doses range from 50 to 400 mg every 1-4 week. Bhasin, et al, (2001) found that doses below 125 mg a week had little effect on muscle mass and strength.
- **Patches.** They are convenient but cause skin irritation in about 40 percent of men and cause embarrassment around friends and family.
- **Gels and creams.** They typically produce more consistent T levels but must be applied several times a day and often do not produce high enough blood levels of the hormone.
- **Compounded T creams.** They are usually more concentrated than prescription creams and gels, but the Food and Drug Administration has not evaluated them.
- **Oral Testosterone.** Oral testosterone has a short half-life which makes it difficult to

maintain consistent testosterone blood levels. In 2019, the FDA approved the oral testosterone Jatenzo (testosterone undecanoate) taken twice a day. Oral anabolic steroids such as methandrostenolone are toxic to the liver and not recommended for testosterone therapy.

- **Testosterone stimulating drugs.** The drugs clomiphene, anastrozole, and hCG stimulate testosterone production but rarely produce optimal blood testosterone levels and should be avoided.

Exercise, Diet, and Testosterone

Physical inactivity and excess caloric intake promote obesity and create poor metabolic health that disrupts sensitive hormone systems that process carbohydrates, fats, and protein. They also regulate signaling chemicals that help to augment bone and muscle mass. Moderate-intensity aerobic exercise, weight training, weight management, and stress reduction contribute to healthy anabolic hormone regulation (i.e., testosterone, growth hormone, IGF-1, and insulin). Good diet and exercise promote testosterone production, improve androgen receptor activity, and enhance metabolic health. While an improved lifestyle cannot compensate for low testosterone levels, it will help to improve health and quality of life.

An aerobic exercise program is essential for good

metabolic health and hormone control. The American College of Sports Medicine recommends a minimum of 30 min, 5 days/week moderate intensity exercise (e.g., walking) or vigorous intensity aerobic activity for a minimum of 20 minutes 3 days/week (https://journals.lww.com/acsm-msse/pages/articleviewer.aspx?year=2021&issue=08000&article=00026&type=Fulltext). They also recommend resistive exercise to build or maintain muscle mass at least 2days/week.

Testosterone and Master's Sports: Exercise and diet should be part of the overall testosterone management program, particularly in older competitive athletes who cannot take testosterone supplements—even when medically prescribed.

Several years ago, a master's shot-putter from England filed a medical exemption waiver to use testosterone with the International Association of Athletics Federation (IAAF, the international ruling body for track and field). The athlete had a low testosterone level contributing to his diabetes. The IAAF ignored his request, tested him at the Master's World Championships in Spain, and gave him a two-year suspension for using testosterone—even though he was following his physician's advice. Testosterone therapy is not approved for athletes participating in master's sports, and it is doubtful these rules will change anytime soon.

Testosterone and the Metabolic Syndrome

Low testosterone increases metabolic syndrome risk—a group of symptoms that include visceral obesity, hypertension, insulin resistance, high triglycerides, and low HDL-cholesterol (Figure 9-1). Testosterone combined with exercise, weight loss, and improved diet is a powerful therapy for type 2 diabetes, congestive heart failure, and the metabolic syndrome. This treatment improves insulin resistance, blood sugar control, and prevents premature death.

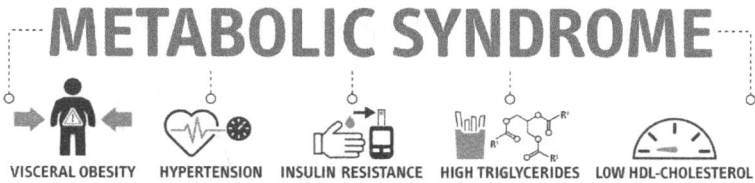

Figure 9-1: The Metabolic Syndrome. Source : Shutterstock.

Testosterone Supplements: Although controversial, many physicians use testosterone supplements to treat aging men with poor metabolic health and low testosterone levels. Data from the TRiUS registry showed that testosterone supplementation in a large group of men receiving testosterone therapy improved metabolic syndrome symptoms, including decreased waist circumference, reduced blood glucose, and decreased blood pressure (Bhattacharya, et al., 2011). Treatment did not affect these symptoms in men without the metabolic syndrome. The study showed that testosterone supplements improved metabolic health in aging men with low testosterone.

Testosterone and other anabolic steroids have powerful effects on protein and fat metabolism. They build muscle, decrease fat, and speed neural conduction. They also have short- and long-term effects on blood sugar metabolism (Linderman, et al., 2020). Users have less body fat than age-matched non-users. Former users had greater total and abdominal fat.

Anabolic steroids reduce insulin sensitivity, promoting abdominal fat deposition (Rasmussen, et al., 2016). These effects appear long-lasting, but they are not inevitable. Long-term studies on former college athletes show that health and longevity after college depend on current exercise levels. Playing college sports does not protect older sedentary adults unless they remained physically active (Lee, et al., 1995). Anabolic steroid users are usually anaerobic athletes. They often become insulin resistant if they do not include aerobic exercise when they retire from competitive sports, stop taking steroids, and become more sedentary.

Testosterone supplements increase muscle mass, strength, and physical vitality in frail older men (Strollo F. et al., 2013). Testosterone works best when combined with an exercise program. The benefits of testosterone therapy increase with dose, but so do the side effects. Individuals need to balance the drugs' benefits with their side effects to boost the quality of life while at the same time minimizing potential health risks.

· · ·

Long Term Testosterone Therapy and Body Composition

For over 25 years, testosterone replacement therapy to combat aging and obesity has been popular in the United States and Europe with many long-term clinical evaluations about treatment benefits and risks. Men treated for at least eight years with testosterone undecanoate showed decreases in waist circumference, body fat, glycated hemoglobin (a measure of blood sugar control), cholesterol, low-density lipoprotein, and prostate enlargement symptoms (Zitzmann, et al., 2013). They showed improvements in sexual function and bone density but no increased heart disease or prostate cancer risk. *Long-term treatment with testosterone in middle-aged men is safe and effective.*

Anabolic Steroids and Recovery from Orthopedic Surgery

Total knee replacement surgery eventually improves mobility and quality of life but requires many rehabilitation months. The process is complicated because severe muscle atrophy delays recovery and impacts surgical outcome. Australian researchers (Hohmann, et al., 2010) found that administering low doses of anabolic steroids (50 mg nandrolone decanoate twice weekly) promoted recovery and increased strength. This study used low doses of anabolic steroids. Greater benefits might have been observed had higher doses (200–300 mg per week) been used (Bhasin, et al,

2001). Other studies in middle-aged adults showed higher doses caused impressive increases in muscle mass and strength and could be administered with minimal side effects (Bhasin et al., 1996, 2001).

Summary

Testosterone therapy in aging men is a valuable tool to improve quality of life and longevity. In men with reduced testosterone levels, testosterone increases body weight, lean body mass, muscle strength, energy levels, mental outlook, and quality of life. The technique has critics so patients should insist that their physicians carefully monitor side effects and poor outcomes. Testosterone therapies allow aging men to participate in vigorous exercise programs with lifesaving effects. These programs would be impossible if patients did not have the physical capacity made possible by testosterone therapy.

Physicians will suspect low testosterone levels if their male patients have decreased sex drive, erection problems, chronic fatigue, depression, increased abdominal fat, and muscle mass and strength loss. Medical considerations include:

- **Patients should get a thorough physical examination.** Men with total testosterone less than 400 ng/dL or free testosterone less than 15 pg/mL may benefit from testosterone therapy.
- **T therapy is for men with low testosterone levels and should not be**

used in high doses to increase athletic performance.

- **Patients should take the testosterone supplement that works best for them.** Options for T therapy include injections, patches, gels, compounded testosterone creams, buccal tablets, pills, and testosterone-boosting drugs.
- **Lose weight.** Excess body fat lowers testosterone by increasing steroid hormone binding globulin.
- **Monitor physical signs that could suggest side effects** including hematocrit, hemoglobin, PSA , blood lipids , and blood pressure. Monitor measures of fertility (i.e., sperm count), to conceive.

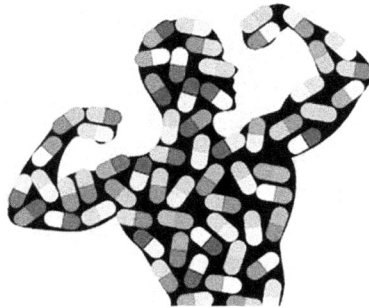

10

DOPING CONTROL AND STATE-SPONSORED DOPING BY THE SOVIET UNION AND RUSSIA

Doping control and athletic drug use have been central topics of discussion during the Olympics since 100-meter gold medalist Ben Johnson tested positive for anabolic steroids during the 1988 games in Seoul, Korea. In track and field alone, superstar Olympic gold medal sprinter Linford Christy, three-time Olympian and the U.S. 100-meter champion Dennis Mitchell, European 200-meter champion Doug Walker, high jump world record holder Javier Sotomayor, shot-putter Randy Barnes, and distance runner Mary Slaney tested positive for anabolic steroids.

The International Olympic Committee (IOC) accused Russia of systematic state-sponsored doping. They stripped Russian athletes of 43 Olympic medals and banned Russian athletes from major sporting events— including the 2021 Tokyo Olympic Games for four years. Nevertheless, Russian athletes competed at Tokyo as the Russian Olympic Committee. The Russian doping program was a continuation of the Soviet

Union's state-sponsored doping program (Kalinski, 2017).

Positive drug tests are rampant in other sports. In recent years, drug scandals have plagued the Tour de France, British and American horse racing, cricket, soccer, basketball, master's track and field, and roller hockey. A Mexican baseball player had a positive test during the 2015 Pan American Games. The most celebrated doping flap involved home run hitter Mark McGuire, who admitted taking androstenedione during his quest in 1998 to break Roger Maris's record of 61 home runs in a single season. He was widely criticized in the press even though the drug was legal in Major League Baseball.

To make matters worse, some doping control experts speculated that athletes could nefariously sabotage competitors by contaminating their food or rubbing cream containing banned substances on their skin. Banned substances could be easily transferred through a handshake or brushing against a competitor. Ben Johnson claimed his sample was sabotaged at the 1988 Olympics. Athletes in Japan and India also have been accused of doping sabotage. Instead of finding ways to avoid getting caught, some athletes are finding ways to get their competitors caught (San Diego Union-Tribune, July 21, 2021).

Dark Side of the Force? To the average person, athletic drug use conjures up images of clean athletes taken over by the dark side of the force. From the perspective of many athletes, drug use is understandable — they do whatever it takes to win and stay competitive.

Prior to the 1992 Olympics, journalist Robert Goldman— author of *Death in the Locker Room* (Elite Sports Medicine Publications)— polled elite athletes about their feelings regarding drugs, sport, and winning. He asked the athletes if they would take a drug that would guarantee them a gold medal but would kill them within two years. Seventy-five percent of the athletes said they would take the drug. The question is known as the *Goldman dilemma* and became an urban legend in sport. Connor, et al. (2013) posed the same question to 212 elite track and field athletes. Only 13 athletes said they would take the drugs if death resulted. Twenty-five athletes said they would take the drugs if there were no consequences.

While changing planes in London recently, one of the authors ran into a world-class sprinter on his way to a competition in Germany. He said, "This doping business is nothing more than a cat and mouse game between WADA and the athletes. Top athletes hire doctors and biochemists to help them get around the regulations. It costs a lot of money, but you must do it to stay in the game. You can't be competitive in world-class sport without taking drugs." Undoubtedly, Olympic officials would not share this position.

The Origins of Sports Drug Testing

Performance-enhancing substance use is as old as sport itself. Ancient Greek athletes used a variety of concoctions such as dried figs, herbs, strychnine, and hallucinogens to improve performance. Inca warriors in South America chewed coca leaves before doing battle in the rarified air of the Andes mountains. At the turn of the 20th century, athletes often breathed supplemental oxygen to improve endurance. Boxers and soccer players got a boost by drinking a cocktail composed of strychnine, brandy, and cocaine. During World War II, some soldiers used amphetamines and anabolic steroids to improve performance on the battlefield.

After World War II, international athletic competitions became cold war surrogates for the battlefield. East and West Bloc athletes squared off on the playing fields, ice rinks, basketball courts, and running tracks. Countries poured hundreds of millions of dollars into athletics hoping to score propaganda points. Victory was the only acceptable outcome for both sides. In this climate of expectations, widespread drug use to improve performance was inevitable.

1960-1968: The excesses of drug use in sport caught up with the athletes. Between 1960 and 1963, the public became disgusted with drug-related deaths in cycling, boxing, and track and field. Many people believed that drug use threatened all sports, undermining the Olympic ideal's very foundations.

The IOC formulated its anti-drug policies. Their basic philosophy was to:

1. Protect the athletes' health
2. Defend medical and sports ethics
3. Provide an equal chance for all competitors

In 1968, the IOC began the first large-scale drug testing at the Grenoble Winter Olympics and the Mexico City Summer Olympics. The early history of athletic drug testing were tenuous times. During the early years, amphetamines and anabolic steroids were the most common banned drugs used by athletes. While amphetamines were easily measured, anabolic steroid assays were more difficult and expensive. Gradually, anabolic steroid detection became more sophisticated. Depending on the steroid, athletes could go off drugs for 2-4 weeks and appear clean during drug testing.

1980s, Random Drug Tests: The obvious answer was random testing. Unfortunately, closed societies would not allow IOC officials to test their athletes randomly as in the Soviet Union. Western countries were not about to randomly test their athletes and give Eastern Bloc athletes an advantage. Doping officials had to rely on surprise tests at competitions (e.g., Pan American Games in Caracas in 1974). When athletes learned of the drug tests, many attempted to leave the athletes' village in the dead of night only to be ambushed by an army of reporters and photographers.

Beginning in the late 1980s and coinciding with the end of the Cold War, the IOC instituted random drug testing for all athletes. Doping officials expected athletes to inform the IOC of their location and be prepared to submit a urine sample within 48 hours. A refusal was considered a positive test for banned drugs and many athletes received sanctions, which might range from a 2-year suspension for a first offense to a ban for life for a second offense. Sanctions have been a significant problem because not everyone gets the same penalty for the same offense. While one athlete is banned for life for inadvertently taking a banned substance, others beat the rap helped by a good lawyer or political connections. It is well known that several "legends" of sport, who tested positive for banned drugs, were quietly asked to retire rather than tarnish their reputation and the sport.

Beating the System: Athletes try to stay one step ahead of the drug testers. When drug labs introduced sophisticated tests for detecting anabolic steroids, athletes resorted to taking high doses of naturally occurring testosterone or growth hormone. Scientists developed a technique to detect supplemental testosterone by measuring one of its urinary metabolite levels—epitestosterone. Typically, testosterone and epitestosterone exist in a 1:1 ratio. However, when athletes take supplemental testosterone, the testosterone/epitestosterone ratio increases. Sophisticated athletes have learned to beat this test by taking epitestosterone injections. While epitestosterone is not used medically as a drug, it is available from chemical supply companies. It also is on the banned substance list.

Growth hormone was a severe problem for doping control laboratories because it could not be measured in urine. Scientists have developed a technique to measure supplemental growth hormone in the blood. To make matters even more difficult, blood samples were not allowed as part of the doping control process. Blood sampling is now routine, so athletes can no longer flagrantly take growth hormone because it is now detectable.

Despite extensive efforts to eradicate doping from sport, roughly 50 percent of elite athletes continue using performance-

enhancing drugs, even in the face of biological passports, random drug tests, and in-competition tests. Ulrich, et al. (2018) surveyed 2167 elite athletes at major athletic competitions in South Korea and Qatar using a randomized response technique that guaranteed anonymity. Fifty percent of athletes said they used banned substances within 12-months of the survey and 70% used supplements.

Doping control labs are not living in a vacuum. They make a serious effort to keep up with current athletic practices. Dr. David Cowan, founder and former director of the Drug Control Center in London, said, "We subscribe to the major bodybuilding magazines in the United States and Europe to get the latest information on what drugs are popular with athletes." The cat and mouse game between the drug testing labs and the athletes have resulted in an ever-widening array of banned substances. Also, WADA bans drugs used to cover up the detection of other drugs.

Drug Testing 101

After an athlete takes a drug, their body breaks it down and changes its chemical structure — forming byproducts called metabolites. Scientists determine that an athlete has taken banned drugs by searching for their metabolites in the urine. For example, when a person takes cocaine, the body breaks down the drug and a metabolite called benzoylecgonine shows up in the urine.

Doping Control Procedures

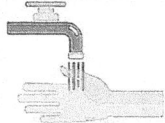

1. Wash hands without soap

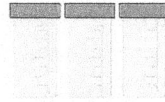

2. Choose vessel

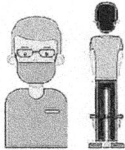

3. Provide sample

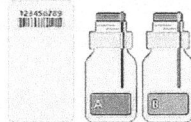

4. Choose sample collection kit

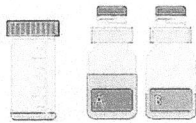

5. Split sample

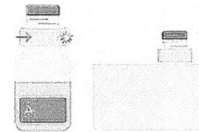

6. Seal sample

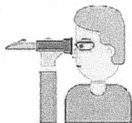

7. Measure specific gravity of sample

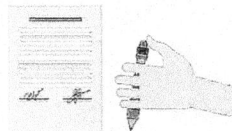

8. Sign form

Figure 11-1 Doping control sample collection procedures

Figure 11-1 shows the procedures for collecting samples, in or out of competition following an 8-step protocol:

1. Athletes wash their hands to prevent sample contamination
2. The athlete chooses two sample vessels
3. The athlete provides a sample under the supervision of a doping control technician
4. The athlete chooses a sample kit (includes labels and caps)
5. The doping control technician pours the sample into A and B sample vials
6. The athlete seals the vials
7. The technician checks the samples for specific gravity to ensure it is not diluted
8. The athlete signs an affidavit certifying the legitimacy of the procedure

Accredited Laboratories: The IOC has many accredited laboratories throughout the world, a comprehensive review process required each year to ensure exacting standards. Samples are generally sent to the nearest accredited lab from the competition, even with athletes from different countries. Doping control officers usually send samples from athletes selected for random tests to the nearest lab in the country where they are training.

World Anti-Doping Agency (WADA; https://www.wada-ama.org)**:** Anabolic drugs are the most commonly detected banned substances. WADA sets the standards for drug testing in Olympic sports. They test for drugs that affect skill, strength, endurance, and recovery. Anabolic steroids and growth hormone are the drugs of choice for high powers sports athletes. Endurance athletes are more likely to be involved in blood doping, either through transfusions or erythropoietin, which stimulates red blood cell production. Athletes in contact sports often use growth hormone to speed recovery. *Hormones account for two-thirds of doping violations in sports.* The agency is interested in substances that enhance performance, harm health, and violate the spirit of sport.

One of the authors (Fahey) served as doping control coordinator for one of the men's soccer venues at the 1984 Olympics. The urine collection methods used are virtually unchanged today. In soccer, representatives from each team, a representative from Fédération Internationale de Football Association (FIFA; https://www.fifa.com), and doping control would randomly select four players for drug testing. When the game ended, doping control personnel would inform the athlete he had one hour to report to the doping control center. Athletes and an assigned escort reported to the doping control station where the athlete selected urine sample bottles, labels, and seals from a box. They signed a form at each stage of the test, certifying the fairness of the procedure. The sample was further divided into "A" and "B" samples and sent to the lab for analysis.

In individual sports (e.g., track and field, gymnastics, and swimming) WADA tests all medal winners and one other competitor randomly chosen after completing the event. In these sports, the procedures are identical as in soccer. Athletes are also subject to out-of-competition random tests. Elite athletes must inform WADA of their location if they venture from home. Athletes competing in sanctioned competitions must submit to urine or blood tests.

After the sample arrives at the lab, technicians analyze it using a precise and expensive instrument called a mass spectrometer. The "mass spec" compares various substances found in the sample from a known tracing to each metabolite to identify it. When scientists detect the tracing of a banned substance or its metabolites, they know that the person most likely took the illegal drug. Scientists have developed precise methods for detecting most drugs on WADA's banned list.

Doping personnel begins the drug assays by measuring the "A" urine sample. If the sample is positive for a drug, technicians repeat the test using the "B" sample. Both the "A" and "B" samples must show evidence of a banned drug to declared the test positive.

Several banned substances—such as growth hormone (GH), erythropoietin (EPO), and human chorionic gonadotrophin (hCG)—have been difficult to measure. More sophisticated tests have made it increasingly difficult for athletes to use these substances.

Athlete Biological Passport (ABP): The World Anti-Doping Agency (WADA) initiated a program called the *Athlete Biological Passport (ABP)*, which establishes baseline levels for an athlete's blood profile. Athletes who show unusual changes in hormone blood levels or substances influenced by hormone changes could be penalized. WADA performs random drug tests and spot checks on elite athletes at major national and international competitions.

The program includes hematological and steroid modules. The hematological module examines factors that might enhance oxygen transport such as drugs that promote erythropoiesis (blood boosting) and blood biomarkers potentially altered by banned substances (e.g., hematocrit). The steroid model monitors for exogenously administered steroids and other anabolic agents such as SARMS (https://www.wada-ama. org/en/media/news/2021-08/wadas-athlete-biological-passport-an-important-tool-for-protecting-clean-sport).

A positive test occurs when urine or blood levels for a banned substance exceeds a specific standard to determine doping substances found naturally in the body. For example, a sudden rise in hematocrit (percent cells in the blood) might suggest testosterone use even if testosterone levels are normal. Since 2008, WADA has sanctioned over 180 athletes because of abnormal biological passports.

Anabolic Steroids and Bodybuilding Supplements

Ron Maughan and colleagues (2005) reported that over 25% of bodybuilding supplements sold on the Internet contained banned drugs, and not much has changed over the past two decades. A study from the Institute of Pharmacological Science at King's College London (Kicman et al., 2014) found 23 of 24 bodybuilding supplements tested contained banned substances, with several products containing doses high enough to trigger significant anabolic effects. Athletes must take responsibility for what they consume. Claiming they inadvertently took tainted supplements is not enough to avoid sanctions.

WADA and Drug Use Exemptions

WADA maintains a list of substances banned during and out of competition for Olympic sports athletes (https://www.wada-ama.org/prohibitedlist). Athletes may apply for an exemption if they can demonstrate a medical need for the drug.

Hacked emails between American sports officials and WADA showed these exemptions were granted haphazardly and inconsistently. Controversy arose over exemptions granted to Bethany Mattek-Sands, who won the women's doubles tennis gold medal at the 2016 Rio Olympics. She had applied to use the banned substance DHEA, a testosterone precursor. Her application was approved by the International Tennis Federation but rejected by WADA.

The WADA exemption process is a vexing problem in master's athletics. Sports governing bodies sanctioned several champion male and female track and field athletes in open and master's divisions for taking banned substances prescribed legitimately for medical reasons. Several athletes applied had for medical exemption through WADA. WADA routinely rejects applications for exempting testosterone. The athletes must choose between participating in their sport and maintaining good health.

Drugs and Practices Banned by WADA

The IOC bans hundreds of drugs divided into five categories. Many common, over-the-counter medications used to treat flu, motion sickness, asthma, and pain contain banned substances.

1. Stimulants: These drugs stimulate the brain and nerves. Amphetamines, the most used illegal stimulant, increase alertness and confidence, prevent fatigue, and give athletes a sense of well-being. Many familiar substances found in foods and over-the-counter drugs contain more mild stimulants such as caffeine, pseudoephedrine, and ephedrine. Using potent stimulants like amphetamines is prohibited, and any amount detected during drug testing is a doping offense. WADA no longer bans caffeine, even though many studies show it improves athletic performance. The National Collegiate Athletic Association (NCAA) still prohibits caffeine above 15 micrograms per milliliter of urine.

2. Narcotics: Banned narcotics include morphine, heroin, methadone, and pethidine. The weaker narcotics codeine, dihydrocodeine, and diphenoxylate, are permitted provided their use is declared *before* the competition.

While narcotics do not improve performance, they can mask pain and lead to severe injury or death during competition. These drugs are addictive and have serious side effects. Because the IOC's philosophy is to ban substances that impair health, they placed narcotics on the doping list.

3. Anabolic Drugs: Anabolic agents include testosterone, oxandrolone, methyltestosterone, and stanozolol that are chemically like testosterone but are not produced naturally by the body. Testosterone precursors androstenedione and dehydroepiandrosterone (DHEA), also are on the banned list. The US Food and Drug Administration prohibited the sale and use of androstenedione as part of the 2004 Anabolic Steroid Control Act, but DHEA is widely available on the Internet and is popular with middle-aged and older adults. Beta-2 agonists to treat asthma are anabolic and have been placed on the doping list. These drugs include clenbuterol, salbutamol, and salmeterol.

Anabolic steroids are the most common drug appearing in positive drug tests. Athletes often attempt to take short-acting testosterone preparations so they can present near-normal testosterone/epitestosterone ratios if doping control officials test them on short notice. Deceased University of California, San Francisco Medical School professor Harmon Brown M.D., hormone specialist and track and field coach (deceased), said:

> "Athletes are deluding themselves when they take small doses of short-acting testosterone to beat the drug tests — their natural production of testosterone shuts down, so they haven't gained anything."

4. Selective Androgen Receptor Modulators (SARMs): These anabolic drugs that selectively bind to receptors in specific skeletal muscle tissues. Most anabolic steroids bind with receptors throughout the body, which trigger many of their side effects. SARMs that bind with androgen receptors in muscle have little or no effect in other tissues, so they produce fewer side effects. While testosterone binds with receptors in muscle, it also binds with receptors in other tissues that impact sperm quality, skin oiliness, and blood pressure. The FDA does not currently approve the medical use of SARMs, but they are available offshore on the Internet. Because they selectively bind to muscle receptors, they do not have the androgenic side effects as do testosterone and other anabolic steroids. SARMs are on the banned drug list. They might be useful treatment options in cancer, prostate enlargement, and hypogonadism (Bhasin, et al., 2021).

In 2011, the Swiss Laboratory for Doping Analyses in Geneva reported the first positive doping tests for a SARM drug, which WADA had banned in 2005. Because they can boost muscle performance with fewer side effects than traditional anabolic steroids, they will become more popular with athletes, yet more scrutinized by WADA.

5. Diuretics: Athletes in weight class sports wrestling, boxing, judo, and weightlifting sometimes use diuretics. Diuretics can cause severe dehydration, sometimes but rarely resulting in illness or death. These drugs severely limit temperature regulation and lead to heat injury and heart rhythm disturbances.

Some athletes attempt to use diuretics or drink large quantities of water to "flush out" their urine to avoid testing positive during drug testing. The testing lab determines urine concentration (specific gravity) at the collection site to control this problem and obtains another sample if the first is diluted. Diuretics do not work—they are on the banned list and easily detected in urine and should not be used.

6. Peptide and glycoprotein hormones: These drugs include growth hormone, insulin-like growth factor (IGF-1), and erythropoietin (EPO). The later hormone increases red blood cell production (essential for transporting oxygen), while the former hormones build tissue, and WADA uses sophisticated tests to measure these substances and detect them.

Prescription growth hormone is expensive, so some elite athletes use inexpensive generic growth hormone available on the Internet. It is highly anabolic and, at least in the short term, promotes fat loss. Growth hormone can cause abnormal bone growth, peripheral neuropathy, and disturbances in blood glucose regulation. Purchasing hormones on the Internet is risky. Some of it is counterfeit and contaminated.

EPO improves oxygen transport to the tissues but increases hematocrit and blood pressure, leading to headaches, stroke, heart attack, and blood clots. Scientists and physicians attributed suspicious athlete's deaths to EPO, particularly among cyclists. *In Belgium alone in the late 1980s, EPO use was suspected in 17 deaths among competitive cyclists.*

7. Prohibited Methods: These include blood doping and manipulating urine samples. For example, the drug probenecid is banned because it temporarily blocks the kidneys from excreting anabolic steroids into the urine. Substituting someone else's urine is also prohibited.

Blood Doping: This technique removes athletes' blood, stores it, and then reinfuses it back into the body, which increases endurance dramatically. This technique was popular with endurance athletes about thirty years ago. However, EPO has the same effect, so blood doping was unnecessary— until WADA developed effective EPO detection tests. Blood doping is again popular with many endurance athletes.

8. Classes Subject to Restrictions: The regulations ban beta-blockers (slow the heart rate and decrease cardiac contractility), alcohol (in small doses can decrease hand tremors), corticosteroids, and marijuana under certain circumstances. For example, beta-blockers in archery and shooting are banned because the drugs help steady the athlete's movement patterns. A heartbeat can cause enough movement to disrupt their aim. Beta-blockers lower heart rate, so they might be an advantage in those sports. In running or basketball, beta-blockers decrease performance because they impair cardiac output, preventing the heart from achieving its maximum capacity to pump blood.

The regulations ban alcohol and marijuana because they go against the Olympic ideal of athletes as model citizens. In the 2002 Salt Lake City Winter Olympics, a snowboarder involved in a marijuana scandal was let off the hook when he claimed he inhaled the marijuana via secondhand smoke.

Syringes Banned at the Olympics: Many Olympic and professional athletes who tested positive for banned substances pleaded that they received vitamins or painkillers containing illegal drugs. The Medical Commission of the International Olympic Committee declared that they must approve all injectable substances. They made this regulation because cyclists often left trash with syringes at race sites, which gave the sport a bad image and sent the wrong message regarding drugs in sport. The international cycling, rowing, and gymnastics federations recently issued similar bans on syringes.

THOMAS D FAHEY & FRANK I KATCH

Future of Drug Testing in Sports

Drug use is inevitable in anything as competitive and potentially lucrative as sports. Elite athletes in football, soccer, horse racing, boxing, and baseball compete for millions of dollars, some with contracts in the hundreds of millions. In track and field, swimming, and other less financially rewarding sports, the competitive culture makes drug use almost irresistible. In such climates, drug testing is justifiable to maintain a level playing field.

Athletes who take drugs such as anabolic steroids have an advantage over those who do not. Also, anabolic steroids provide long term advantages, even after they stop taking the drugs. Perhaps the random drug testing programs used in many sports will stem drug use among elite athletes. We doubt it, but only time will tell.

Drug testing at lower levels of sport presents a unique conundrum. Most high school and college sports programs barely have enough money to survive. During the past 20 years, most programs have seen the steady erosion in athletic opportunities. Financially strapped school systems try to balance the budget by cutting sports and hiring poorly paid and trained part-time coaches. *Drug use is the least of their problems. Administrators and coaches could use the money devoted to drug programs for equipment, quality coaching, and drug education.*

For older athletes, drug testing may have negative long-term health consequences. Many physicians and physiologists believe that supplemental hormone therapy is essential in many older people for heart disease prevention and muscle and bone loss (Bhasin, et al., 2021). Throughout the world, anti-aging and wellness clinics treat physical deterioration with growth hormone and testosterone. Under the current doping regulations, older athletes cannot participate in these medical programs.

Drug testing will continue to be a can of worms for many years to come. *Officials must constantly balance the desire for fairness and healthy athletic participation with the reality of financial limitations and control effectiveness.*

State-Sponsored Doping Research in the Former Soviet Union and Russia

We obtained information on State-sponsored doping in the Soviet Union from personal communications with Dr. Michael Kalinski, former Chair of Biochemistry at the University of Kyiv in Ukraine and former professor and Chair at Kent State and Murray State Universities. Dr. Kalinski smuggled a top-secret doping protocol from the Soviet Union when he immigrated to the United States in 1991. The State Central Institute of Physical Culture in the Soviet Union had published a highly classified document that outlined the state-sponsored Soviet research on steroids and recommendations for their use in sports (Kalinski, M., 2003).

After World War II, the former Soviet Union participated in the Olympic Games beginning with the Helsinki games in 1952, and soon achieved a dominant position in these sporting competitions. The success of Soviet athletic programs was astounding. It was one of the most successful sports programs of all time. At the Helsinki games, Soviet athletes did exceptionally well in weightlifting, winning three gold, three silver, and one bronze-medal.

Following the Helsinki Olympic Games, the United States Olympic weightlifting coach, Bob Hoffman, accused the Soviet weightlifters of taking hormones to increase strength. This public charge was corroborated by a Russian team physician and United States weightlifting physician, Dr. John Ziegler, during the 1954 World Weightlifting Championships in Vienna. Rumors during the 1956 Olympic Games in Melbourne, Australia accused competitors in the weightlifting and throwing events of anabolic steroid use.

Major Soviet Scandal: One of the most damaging Soviet scandals occurred in 1984 at the International Athletics Meet in Paris. Tatiana Kazankina (Figure 11-2), one of the best track and field athletes from the Soviet Union, was suspended for life for refusing to submit to a drug test for anabolic-androgenic steroids.

Long-standing suspicions of testosterone use by the Soviet athletes were commonplace in the Western literature. But even with scandals involving Soviet athletes caught doping, not one journalist or official was able to obtain documentation of State collusion.

Suspicion of anabolic-androgenic steroid use by athletes in the former USSR had been rampant as early as the 1960s. Although anecdotal reports continued, unproven reports of steroid abuse by specific Soviet athletes cannot be considered proof of State sponsored research and conspiracy. Athletic success in Olympic games provided extensive privileges in the USSR for the elite athletes, coaches, scientists, and sport officials. These privileges included prestige at the state level, expensive gifts, cars, apartments, state stipends, increased salaries, and extensive travel abroad.

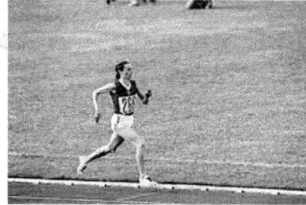

Figure 11-2 Tatiana Kazankina. Wiki Commons

The security measures that could be used routinely in totalitarian societies are difficult to appreciate in Western countries. During the 1940s through the 1980s, authorities in those totalitarian countries would have punished any scientist, journalist, athlete, or coach who published revelations about steroid use in elite sport. One of us (FK) attempted to give a small monetary gift for three young children of a top scientist who was attending a sports medicine conference in Athens, Greece. He politely said he would be jailed and forfeit his prominent scientific appointment if he was caught with American paper currency, no matter the amount.

Classified Document Revealed. In 1972, the State Central Institute of Physical Culture published a classified document that outlined the Soviet research program on steroids and recommendations for steroid use in sports. The document contains scientific reports providing the times and dosages for androgenic-anabolic steroids in human subjects (athletes) and data from experiments conducted at the Research Laboratory of Training Programming and Physiology of Sports Performance of the State Central Institute of Physical Culture in Moscow. It contains these subsections: "Introduction," "Anabolics and Endurance," "Anabolics and Strength," "Anabolics and Sport Performance," "Anabolics and Sports Results," "Dosages of the Anabolics," "Possible Adverse Effects," "Control of Use" (Fahey, et al., 2014).

There is no evidence in the research reports that treating the athletes with anabolic-androgenic steroids adhered to human treatment guidelines for research (e.g., informed consent or institutional review). Obvious from the State Central Institute of Physical Culture's report, experiments with anabolic-androgenic steroids with athletes had occurred in the former USSR by 1971 to 1972 or earlier. Dr. Kalinski published papers summarizing the report's contents and lectured extensively around the world (including the American College of Sports Medicine) about organized studies and anabolic steroid use. Here is how Dr. Kalinski described the doping program in the USSR (Fahey, et al., 2014):

> "Central government departments issued orders to organize, finance, and administer research on performance-enhancing drugs and supplements and oversee their use. Research into the medical and biological aspects of sport was an integral part of the athletic agenda in the former Soviet Union. It was conducted in over 28 State Institutes of Physical Education and State Research Institutes of Physical Culture. It is unlikely that crucial decisions about financing and implementation of research programs on androgenic-anabolic steroids by the State

Central Institute of Physical Culture in Moscow were made without government officials' knowledge and consent.

Some may argue that androgenic-anabolic steroid use is widespread, and the West's situation did not differ from the Soviet Union. There is, however, an essential difference between East Germany, the former USSR, and Western countries. In the West, governments did not finance human subject research on steroids to enhance athletic performance. Use of these substances is prohibited and discouraged. Athletes who use steroids are doing so on their own initiative, without government agencies' support or consent.

The document from the State Central Institute of Physical Culture clarified there was a different situation in the USSR, — a government sponsored scientific effort, which did not follow the accepted norms for treatment of human subjects. By governmental agencies circulating the research report among elite State Sports Institutions in the former Soviet Union, sports officials, coaches, and athletes were advised, recommended, and encouraged to use androgenic-anabolic steroids. In East Germany, for example, reports released after the reunification of Germany showed that taking anabolic-androgenic steroids was mandatory for any athletes wanting to participate in the 1988 Seoul Olympics.

The classified document described in this article proves the existence of state-sponsored studies on the effect of anabolic-androgenic steroids on athlete's morphological, biochemical, physiological variables and athletic performance conducted in the former Soviet Union. The studies were performed in the Research Laboratory of Training Programming and Physiology of the Sport Performance at the State Central Institute of Physical Culture in Moscow. They could not have been enacted and financed without government orders. The document made recommendations for steroid use for different sports, particularly for elite athletes specializing in endurance and strength-dependent sports. Ethical considerations were not important: coaches did not obtain informed consent, and they recommended high doses of anabolic steroids for weightlifters and high-power athletes.

The State Central Institute of Physical Culture in Moscow secretly circulated the results and recommendations obtained from state-sponsored studies on androgenic-anabolic steroids to elite sport institutions in the USSR. This information was classified and accessible only to selected professionals."

International Sanctions Against Russia and its Athletes

State-sponsored doping did not cease with the end of the Cold War. Some countries, most notably Russia, took state-sponsored doping to new levels. The IOC uncovered a broad conspiracy to promote doping in Russian athletes during the 2014 Sochi, Russia Winter Olympics (Figure 11-3). The conspiracy included systematically manipulating doping tests, covering up positive tests, and state-sponsored illegal drug use at the grassroots level.

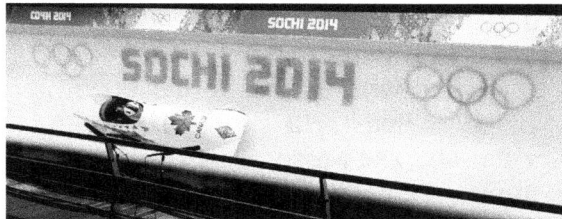

Figure 11-3 The Sochi Winter Olympics was the site of a major doping scandal. Shutterstock

Following the Sochi games, officials from the IOC uncovered a conspiracy to cover up athletes' positive tests in 31 sports. The result was extreme: Russia was regarded as "non-compliant" to WADA's doping code and banned most Russian athletes in the Olympics and Para-Olympics at Rio de Janeiro in 2016. The sanctions were extended to the Olympic Games in Tokyo in 2021 but subsequently modified.

Other countries also are involved. Doping control is under the auspices of doping control labs in different countries. The records are often not transparent, which increases the chances for systematic abuse. Systematic violations of international doping regulations will not end soon. As of 2021, Russia is banned from participating in various international sports because of non-transparent drug testing programs. In December 2019, WADA issued a report that accused Russia of doctoring doping compliance documents and has recommended suspending athletes for another four-years from international sport— including the 2021 Olympics in Tokyo.

Dr. Kalinski summarized the Russian violations (Kalinski, 2017):

1. "An institutional conspiracy existed across summer and winter sports athletes who participated with Russian officials within the Ministry of Sport, Russian Anti–Doping Agency, and the Moscow Laboratory to manipulate doping controls.
2. The summer and winter sports athletes were not acting individually but within an organized infrastructure.
3. This systematic and centralized cover-up and manipulation of the doping control process evolved through 2020.
4. Swapping Russian athletes' urine samples further confirmed irregularities at the Sochi Winter Olympics, which continued at the Moscow Laboratory for elite summer and winter athletes.
5. Knowledge of the Russian doping conspiracy was based on immutable facts. WADA

established that the conspiracy was perpetrated between 2011 and 2015.

6. Over 1000 Russian athletes competing in summer, winter, and Paralympic sports, were involved or benefited from sample manipulations to conceal positive doping tests. The conspiracy involved 600 (84%) summer athletes and 95 (16%) winter athletes.

7. Fifteen Russian athlete medal winners were identified out of the 78 on the London Summer Olympic Games Washout Lists. Ten of these athletes had their medals stripped.

8. Following the 2013 IAAF Moscow World Championships, Russian doping technicians swapped four athletics athletes' samples. Additional target testing is in progress.

9. Sochi Winter Olympic Games: Sample swapping was established by two female ice hockey players' samples with male DNA.

10. Tampering with original sample established by two (sports) athletes, winners of four Sochi Olympic Gold medals, and a female silver medal winner who exhibited physiologically impossible sodium readings.

11. Twelve medal-winning athletes from 44 examined samples had scratches and marks on the inside of the caps of their B sample bottles, indicating tampering.

12. Urine samples from 6 of 21 Paralympic medal winners at Sochi showed evidence of tampering.

13. The IOC stated the report showed, "There

was a fundamental attack on the integrity of the Olympic Games and on sport in general."

Financially Punishing Sanctions: State-sponsored doping programs in the USSR, East Germany, and Russia cast a pall over the Olympic sports image. To their credit, sanctions against the Russian Olympic team at Rio de Janeiro and Tokyo sent a stern message that state-sponsored doping would not be tolerated. This move was financially punishing to the Olympic movement but was necessary to maintaining the sanctity for all of the Olympic programs worldwide.

Summary

Doping control and athletic drug use have been central topics of discussion during the Olympics since 100-meter gold medalist Ben Johnson tested positive for anabolic steroids during the 1988 games in Seoul, Korea. Following World War II, international athletic competitions became the cold war surrogates to the battlefield. East and West squared off on the playing fields, ice rinks, basketball courts, and running tracks. Performance-enhancing drugs became tools in the East and West to advance athletic prowess.

Doping control has progressed from *in-competition* drug tests to sophisticated *out-of-competition* random tests. The World Anti-Doping Agency added a "biological passport" in 1999 to detect doping agents by changes in hematocrit and hemoglobin. Doping categories include stimulants, narcotics, anabolic drugs, selective androgen receptor modulators (SARMs), diuretics, peptide and glycoprotein hormones, prohibited methods, and classes subject to restrictions.

Irregularities at the Sochi Olympics cast a pall over doping control, leading to suspending Russian Federation athletes from the Rio de Janeiro and Tokyo Olympics. An investigation determined that athletes were part of a state-sponsored program involving positive test coverups and switching and tampering with urine samples. The IOC deemed their actions "A fundamental attack on the integrity of the Olympic Games and on sport in general." Not surprisingly, the Court for Arbitration of Sport reduced sanctions against Russia for the Tokyo Summer Games in 2021 and Beijing Winter Games in 2022.

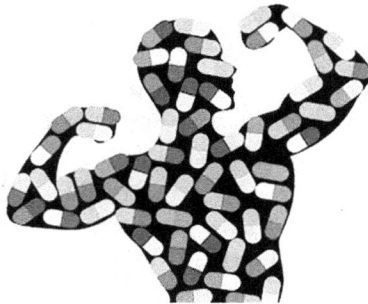

11

ANABOLIC STEROIDS, ETHICS, AND THE LAW

Laws against anabolic steroid abuse in many countries have placed athletes who use steroids in legal jeopardy. In 1990, the United States Congress passed the Anabolic Steroid Control Act, effective February 21, 1991. The Steroid Act classified 27 anabolic steroids as Schedule III substances. The law gave the U.S. Drug Enforcement Agency power to restrict the importation, exportation, distribution, and dispensing of anabolic steroids. On March 11, 2004, Congress amended it (S.2195) to include the "pro-hormone" androstenedione—a pro hormone to testosterone, which makes this drug an "indirect" anabolic steroid. The law prohibited physicians from prescribing anabolic steroids to athletes for enhancing athletic performance.

Former President George Bush mentioned anabolic steroids use in his State of the Union address in 2004:

> "To help children make right choices, they need good examples. Athletics play such an

important role in our society, but, unfortunately, some in professional sports are not setting much of an example. Using performance-enhancing drugs like steroids in baseball, football, and other sports is dangerous, and it sends the wrong message — there are shortcuts to accomplishment, and performance is more important than character. So, tonight I call on team owners, union representatives, coaches, and players to take the lead, to send the right signal, to get tough, and to get rid of steroids now."

Drug scandals plague sport at almost every level. Allegations of drug use by professional and Olympic athletes in the BALCO affair, Russian athletes at the Sochi Olympics, and athletes competing in the Tour de France are the latest incidents in the long history of drug use in sport. Notorious sports doping incidents include:

- The institutionalized sports drug programs in Russia, USSR, East Germany, and China (Figure 10-1; Ilona Slupianek GDR tested positive for steroids 1977).
- The massive exodus of athletes from the Pan American Games in 1983 to avoid drug testing.
- Ben Johnson's steroid disqualification from the 1988 Olympic Games (Figure 10-2).
- The institutionalized cover-up of American athletes who tested positive for banned substances by the USOC.
- Widespread use of erythropoietin (EPO) and

blood doping by athletes in the Tour de France and Nordic ski racing. Lance Armstrong banned for life in 2005 after admitting to using EPO and testosterone (Figure 10-3).

- The Balco scandal in the U.S. involved leading Olympic and professional athletes. Track and Field superstar Marion Jones (Figure 10-4) implicated in the Balco scandal, was disqualified from the 2000 Olympics and 2001 World Championships when she admitted using anabolic steroids.

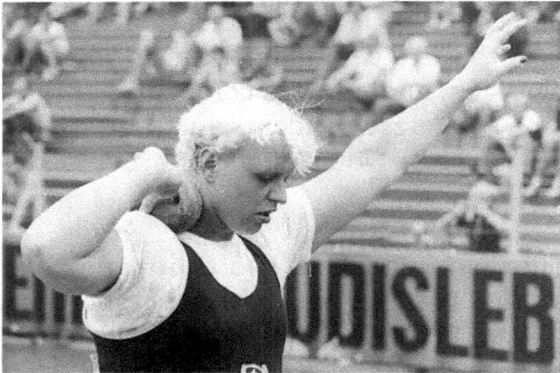

Figure 10-1: Ilona Slupianek. Source: German Federal Archive, Wiki Commons.

- Anabolic steroid use in baseball and American football.

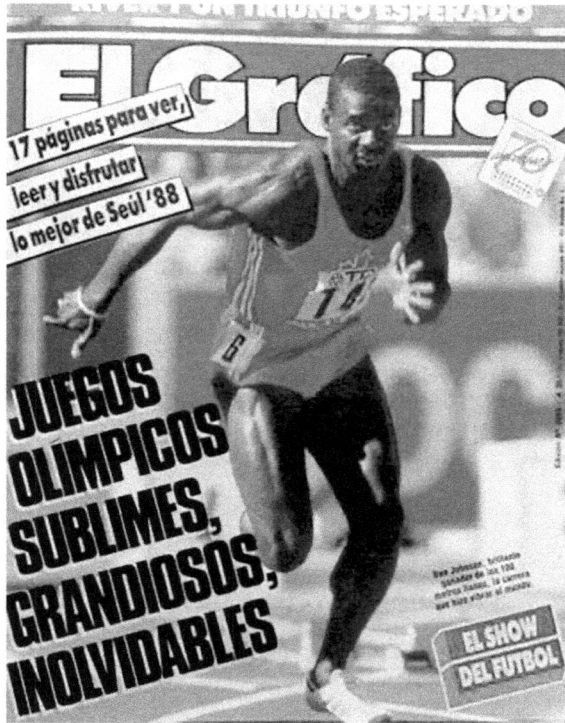

Figure 10-2: Ben Johnson; Source: *El Gráfico,*
Wiki Commons.

- Contaminated over-the-counter food
  supplements with anabolic steroids.
- Systematically using banned substances by
  Russian athletes resulting in whole-team
  suspensions in 31 sports in 2016 and 2021.
  Figure 10-5 summarizes false doping reports
  submitted by the Russian Doping Control
  Laboratory uncovered by the McLaren report
  (2016).

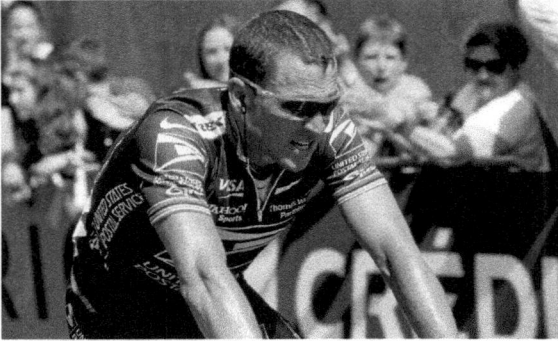

Figure 10-3: Lance Armstrong. Source:
de:Benutzer:Hase, Wiki Commons

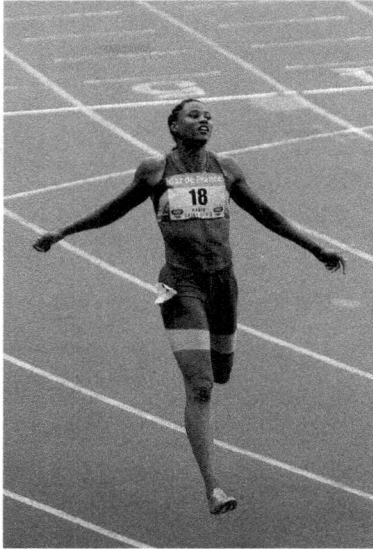

Figure 10-4: Marion Jones. Source: https://www.
flickr.com/photos/tfa/ Thomas Faivre-Duboz.

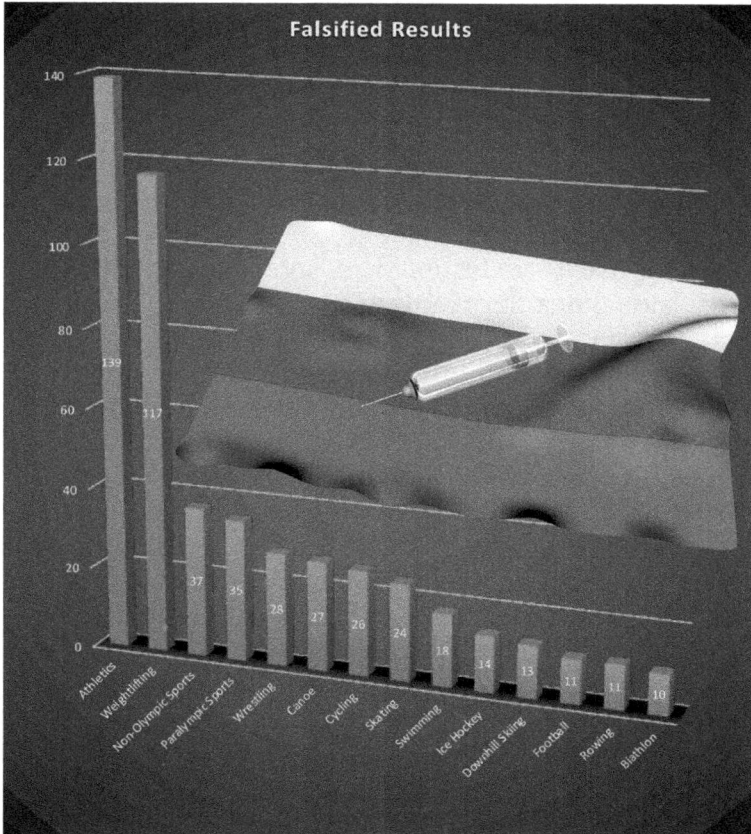

Figure 10-5: False doping reports submitted by the Russian Doping Control Laboratory. Source: Produced from McLaren Report data, 2016.

These drug controversies involved athletes taking prohibited substances to maximize performance and the sports hierarchy's attempts to stop them.

. . .

Widespread Scandals: In late 2020, the Court for Arbitration of Sport reduced sanctions against Russia for the Tokyo Summer and Beijing Winter Games. Russians competed as the Russian Olympic Committee with sanctions to prohibit displaying the Russian flag or playing the Russian national anthem during gold medal ceremonies.

Drug use is widespread in sports, but politicians, professional health organizations, and athletic administrators want to prevent athletes from using them. Other scientists and ethicists argue that we are losing the war on drugs and sport and needlessly squandering resources that could be devoted to the sports themselves. The issues surrounding prohibiting steroid use in amateur, Olympic, and professional sports are complex and include steroids and the "level playing field," anabolic steroid health risks, unnaturalness of anabolic steroids, 4th Amendment and drug testing, balance between the goals of athletes versus the goals of society, and institutional responsibility for preventing drug use in sport.

Reforming the Rules Needed: The rules should ban anabolic steroids from sports but not for the reasons cited by politicians, physicians, sports administrators, and the media. While steroids help athletes improve their performance, they are contrary to the goals of sport in the society. *The harm caused to society by allowing the widespread use of drugs by people who have no chance of excelling in sports overshadows the benefits of allowing a few elite athletes to use drugs to prepare them for competition.*

University of Texas, Austin historian John Hoberman discussed the ambivalence and inconsistency in America regarding the widespread use of per-formance-enhancing drugs and drug testing athletes in his book *Testosterone Dreams: Rejuvenation, Aphrodisia, Doping* (2004). Since the 1880s, Hucksters promoted testicular extracts to increase vitality and sexual po-tency. Testosterone was synthesized and used clinically beginning in 1934 to treat male and female sexual problems and later, to promote muscle growth and strength. Hoberman said that while drug use was frowned upon in amateur sports, elite sports accepted it (or looked the other way). Incidents that turned the tide of public opinion included Ben Johnson's steroid disqualification in the 1988 Olympics, Mark McGuire's alleged use of androstenedione (a legal supplement at the time), and the BALCO drug scandal. These inci-dents conflicted with sacred traditions and American folklore including Babe Ruth's season home run record and the myth surrounding Olympic athletes' amateur purity.

The BALCO Scandal

The BALCO scandal involved systematic doping of Olympic and professional athletes through the Bay Area Laboratory in Burlingame, California (BALCO). The company sold supplements and provided urine and blood tests to help athletes maintain "metabolic bal-ance." The South San Francisco Bay Area was a hotbed for world-class Olympic athletes particularly in track and field. Some of the best strength athletes in the world lived within 20 miles of each other. The area also was home to the San Francisco Giants and Oakland A's baseball teams and San Francisco 49ers and Oakland Raiders football teams.

The lab marketed undetectable "designer steroids," erythropoietin (blood booster), human growth hormone, modafinil (stimulant that increases mental focus), and testosterone cream. Testosterone levels were closely monitored to avoid detection. BALCO employed several notable athletes who recruited an impressive client list of elite professional and Olympic athletes.

A sample of "the cream"— BALCO's designer steroid— was anonymously sent to the UCLA Olympic Analytical Laboratory and information detailing the BALCO program. The lab developed a chemical method to analyze the substance— the designer steroid *tetrahydrogestrinone*. The revelation became a national scandal publicly investigated by the Federal government. Twenty of 550 previously collected urine samples tested positive for *tetrahydrogestrinone*.

The scandal resulted in severe sanctions for many notable track and field athletes. Before the scandal, Major League Baseball did not specifically prohibit steroids. The scandal triggered strict anti-doping rules in Professional Baseball including a 50-game suspension for a first offense. Several of the laboratory principles received prison sentences of 3-4 months.

Anabolic Steroids, Public Expectations, and Lure of Success and Money

WWII General George Patton said:

66 "Americans love a winner and will not tolerate a loser. Americans play to win all the time. That's why Americans have never lost and will never lose a war."

His quote reflects a widespread view about sports and war.

The public embraces performance-enhancing substances to help people excel in school, the workplace, and the bedroom. Millions consume the mood stabilizer Prozac and mind enhancer modafinil (Provigil). Symphony conductors and public speakers often take beta-blockers or tranquilizers to reduce anxiety before performances or lectures. These drugs increase productivity, mental focus, and perhaps income, but few people fault those who use them. Few denounce mountain climbers for using supplemental oxygen, yet climbers could not accomplish record-setting climbs without it. Drugs to treat erectile dysfunction have boosted sexual performance in an entire generation of aging men.

Geriatrics and quality of life enhancement in older patients are the fastest growing areas in medicine. Many physicians prescribe testosterone and growth hormone to aging patients to improve sexual capacity, vitality, and physical fitness. Few of these patients need hormone replacement therapy (HRT) to compensate for hormone deficiencies. Rather, they take hormones to improve quality of life. Should athletes be deprived of medical treatments used by ordinary people that retard aging effects and improve physical performance? An examination of drug tests in sports shows that positive tests occur regularly in master's athletes competing in track and field and CrossFit Games.

Public expectations add to the inconsistency. Spectators pay to see elite athletes playing at the top of their game. Pro football linemen from the 1950s often weighed less than 240 pounds, while the average lineman in 2021 weighs over 320 pounds. Division I football linemen increased in size and strength by over 20 percent in the last 20 years. While players from 25 years ago were great athletes, they did not have the crowd appeal of today's lightning-fast behemoths. People want to see larger-than-life bodybuilders, hitters pounding the ball over the center field wall, and sprinters and swimmers running and swimming faster than ever. New training methods, improved sports nutrition, and effective supplements and drugs have pushed performances to higher levels.

The economic incentive to use steroids is almost irresistible in some sports. Players make considerably greater salaries than the average person, so the public holds them to a moral standard higher than ordinary people. This phenomenon was described by Harvard Law professor Paul Weiler:

> "In 1947 the average baseball player earned $11,000 a year, a little over four times the pay of the average American worker. In 1967, the average player earned $19,000, about 3.5 times the $5,500 average for workers. In 1973 baseball salaries jumped to $36,000, but workers experienced a large gain (to $9,500), leaving the player-worker ratio still a little

under the 1947 level. However, by 1999 the average baseball player was earning $1.57 million, while the average worker earned just $28,000: a ratio of 56 to one. In 2020, the average Major League baseball player made $1.4 million per year while the average American full-time worker made $48,672— a ratio of about 28 to one."

One could argue that pro athletes are losing ground compared to athletes in 1999, but their salaries are more than most people dream about. Elite athletes are cultural icons with enormous influence on the behavior of ordinary people. The purity of pro and Olympic athletes is part of the popular tradition and folklore.

Business executives often take Prozac or modafinil to increase productivity and performance. Students consume "smart drugs" before taking entrance exams to pursue careers in education (Graduate Record Exam), medical school (MCAT), law school (LSAT) and many other professional opportunities (including specialties in military services). Yet, athletes cannot take steroids to break legendary athletic records. Steroids violate our perceptions and illusions about sport, which is the real reason the rules ban them from athletic competitions.

The Level Playing Field Myth

Elite athletic competitions in Olympic sports, professional baseball, football, basketball, and hockey are contests between genetically gifted individuals who train hard and have access to the latest training and nutrition information .

The Human Genome Project, completed in 2003, identified the human gene sequences. Most genes have variants called polymorphisms that cause individual differences in every human characteristic, including intelligence, susceptibility to disease, reaction to drugs, muscle strength, and appearance (www. genome.gov/human).

Researchers discovered more about genes in the last 10 years than during our entire history. Athletic performance has a strong genetic component. Scientists have identified over 800 genes linked to endurance, strength, power, fat deposition, and fat use.

Heritage Family Study: A massive research project has explored the role of genetics in weight loss, diet, and exercise. People showed highly variable responses when following the same diet or exercise program. Some people make 50% improvements in response to training, while others improve only 2 to 3% (Bouchard, et al., 1999). Creating changes in fitness components and fatness levels are more difficult in non-responders.

People without key gene variants cannot achieve elite levels of performance. Athletic officials continue to propagate the myth that anyone can be a champion if they only worked and trained hard enough. A statement by Juan Antonio Samaranch, past president of the International Olympic Committee, is a typical sentiment about this important issue:

" "Doping is not only a danger for the health of athletes, and it also constitutes a form of cheating which we cannot accept. Such behavior makes a mockery of the very essence of sport, and our most sacrosanct ideals: the inner desire to surpass one's own limits, the social need to compete with others, to find one's identity within society and to develop at all levels."

Is it a level playing field when genes give some people superior athletic ability than others?

The Transgender Controversy: Controversies regarding transgender athletes have added to the confusion about testosterone and sports performance. A literature review by Handelsman, et al. (2018) reported that testosterone gives men an 8 to 12 percent competitive advantage due to greater circulating hemoglobin, muscle mass, and strength. In 2015, the International Olympic Committee ruled that transgender athletes may compete under these two conditions:

1. Those who transition from female to male are eligible to compete in the male category without restriction.
2. Those who transition from male to female are eligible to compete in the female category under these conditions: First, the athlete has declared that her gender identity is female. The declaration cannot be changed, for sporting purposes, for at least four years. Second, the athlete must demonstrate that

her total testosterone level in serum has remained below 10 nmol/L (288 ng/dL) for at least 12 months before her first competition (with the requirement for any longer period based on a confidential case-by-case evaluation, considering whether 12 months is a sufficient length of time to minimize any advantage in women's competition).

A main concern with these conditions is that exposure to testosterone causes long-term and perhaps permanent physiological changes. Anabolic steroids combined with training increase muscle satellite cells, androgen receptor density and sensitivity, and myelin density surrounding motor nerves. These changes persist long after reductions in testosterone levels. *An athlete transitioning from male to female will have more muscle satellite cells, myelin development, and androgen receptors because of earlier exposure to higher testosterone levels, which will provide life-long benefits.*

Is Steroid Use in Sport Ethical? Two notable bioethicists—Norman Fost, Director of the Medical Ethics Program at the University of Wisconsin Medical School, and Julian Savulescu, Chair in Practical Ethics at Oxford University, alluded to the fallaciousness and hypocrisy inherent in the level playing field argument (Fost, N, 2004; Savulescu, et al., 2004; Savulescu, et al., 2013).

Fost rejected that athletes are coerced to use steroids to succeed. Steroids, along with weight training, confer an advantage, but athletes are free not to participate. American football also requires back-breaking work, hours in the weight room, and chronic pain from contact that can last a lifetime. *Athletes who say they are coerced to use steroids fail to distinguish an opportunity from a threat.* They also are free not to use space-age weight machines, food supplements that work like drugs, mental techniques designed to improve focus, downhill running tracks, and plyometric benches.

Sam Shuster, from the University of Newcastle upon Tyne Medical School in the United Kingdom, is a contrarian (Shuster, 2012). He believes that over concern about melanoma has needlessly kept people out of the sun. He also believes that the rules should not sanction athletes for taking performance-enhancing drugs. Shuster argues that anabolic steroids do not differ from performance enhancing speed suits in skiing, shaving body hair in swimming, or Lasik eye surgery to improve accuracy in archers, golfers, and shooters. Shuster concluded there is little proof that drugs provide a competitive advantage, so it is wrong and immoral to punish athletes for using them.

Fost agreed that steroids are unnatural, but so are running shoes, weight machines, and athletic fluid replacement beverages. Why not insist that athletes lift rocks instead of training on high-tech weightlifting machines? *There is no moral distinction between natural and artificial performance aids.*

Ben Johnson: In the 1988 Olympics in Seoul, Ben Johnson forfeited his gold medal for steroid use. He was called a cheater for taking advantage of his opponents. The sweetheart in that Olympics was swimming star Janet Evans who won because she wore a "speed suit" developed by American engineers kept secret from the East Germans. Evans used a performance aid nobody else had. Johnson used steroids available to anyone and probably used by most athletes who competed in the Games. Johnson's problem was that he failed a drug test—not that he had created an unequal competition.

Rich vs Poor Countries: Fost argued that while steroids provide a competitive advantage, so does weight training, good nutrition, coaching, and equipment. The United States, Russia, Britain, and China spend millions of dollars sponsoring elite athletes. Sierra Leone in Africa has difficulty providing track shoes to their athletes. In third world countries, socioeconomic status is highly related to height, weight, body mass index, fat mass, and lean body mass, all important to athletic success.

Technological Advances: Advances in technology always have been part of sports. People used shoes to help them run on rocky, uneven surfaces, added spikes to increase traction, and used high tech components to lighten their weight. In the 1940s, Cornelius "Dutch" Warmerdam broke the 15-foot (4.57 m) barrier in the pole vault with a bamboo pole and dominated the event for ten years. Bamboo was an improvement on rigid poles made from pine. Today, 15-feet is not even a good high school vault. Advances in pole technology have enabled pole-vaulters to exceed 20 feet (6.10 m). The best vaulting poles are so expensive that they are unavailable to most athletes. Is this a level playing field?

East African distance runners dominate the sport because they have a greater running economy and higher fractional maximal oxygen consumption utilization, possibly because of higher hemoglobin levels and mitochondrial density than people in other parts of the world. Hemoglobin and mitochondria are essential factors in oxygen metabolism. Savulescu and Foddy (2004) cited the case of Finnish skier Eoro Maentyranta.

> "In 1964, he won 2 gold medals. Then it was found his genetic mutation meant that he "naturally" had 40 to 50 percent more red blood cells than average. Was it fair he had a significant advantage given to him by chance? Why not match running competitions by hematocrit (percent cells in the blood) and mitochondrial content just as they do by gender? Yet, when athletes take the drug EPO (erythropoietin) to increase their blood count, they are called cheaters."

Jamaican Bobsled Team: Bobsledding is another good example where technology gives athletes advantages over others. Nobody complained when the famous but rag-tag Jamaican bobsled team, shown in the film *Cool Runnings (www.youtube.com/watch?v=2jBgeK-vjHk)*, competed and lost using second-rate equipment against Swiss and Austrian teams using technologically advanced sleds. Had the Jamaicans tested positive for steroids, there would have been an international uproar.

New York Yankees: Similar inequities exist in professional baseball and American football. According to Forbes, "Big markets such as New York, Boston and Chicago offer more revenue opportunities than Kansas City, Minneapolis or Tampa. As of August 2021, the Yankees are valued at $5 billion and produced more than $683 million in revenue in 2019. The Miami Marlins, in 30th place, are valued at $980 million with 2019 revenue of $222 million." Major League baseball has a revenue-sharing plan. Still, this does not "level the playing field" in the ability to hire the best players and create the optimal training environment.

People invented sports, and sports rules change frequently. Home run hitters Barry Bonds and Mark McGuire, who allegedly used performance-enhancing substances, electrified a dying game on their stellar exploits. These highly skilled athletes used supplements to help them prepare to play their best, and they succeeded marvelously. Rule changes have accommodated the forward pass, fiberglass poles, starting blocks, and the Fosbury flop. Anabolic steroids are in this same tradition.

There is no level playing field in sports, and there never has been. Steroids represent a training innovation that is no more unnatural than weight machines, sports drinks, running shoes, or fiberglass poles. Savulescu and Foddy (2004) stated:

"Performance enhancement is not against the spirit of sport; it is the spirit of sport. To be better is to be human. Athletes should be given this choice. Their welfare should be paramount. However, taking drugs is not necessarily cheating. The legalization of drugs in sport may be fairer and safer."

Anabolic Steroids are Unhealthy

Taking anabolic steroids in effective doses is unhealthy, but are the health risks any higher than playing some sports? The IOC, politicians, media, and athletic administrators cite the anabolic steroids' health risks as a major reason to ban the drugs. The media has whipped up a frenzy about steroids not based on scientific fact. Steroids have side effects, but most are reversible and generally mild. For some irrational reason, the press distorts and overstates them. They continue to dwell on the evils of steroids when much of the information is patently false.

Betterman summarized the difficulty conducting objective research on steroids (Reilly and Orme, 1997):

"Several athletes I have worked with have accused sports scientists of using only selective evidence to show that steroids are dangerous. We cite random observations for evidence of adverse side effects. But we require strictly controlled studies for evidence that the drugs boost performance. Scientists cannot have it both ways. They must look at the pluses and minuses of these drugs objectively."

Athletes often have trouble obtaining accurate information from physicians and scientists about anabolic steroid side effects. *Steroids are so politicized that it is impossible to get an honest assessment of their risks even from some health experts.* Their typical reaction is to advise athletes to stay away from steroids because they are illegal and dangerous. There is an extensive list of side effects of anabolic steroid use including acne, testicular atrophy, arteriosclerosis, prostate and liver cancers, and psychiatric disturbances.

Are Steroids More Dangerous than American Football or Downhill Skiing? *In most people, steroids do not pose a deadly risk.* People have used anabolic steroids since the 1930s, yet only one epidemiological study shows a link between steroids and premature death, and this study included only nine subjects. *Steroids have side effects, but the risks are small compared to the risks in many sports.*

Legions of former American football players are permanently disabled from playing the sport. Mez, et al. (2007) found that 110 of 111 deceased NFL players showed permanent brain damage. Gymnasts, downhill skiers, divers, lacrosse and rugby players, bike racers, boxers, wrestlers, equestrian athletes, and kayakers take risks that far exceed those posed by steroids. Should we ban these sports because they are dangerous and harmful to their health?

The risks posed in these sports far exceed those from taking anabolic steroid drugs. Competent adults who make rational decisions about playing crippling sports can make an informed choice about taking anabolic steroids that have relatively mild side effects.

Should Anabolic Steroids be Permitted in Sports?

Elite athletes are role models to millions of people with various athletic talents worldwide who will never achieve Olympic or professional levels in sport. Rules banning steroid use in sports are justified because they serve society's greater good.

Two questions are critical:

1. Do the actions of professional athletes significant impact the general population?
2. Is there a demonstrated special need to single out professional athletes for warrantless searches? The answer to both questions is yes.

Athletes Play an Essential Role in Society: Children and adults look up to athletes and emulate their behavior, but most young athletes will never play professional or Olympic sports (Table 11-1).

Student Athletes	Men's Basketball	Women's Basketball	Football	Baseball	Men's Ice Hockey	Men's Soccer
High School Student Athletes	538,676	433,120	1,086,627	474,791	35,198	410,982
High School Senior Student Athletes	153,907	123,749	310,465	135,655	10,057	117,423
NCAA Student Athletes	17,984	16,186	70,147	32,450	3,964	23,365
NCAA Freshman Roster Positions	5,138	4,625	20,042	9,271	1,133	6,676
NCAA Senior Student Athletes	3,996	3,597	15,588	7,211	881	5,192
NCAA Student Athletes Drafted	46	32	254	678	7	101
Percent High School to NCAA	3.3%	3.7%	6.5%	6.8%	11.3%	5.7%
Percent NCAA to Professional	1.2%	0.9%	1.6%	9.4%	0.8%	1.9%
Percent High School to Professional	0.03%	0.03%	0.08%	0.50%	0.07%	0.09%

Table 11-1: Only. a fraction of athletes will ever play professional or Olympic sports. Athletes should follow their dreams, but they must be realistic and not use anabolic steroids to attain what for most is unattainable.

In 2020, nearly 3 million children played Little League baseball in the U.S., but only 750 athletes played in the major leagues on opening day. The prospects for becoming a professional basketball player in the National Basketball Association are less because team rosters are smaller. Only three athletes can compete in individual Olympic sports— if they meet minimum qualifying standards. In weightlifting, only three American males and females in all weight categories competed in the 2012 London Olympics because the U.S. team did not have enough athletes who met the performance standards. Most children have a better chance to win the lottery than to play elite sports.

There is no level playing field with athletic excellence. Elite athletes have genetic prerequisites. The average person without these genes has no chance to play pro baseball or compete in the Olympics— no matter how hard they train. Nevertheless, people see the money, fame, and glory heaped on athletic stars and want to be one of them.

High school and college athletes—and non-athletes —will use steroids if they think the drugs will improve performance. They say to themselves, "Barry Bonds broke the home run record, and he allegedly took steroids. If I take steroids, I can be more like Bonds." Instead of developing life-long habits associated with a healthy lifestyle, they take drugs with dangerous side effects.

As former coaches, both of us have witnessed athletes ruined by taking steroids in high school. Many do well in high school but fail to transition to college. Typically, they succeeded in high school because they were stronger and more powerful than the competition. They never developed the technique to compete at a higher level and found it challenging to relearn basic skills in college. Also, many failed random drug tests and lost their ability to compete in college.

Sport and exercise play important roles in society. It improves metabolic health, instills a sense of community, fosters a competitive work ethic, and promotes cooperation. While these benefits are debatable, they represent core societal values. *Except for improved metabolic health, the values of sport to society are difficult to demonstrate experimentally. Like religion, they are a matter of faith rather than science.*

Sport and Family Values: As a society, we value Babe Ruth's 60 home runs, Willie Mays' overhead basket catches, Michael Phelps' 20 Olympic gold medals, fathers and sons playing catch on the front lawn, families watching their kids play soccer, or friends watching the Olympics or football games on television. Somehow, taking steroids ruins these images, and sport loses some of its wholesomeness. It does not matter that taking steroids is no more unnatural than training on weight machines, wearing support clothing in weightlifting, or using ultra-light running shoes. It also does not matter that banning steroids interferes with the rights of individual athletes to be as good as they can be. Society simply will not support steroid use.

Every Sport Has Rules. As an example, the American football field is 100 yards, a discus weighs 2 kg, the height of the basketball hoop is 3.05 m, and players are allowed two serves for each point in tennis. Why not increase the length of the field to 140 yd or raise the basket to 4 m? Sports organizations establish rules, and players abide by them— even if the rules are arbitrary and sometimes ambiguous.

Most sports have rules against taking steroids, so athletes must abide by them. If they do not, they must be sanctioned just as they would be for breaking other rules. For example, in football, a team is penalized 5 yards when a player is offsides. If a baseball player abuses the umpire, he can be ejected from the game, fined, or suspended. Under the doping regulations, athletes who break the rules and take illegal drugs receive suspensions.

Sport has a special status in our society. Children and adults look up to elite athletes and emulate their behavior. As of 2020, only 19,492 men have ever played Major League Baseball (1875-2020; www. baseball-almanac.com), and approximately 25,000 men have played professional football since 1920 (http://www.profootballresearchers.org). *The rights of a handful of elite athletes are of little consequence compared to the harm their drug use does to our perceptions about the value and wholesomeness of sport.*

Anabolic steroids provide short-term and long-term advantages to athletes who use them. *Current sanctions for using anabolic steroids do not go far enough because the drugs have long-term effects on muscle satellite cells, capillary density, androgen receptors, and nerve myelination that provide advantages when the athletes no longer take the drugs (Bhasin, et al., 2021).*

Drug Testing and the Law

. . .

Athletes expect privacy while under the protection, guidance, and supervision of organized sport. The Fourth Amendment of the U.S. Constitution states,

> "The right of the people to be secure in their persons, houses, papers, and effects, against unreasonable searches and seizures, shall not be violated, and no warrants shall issue, but upon probable cause, supported by oath or affirmation, and particularly describing the place to be searched, and the persons or things to be seized."

In the summer of 2005, Senator John McCain [deceased 2018; R-AZ] introduced S.1114, the Clean Sports Act of 2005. The bill included four main components:

- Mandated that professional sports teams conduct drug testing of their players.
- Required public disclosure of the names of athletes who test positive for banned substances.
- Athletes who test positive will be suspended for at least two years for the first violation and a lifetime ban for the second violation.
- Treated violations of this Act as unfair or deceptive acts or practices under the Federal Trade Commission Act.

The bill did not pass and was removed from further consideration. Marvin Miller, former executive director of the Professional Baseball Players Association, said that the law is unconstitutional because players will be tested without probable cause they are using performance-enhancing drugs (https://www.mlbplayers.com/marvin-miller):

> "An employer can do this, and a union can agree to do this, as part of collective bargaining, but Congress can't. No government agency can conduct a search without first going to court and swearing before a judge that there's a probable cause to believe that player 'X' is guilty. Until the judge gives that order, the person can't be searched."

Workers employed in occupations affecting public safety—airline pilots, railroad engineers, and truck drivers who transport goods on interstate highways—may be drug tested and are exceptions to the Fourth Amendment with their job. Athletes do not meet that criterion, so drug testing is a matter of collective bargaining. College and Olympic athletes are tested routinely because they are members of organizations that require it as a prerequisite for membership and participation in their events.

The NCAA and WADA. These organizations test College and Olympic athletes without probable cause, but they agree to year-round drug testing through membership in the governing bodies of their respective sports. Supporters of the bill contend that Congress has the power to mandate drug testing because maintaining purity in sport is in the national interest. Keith Ausbrook, chief counsel for the House Government Reform Committee, speaking for the bill said, "We think the record shows there's compelling interest in doing it to protect the integrity of the game and protect the health of players and children who look up to them. (https://www.nytimes.com/2005/06/02/sports/baseball/steroid-tests-ignore-the-4th-amendment.html)

Legal Cases: Three cases, Ferguson v Charleston (532 U.S. 67), Chandler v. Miller (520 U.S. 305), and Vernonia School Dist. 47J v. Acton (515 U.S. 646), are germane to government-mandated drug tests for professional athletes. In Ferguson, the Medical University of South Carolina instituted a testing program in cooperation with the Charleston police to identify and prosecute expectant mothers who tested positive for cocaine. They did not obtain informed consent from the patients. The court ruled, "While state hospital employees, like other citizens, must provide the police with evidence of criminal conduct that such employees inadvertently acquire in routine treatment, such employees have a special obligation to make sure that the patients are informed about their rights under the Federal Constitution's Fourth Amendment--as standards of knowing waiver require--when such employees undertake to obtain such evidence from patients specifically to incriminate those patients."

In Chandler, a Georgia statute required a drug test before candidates could run for state office. The Libertarian Party nominees sued in the District Court. The District Court and later the Eleventh Circuit Court ruled against the petitioners based on precedents involving student-athletes (Vernonia School Dist. 47J v.

Acton 515 U.S. 646), Customs Service employees (Treasury Employees v. Von Raab, 489 U.S. 656), and railway workers, (Skinner v. Railway Labor Executives' Assn. 489 U.S. 602). While the Court ruled in Chandler that the urine tests were searches, "the statute served 'special needs,'" interests other than the ordinary needs of law enforcement." Balancing the individual's privacy expectations against the State's interest in the drug-testing program, the court held the statute, as applied to petitioners, followed the Fourth and Fourteenth Amendments. The U.S. Supreme Court overturned these decisions ruling that, "Georgia's requirement that candidates for state office pass a drug test does not fit within the closely guarded category of constitutionally permissible suspicionless searches."

Supreme Court: The Supreme Court's ruling in Vernonia School Dist. 47J v. Acton has applicability to the question of professional athletes' Fourth Amendment rights. The Vernonian School District is a small collection of schools in Vernonian, Oregon. Due to a burgeoning drug problem the school district initiated a drug-testing program for athletes in 1989 with the parental groups' advice and consent. The purpose of the program was "to prevent student athletes from using drugs, to protect their health and safety, and to provide drug users with assistance programs."

In 1991, a seventh-grade student named James Acton, could not participate on the football team because his parents refused to sign the drug testing consent form. The parents sued on behalf of their son, but the District Court ruled that the claim was without merit and dismissed the action. The U.S. Court of Appeals for the Ninth Circuit reversed the decision, holding that the drug testing policy violated the Fourth and

Fourteenth Amendments of the U.S. Constitution and Article I of the Oregon Constitution. The U.S. Supreme Court ruled that the school district athletic drug testing policy was acceptable because "the Policy furthered the government's responsibilities, under a public school system, as guardian and tutor of children entrusted to its care. For their own good and that of their classmates, public school children must often wear masks to protect against viral transmission, submit to various physical examinations, and receive vaccinations against diseases.

Vaccinations: In the 1991-1992 school year, all 50 States required vaccinations against diphtheria, measles, rubella, and polio for all public-school students. Students within the school environment expect more privacy than members of the population generally. . . Legitimate privacy expectations are even less regarding student athletes. By choosing to "go out for the team," they voluntarily subject themselves to regulation even higher than that imposed on students generally. Somewhat like adults who participate in a tightly regulated industry (e.g., airline pilots), students who voluntarily participate in school athletics have reason to expect intrusions upon normal rights and privileges, including privacy. "

How Do These Legal Rulings Relate to Professional Sports? In Vernonia (Vernon School District. 47J v. Acton 515 U.S.646), the Court allowed random drug testing after demonstrating a serious drug problem in the school district. We agree with Glassman (2002), who wrote, "In the absence of finding of a special need, no school district should be able to extend suspicionless drug testing to include participants in non-athletic extracurricular activities." In Vernonia, "Students have a decreased expectation of privacy while under the protection, guidance, and supervision of the public school system."

We pose this question: Is the same true for professional athletes?

Summary

Anabolic steroids have infamously captured the imagination of athletes, coaches, sports organizations, physicians, the media, and sports fans. They improve performance but sometimes have catastrophic side effects and delegitimize sport. The money and glory available in big-time sport make steroids and other ergogenic aids difficult to resist. *We believe the needs of society must take precedence over the need for a few athletes for success. The efforts to eliminate or restrict the use of steroids in sport must continue.*

THOMAS D FAHEY & FRANK I KATCH

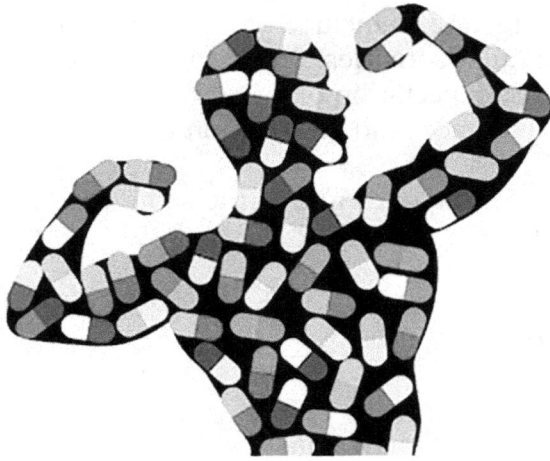

EPILOGUE

A nabolic steroids are the most controversial topics in sports today. People suspect athletes of using steroids every time they break a record, appear bigger or stronger than normal, or react angrily on the playing field. This attitude has taken some of the wonder out of sports and turned millions of fans into cynics.

Sport plays an almost sacred role in society. Parents look forward to their children playing sports during childhood and adolescence. Geographical regions root for the local professional, college, or high school team. Parents take pride in teaching children how to kick a soccer ball, swing a baseball bat, or ski down a hill. Anabolic steroids have taken some of the luster out of our love of sport.

Steroids are part of the scientific sports revolution. Advances in technique, training methods, equipment, sports nutrition, and knowledge about physiology and biomechanics have increased sports performances to levels unheard of twenty or thirty-years ago. The benefits of steroids are no more profound than advances in other sports science areas.

Nevertheless, steroids have tarnished the sacred role sports play in society, which is the real reason the public, politicians, and sports officials take such a dogmatic stance against them.

Scientific studies involving testosterone and other anabolic steroids help us understand the mechanisms behind muscle physiology and adaptations of the body to exercise. Research helps us all to better understand muscle physiology, metabolism, and disease.

Older adults often take testosterone to promote longevity, increase energy levels, boost libido, and maintain muscle and bone mass. Unfortunately, the steroid-sports controversy has interfered with the medical uses for the drugs. Political considerations severely limit their availability and use.

Doping control in amateur and professional sports has restricted steroid use in sports. Nevertheless, athletes will always try to find an edge because of financial rewards and the competitiveness in sport. The cat and mouse game between athletes and doping officials will continue.

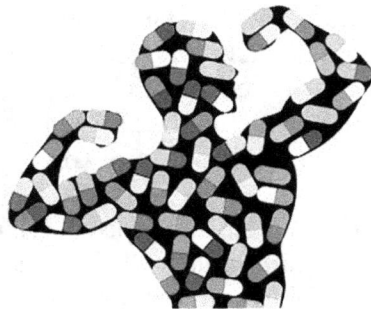

REFERENCES

ORIGINAL PAPERS AND ABSTRACTS AVAILABLE ON
EBOOK VERSION

References: Position Statements on Anabolic Steroids from Professional Organizations

Advisory Panel on Testosterone Replacement in M. Report of National Institute on Aging Advisory Panel on Testosterone Replacement in Men. *J Clin Endocrinol Metab.* 86:4611, 2001.

American College of Obstetricians and Gynecologists. ACOG committee opinion no. 484: Performance enhancing anabolic steroid abuse in women. *Obstet Gynecol.* 117:1016, 2011.

American College of Sports Medicine. Position statement on anabolic-androgenic steroids in sports. *Med Sci Sports.* 9:xi, 1977.

Andrology A.S. Testosterone replacement therapy for male aging: ASA position statement. *J Androl.* 27:133, 2006.

Association A.M. Medical and non-medical uses of

anabolic-androgenic steroids. Council on scientific affairs. *JAMA*. 264:2923, 1990.

Bhasin S. et al. Testosterone therapy in men with hypogonadism: An Endocrine Society clinical practice guideline. *J Clin Endocrinol Metab*. 103:1715, 2018.

Bhasin, S. et al. Anabolic-androgenic steroid use in sports, health, and society. *Med. Sci. Sports Exerc*. 53: 1778-1794, 2021.

Böttiger Y. et al. *Swedish clinical guidelines on the abuse of anabolic androgenic steroids (AAS) and other hormonal drugs*. Stockholm: Anti-doping hotline, Karolinska University Hospital,; 2013.

CONTROL S.C.O.I.N. et al. Abuse of anabolic steroids and their precursors by adolescent amateur athletes. In: UGP Office editor, 2004.

Crawley F.P. et al. Health, integrity, and doping in sports for children and young adults. A resolution of the European Academy of Paediatrics. *Eur J Pediatr*. 176:825, 2017.

Davis S.R. et al. Global consensus position statement on the use of testosterone therapy for women. *Climacteric*. 22:429, 2019.

Dean J.D. et al. The International Society for Sexual Medicine's process of care for the assessment and management of testosterone deficiency in adult men. *J Sex Med*. 12:1660, 2015.

Dimopoulou C. et al. EMAS position statement: Testosterone replacement therapy in the aging male. *Maturitas*. 84:94, 2016.

Hoffman J.R. et al. Position stand on androgen and human growth hormone use. *J Strength Cond Res*. 23:S1, 2009.

Kersey R.D. et al. National Athletic Trainers' Association position statement: Anabolic-androgenic steroids. *J Athl Train.* 47:567, 2012.

Kwong J.C.C. et al. Testosterone deficiency: A review and comparison of current guidelines. *J Sex Med.* 16:812, 2019.

Maughan R.J. IOC Medical and Scientific Commission reviews its position on the use of dietary supplements by elite athletes. *Br J Sports Med.* 52:418, 2018.

Maughan R.J. et al. IOC consensus statement: Dietary supplements and the high-performance athlete. *Int J Sport Nutr Exerc Metab.* 28:104, 2018.

Maughan R.J. et al. IOC consensus statement: Dietary supplements and the high-performance athlete. *Br J Sports Med.* 52:439, 2018.

Mitchell G.J. *Report to the Commissioner of Baseball of an independent investigation into the illegal use of steroids and other performance enhancing substances by players in Major League Baseball.*: DLA PIPER US LLP2007.

Neuberger J. Editorial: Showing due diligence--the lessons from anabolic steroids. *Aliment Pharmacol Ther.* 41:321, 2015.

National Federation of High Schools. Position statement on anabolic, androgenic steroids. 2012. https://www.osaa.org/docs/health-safety/steriods.pdf

Park H.J. et al. Evolution of guidelines for testosterone replacement therapy. *J Clin Med.* 8:2019.

Pope H.G., Jr. et al. Adverse health consequences of performance-enhancing drugs: An endocrine society scientific statement. *Endocr Rev.* 35:341, 2014.

Endocrine Society. Position statement: Steroid abuse. In. Washington D.C.: Endocrine Society; 2008. Thieme D. et al. *Doping in sport.* Springer; 2010.

Ventimiglia E. et al. Validation of the American Society for Reproductive Medicine guidelines/recommen-

dations in white European men presenting for couple's infertility. *Fertil Steril.* 106:1076, 2016.
Weiss R.V. et al. Testosterone therapy for women with low sexual desire: A position statement from the Brazilian Society of Endocrinology and Metabolism. *Arch Endocrinol Metab.* 63:190, 2019.

References: The Epidemiology of Anabolic Steroids

Abrahin O.S. et al. Prevalence of the use of anabolic-androgenic steroids in Brazil: A systematic review. *Subst Use Misuse.* 49:1156, 2014.
Agullo-Calatayud V. et al. Consumption of anabolic steroids in sport, physical activity and as a drug of abuse: An analysis of the scientific literature and areas of research. *Br J Sports Med.* 42:103, 2008.
Ahmed M.H. et al. Knowledge of and attitudes toward the use of anabolic-androgenic steroids among the population of Jeddah, Saudi Arabia. *J Microsc Ultrastruct.* 7:78, 2019.
Alsaeed I. et al. Usage and perceptions of anabolic-androgenic steroids among male fitness centre attendees in Kuwait--a cross-sectional study. *Subst Abuse Treat Prev Policy.* 10:33, 2015.
Althobiti S.D. et al. Prevalence, attitude, knowledge, and practice of anabolic androgenic steroid (AAS) use among gym participants. *Mater Sociomed.* 30:49, 2018.
Angell P. et al. Anabolic steroids and cardiovascular risk. *Sports Med.* 42:119, 2012.
Anshel M.H. et al. Examining athletes' attitudes toward using anabolic steroids and their knowledge of the possible effects. *J Drug Educ.* 27:121, 1997.
Association A.M. Medical and non-medical uses of ana-

bolic-androgenic steroids. Council on Scientific Affairs. *JAMA.* 264:2923, 1990.

Avilez J.L. et al. Use of enhancement drugs amongst athletes and television celebrities and public interest in androgenic anabolic steroids. Exploring two Peruvian cases with google trends. *Public Health.* 146:29, 2017.

Berning J.M. et al. Anabolic androgenic steroids: Use and perceived use in non-athlete college students. *J Am Coll Health.* 56:499, 2008.

Blashill A.J. et al. Sexual orientation and anabolic-androgenic steroids in U.S. Adolescent boys. *Pediatrics.* 133:469, 2014.

Bolding G. et al. Use of anabolic steroids and associated health risks among gay men attending London gyms. *Addiction.* 97:195, 2002.

Bolding G. et al. HIV risk behaviours among gay men who use anabolic steroids. *Addiction.* 94:1829, 1999.

Bonnecaze A.K. et al. Characteristics and attitudes of men using anabolic androgenic steroids (AAS): A survey of 2385 men. *Am J Mens Health.* 14:1557988320966536, 2020.

Borjesson A. et al. Men's experiences of using anabolic androgenic steroids. *Int J Qual Stud Health Well-being.* 16:1927490, 2021.

Brady J.P. et al. Machismo and anabolic steroid misuse among young Latino sexual minority men. *Body Image.* 30:165, 2019.

Brand R. et al. Using response-time latencies to measure athletes' doping attitudes: The brief implicit attitude test identifies substance abuse in bodybuilders. *Subst Abus Treat Prev Pol.* 9:36, 2014.

Christoffersen T. et al. Anabolic-androgenic steroids and the risk of imprisonment. *Drug Alcohol Depend.* 203:92, 2019.

Christou M.A. et al. Effects of anabolic androgenic steroids on the reproductive system of athletes and recreational users: A systematic review and meta-analysis. *Sports Med.* 47:1869, 2017.

Cohen J. et al. A league of their own: Demographics, motivations and patterns of use of 1,955 male adult non-medical anabolic steroid users in the united states. *J Int Soc Sports Nutr.* 4:12, 2007.

Coomber R. et al. The supply of steroids and other performance and image enhancing drugs (PIEDs) in one English city: Fakes, counterfeits, supplier trust, common beliefs and access. *Perf Enhanc Health.* 3:135, 2014.

Cordaro F.G. et al. Selling androgenic anabolic steroids by the pound: Identification and analysis of popular websites on the internet. *Scand J Med Sci Sports.* 21:e247, 2011.

Cornford C.S. et al. Anabolic-androgenic steroids and heroin use: A qualitative study exploring the connection. *Int J Drug Policy.* 25:928, 2014.

Curry L.A. et al. Qualitative description of the prevalence and use of anabolic androgenic steroids by united states powerlifters. *Percept Mot Skills.* 88:224, 1999.

Darke S. et al. Sudden or unnatural deaths involving anabolic-androgenic steroids. *J Forensic Sci.* 59:1025, 2014.

Denham B.E. Anabolic-androgenic steroids and adolescents: Recent developments. *J Addict Nurs.* 23:167, 2012.

Dodge T. et al. The use of anabolic androgenic steroids and polypharmacy: A review of the literature. *Drug Alcohol Depend.* 114:100, 2011.

Dotson J.L. et al. The history of the development of

anabolic-androgenic steroids. *Pediatr Clin North Am.* 54:761, 2007.

Dunn M. et al. The epidemiology of anabolic-androgenic steroid use among Australian secondary school students. *J Sci Med Sport.* 14:10, 2011.

DuRant R.H. et al. Use of multiple drugs among adolescents who use anabolic steroids. *N Engl J Med.* 328:922, 1993.

Fahey, T.D. and G.D. Swanson. A model for defining the optimal amount of exercise contributing to health and avoiding sudden cardiac death. *Medicina Sport* 12: 124-128, 2008.

Fahey, T., et al. Sport and exercise physiology: performance-enhancing substances - anabolic steroids in *Sports Science and Physical Education,* (Georgescu L, ed), in *Encyclopedia of Life Support Systems (EOLSS),* Developed under the Auspices of the UNESCO, EOlSS Publishers, Oxford, UK, 2014.

Fauner M. et al. Estimated consumption of anabolic steroids among athletes in Denmark. *Nord Med.* 110:23, 1995.

Fayyazi Bordbar M.R. et al. Frequency of use, awareness, and attitudes toward side effects of anabolic-androgenic steroids consumption among male medical students in Iran. *Subst Use Misuse.* 49:1751, 2014.

Fink J. et al. Anabolic-androgenic steroids: Procurement and administration practices of doping athletes. *Phys Sportsmed.* 47:10, 2019.

Frankle M.A. et al. Use of androgenic anabolic steroids by athletes. *JAMA.* 252:482, 1984.

Fuller M.G. Anabolic-androgenic steroids: Use and abuse. *Compr Ther.* 19:69, 1993.

Garevik N. et al. Dual use of anabolic-androgenic

steroids and narcotics in Sweden. *Drug Alcohol Depend.* 109:144, 2010.

Goldstein P.J. Anabolic steroids: An ethnographic approach. *NIDA Res Monogr.* 102:74, 1990.

Hagen A. et al. Bigger, faster, stronger! An overview of anabolic androgenic steroids and their use and impact on the sport industry. *Forensic Research & Criminology International Journal.* 1:00018. DOI: 10.15406/frcij.2015.01.00018, 2015.

Hakansson A. et al. Anabolic androgenic steroids in the general population: User characteristics and associations with substance use. *Eur Addict Res.* 18:83, 2012.

Halliburton A.E. et al. Health beliefs as a key determinant of intent to use anabolic-androgenic steroids (AAS) among high-school football players: Implications for prevention. *Int J Adolesc Youth.* 23:269, 2018.

Harvey O. et al. Support for people who use anabolic androgenic steroids: A systematic scoping review into what they want and what they access. *BMC Public Health.* 19:1024, 2019.

Horn S. et al. Self-reported anabolic-androgenic steroids use and musculoskeletal injuries: Findings from the center for the study of retired athletes health survey of retired NFL players. *Am J Phys Med Rehabil.* 88:192, 2009.

Hupperets P. et al. A retrospective study of the effect of anabolic steroids on the dyshaematopoietic syndrome (preleukaemic syndrome). *Neth J Med.* 26:181, 1983.

Ip E.J. et al. The anabolic 500 survey: Characteristics of male users versus nonusers of anabolic-androgenic steroids for strength training. *Pharmacotherapy.* 31:757, 2011.

Ip E.J. et al. Anabolic steroid users' misuse of non-traditional prescription drugs. *Res Social Adm Pharm.* 15:949, 2019.

Isacsson G. et al. Anabolic steroids and violent crime--an epidemiological study at a jail in Stockholm, Sweden. *Compr Psychiatry.* 39:203, 1998.

Jacka B. et al. Health care engagement behaviors of men who use performance- and image-enhancing drugs in Australia. *Subst Abus.* 1, 2019.

Jasuja G.K. et al. Patterns of testosterone prescription overuse. *Curr Opin Endocrinol Diabetes Obes.* 24:240, 2017.

Kanayama G. et al. Over-the-counter drug use in gymnasiums: An under-recognized substance abuse problem? *Psychother Psychosom.* 70:137, 2001.

Kanayama G. et al. History and epidemiology of anabolic androgens in athletes and non-athletes. *Mol Cell Endocrinol.* 464:4, 2018.

Kerr J.M. et al. Anabolic-androgenic steroids: Use and abuse in pediatric patients. *Pediatr Clin North Am.* 54:771, 2007.

Kimergard A. et al. The composition of anabolic steroids from the illicit market is largely unknown: Implications for clinical case reports. *QJM.* 107:597, 2014.

Kindlundh A.M. et al. Adolescent use of anabolic-androgenic steroids and relations to self-reports of social, personality and health aspects. *Eur J Public Health.* 11:322, 2001.

Kindlundh A.M. et al. Factors associated with adolescent use of doping agents: Anabolic-androgenic steroids. *Addiction.* 94:543, 1999.

Klotz F. et al. Criminality among individuals testing positive for the presence of anabolic androgenic steroids. *Arch Gen Psychiatry.* 63:1274, 2006.

Klotz F. et al. The significance of anabolic androgenic

steroids in a Swedish prison population. *Compr Psychiatry.* 51:312, 2010.

Kochakian C.D. History of anabolic-androgenic steroids. *NIDA Res Monogr.* 102:29, 1990.

Kochakian C.D. History, chemistry and pharmacodynamics of anabolic-androgenic steroids. *Wien Med Wochenschr.* 143:359, 1993.

Kopera H. The history of anabolic steroids and a review of clinical experience with anabolic steroids. *Acta Endocrinol Suppl.* 271:11, 1985.

Korkia P. Use of anabolic steroids has been reported by 9% of men attending gymnasiums. *BMJ.* 313:1009, 1996.

Kotronoulas A. et al. Evaluation of markers out of the steroid profile for the screening of testosterone misuse. Part II: Intramuscular administration. *Drug Test Anal.* 10:849, 2018.

Kouri E.M. et al. Use of anabolic-androgenic steroids: We are talking prevalence rates. *JAMA.* 271:347, 1994.

La Gerche A. et al. Drugs in sport - a change is needed, but what? *Heart Lung Circ.* 27:1099, 2018.

Landy J.F. et al. What's wrong with using steroids? Exploring whether and why people oppose the use of performance enhancing drugs. *J Pers Soc Psychol.* 113:377, 2017.

Laure P. et al. General practitioners and doping in sport: Attitudes and experience. *Br J Sports Med.* 37:335, 2003.

Lee, D.C. et al. Long-term effects of changes in cardiorespiratory fitness and body mass index on all-cause and cardiovascular disease mortality in men: the Aerobics Center Longitudinal Study. *Circulation* 4:2483-490, 2011.

Lee, I.M. et al. Exercise intensity and longevity in

men:The Harvard Alumni Health Study. *JAMA.* 273:1179-1184, 1995.

Lee, I.M. et al. Physical activity, physical fitness and longevity. *Aging Clinical Experiments Res.* 9: 2-11, 1997.

Leifman H. et al. Anabolic androgenic steroids--use and correlates among gym users--an assessment study using questionnaires and observations at gyms in the Stockholm region. *Int J Environ Res Public Health.* 8:2656, 2011.

Lindstrom M. et al. Use of anabolic-androgenic steroids among body builders--frequency and attitudes. *J Intern Med.* 227:407, 1990

Litman H.J. et al. Serum androgen levels in black, Hispanic, and white men. *J Clin Endocrinol Metab.* 91:4326, 2006.

Ljungqvist A. The use of anabolic steroids in top Swedish athletes. *Br J Sports Med.* 9:82, 1975.

Lombardo J.A. Anabolic-androgenic steroids. *NIDA Res Monogr.* 102:60, 1990.

Lood Y. et al. Anabolic androgenic steroids in police cases in Sweden 1999-2009. *Forensic Sci Int.* 219:199, 2012.

Lundholm L. et al. Anabolic androgenic steroids and violent offending: Confounding by polysubstance abuse among 10,365 general population men. *Addiction.* 110:100, 2015.

Lundholm L. et al. Use of anabolic androgenic steroids in substance abusers arrested for crime. *Drug Alcohol Depend.* 111:222, 2010.

Marcos-Serrano M. et al. Urinary steroid profile in ironman triathletes. *J Hum Kinet.* 61:109, 2018.

Mattila V.M. et al. Use of dietary supplements and anabolic-androgenic steroids among Finnish adolescents in 1991-2005. *Eur J Public Health.* 20:306, 2010.

McBride J.A. et al. The availability and acquisition of illicit anabolic androgenic steroids and testosterone preparations on the internet. *Am J Mens Health.* 12:1352, 2018.

McCabe S.E. et al. Trends in non-medical use of anabolic steroids by U.S. College students: Results from four national surveys. *Drug Alcohol Depend.* 90:243, 2007.

McDuff D. et al. Recreational and ergogenic substance use and substance use disorders in elite athletes: A narrative review. *Br J Sports Med.* 53:754, 2019.

Melia P. et al. The use of anabolic-androgenic steroids by Canadian students. *Clin J Sport Med.* 6:9, 1996.

Middleman A.B. et al. High-risk behaviors among high school students in Massachusetts who use anabolic steroids. *Pediatrics.* 96:268, 1995.

Milhorn H.T., Jr. Anabolic steroids: Another form of drug abuse. *J Miss State Med Assoc.* 32:293, 1991.

Millar A.P. Anabolic steroids--a contemporary view. *S Afr Med J.* 85:1303, 1995.

Miller C. Anabolic steroids: An Australian sports physician goes public. *Phys Sportsmed.* 14:167, 1986.

Morgentaler A. et al. The history of testosterone and the evolution of its therapeutic potential. *Sex Med Rev.* 8:286, 2020.

Musshoff F. et al. Anabolic steroids on the German black market. *Arch Kriminol.* 199:152, 1997.

Nagata J.M. et al. Predictors of muscularity-oriented disordered eating behaviors in U.S. Young adults: A prospective cohort study. *Int J Eat Disord.* 2019.

Nakhaee M.R. et al. Prevalence of use of anabolic steroids by bodybuilders using three methods in a city of Iran. *Addict Health.* 5:77, 2013.

Nieschlag E. et al. Endocrine history: The history of

discovery, synthesis and development of testosterone for clinical use. *Eur J Endocrinol.* 180:R201, 2019.

Nilsson S. A study among teenagers in Falkenberg: Frightening abuse of anabolic steroids. *Lakartidningen.* 91:2877, 1994.

Nilsson S. et al. Evaluation of a health promotion programme to prevent the misuse of androgenic anabolic steroids among Swedish adolescents. *Health Promot Int.* 19:61, 2004.

Nilsson S. et al. Trends in the misuse of androgenic anabolic steroids among boys 16-17 years old in a primary health care area in Sweden. *Scand J Prim Health Care.* 19:181, 2001.

Nilsson S. et al. The prevalence of the use of androgenic anabolic steroids by adolescents in a county of Sweden. *Eur J Public Health.* 11:195, 2001.

Parkinson A.B. et al. Anabolic androgenic steroids: A survey of 500 users. *Med Sci Sports Exerc.* 38:644, 2006.

Pereira E. et al. Anabolic steroids among resistance training practitioners. *PLoS One.* 14:e0223384, 2019.

Perko M.A. et al. Associations between academic performance of Division 1 college athletes and their perceptions of the effects of anabolic steroids. *Percept Mot Skills.* 80:284, 1995.

Perlmutter G. et al. Use of anabolic steroids by athletes. *Am Fam Physician.* 32:208, 1985.

Perls T.T. Growth hormone and anabolic steroids: Athletes are the tip of the iceberg. *Drug Test Anal.* 1:419, 2009.

Petersson A. et al. Substance abusers' motives for using anabolic androgenic steroids. *Drug Alcohol Depend.* 111:170, 2010.

Petersson A. et al. Morbidity and mortality in patients testing positively for the presence of anabolic androgenic steroids in connection with receiving medical care. A controlled retrospective cohort study. *Drug Alcohol Depend.* 81:215, 2006.

Petersson A. et al. Convulsions in users of anabolic androgenic steroids: Possible explanations. *J Clin Psychopharmacol.* 27:723, 2007.

Petersson A. et al. Toxicological findings and manner of death in autopsied users of anabolic androgenic steroids. *Drug Alcohol Depend.* 81:241, 2006.

Pineau T. et al. The study of doping market: How to produce intelligence from internet forums. *Forensic Sci Int.* 268:103, 2016.

Pope H.G., Jr. et al. The lifetime prevalence of anabolic-androgenic steroid use and dependence in Americans: Current best estimates. *Am J Addict.* 23:371, 2014.

Pope H.G., Jr. et al. Anabolic-androgenic steroid use among 1,010 college men. *Phys Sportsmed.* 16:75, 1988.

Pope H.G., Jr. et al. Anabolic-androgenic steroid use among 133 prisoners. *Compr Psychiatry.* 37:322, 1996.

Rachon D. et al. Prevalence and risk factors of anabolic-androgenic steroids (AAS) abuse among adolescents and young adults in Poland. *Soz Praventivmed.* 51:392, 2006.

Ribeiro M.V.M. et al. (1)h NMR determination of adulteration of anabolic steroids in seized drugs. *Steroids.* 138:47, 2018.

Richardson A. et al. Anabolic-androgenic steroids (AAS) users on AAS use: Negative effects, 'code of silence', and implications for forensic and medical professionals. *J Forensic Leg Med.* 68:101871, 2019.

Roccella M. et al. New addictions in the third millennium: Anabolic steroids as a substance of abuse. *Minerva Pediatr.* 57:129, 2005.

Runacres, A., et al. Health consequences of an elite

sporting career: long-term detriment or long-term gain? A meta-analysis of 165,000 former athletes. *Sports Med.* 51:289–301, 2021.

Sagoe D. et al. Attitudes towards use of anabolic-androgenic steroids among Ghanaian high school students. *Int J Drug Policy.* 26:169, 2015.

Salva P.S. Anabolic steroids and sports. *JAMA.* 258:1608, 1987.

Salva P.S. et al. Anabolic steroids and growth hormone in the Texas Panhandle. *Tex Med.* 85:43, 1989.

Salva P.S. et al. Anabolic steroids: Interest among parents and nonathletes. *South Med J.* 84:552, 1991.

Sandvik M.R. et al. Anabolic-androgenic steroid use and correlates in Norwegian adolescents. *Eur J Sport Sci.* 18:903, 2018.

Santora L.J. et al. Coronary calcification in body builders using anabolic steroids. *Prev Cardiol.* 9:198, 2006.

Santos A.M. et al. Illicit use and abuse of anabolic-androgenic steroids among brazilian bodybuilders. *Subst Use Misuse.* 46:742, 2011.

Sigurdson A. et al. Use of anabolic-androgenic steroids: We are talking prevalence rates. *JAMA.* 271:347, 1994.

Sjoqvist F. et al. Use of doping agents, particularly anabolic steroids, in sports and society. *Lancet.* 371:1872, 2008.

Skarberg K. et al. Multisubstance use as a feature of addiction to anabolic-androgenic steroids. *Eur Addict Res.* 15:99, 2009.

Smit D.L. et al. Baseline characteristics of the Haarlem study: 100 male amateur athletes using anabolic androgenic steroids. *Scand J Med Sci Sports.* 2019.

Smit D.L. et al. Outpatient clinic for users of anabolic androgenic steroids: An overview. *Neth J Med.* 76:167, 2018.

Solberg S. Anabolic steroids and Norwegian weightlifters. *Br J Sports Med.* 16:169, 1982.

Takahashi M. et al. Telephone counseling of athletes abusing anabolic-androgenic steroids. *J Sports Med Phys Fitness.* 47:356, 2007.

Tamir E. et al. Knowledge and attitude regarding use of anabolic steroids among youth exercising in fitness centers. *Harefuah.* 143:348, 2004.

Tay Wee Teck J. et al. Tracking internet interest in anabolic-androgenic steroids using google trends. *Int J Drug Policy.* 51:52, 2018.

Terney R. et al. The use of anabolic steroids in high school students. *Am J Dis Child.* 144:99, 1990.

Thevis M. et al. Determination of the prevalence of anabolic steroids, stimulants, and selected drugs subject to doping controls among elite sport students using analytical chemistry. *J Sports Sci.* 26:1059, 2008.

Thiblin I. et al. Anabolic steroids and cardiovascular risk: A national population-based cohort study. *Drug Alcohol Depend.* 152:87, 2015.

Thiblin I. et al. Cause and manner of death among users of anabolic androgenic steroids. *J Forensic Sci.* 45:16, 2000.

Thiblin I. et al. Pharmacoepidemiology of anabolic androgenic steroids: A review. *Fundam Clin Pharmacol.* 19:27, 2005.

Thompson P.D. et al. Use of anabolic steroids among adolescents. *N Engl J Med.* 329:888, 1993.

Thorlindsson T. et al. Sport and use of anabolic androgenic steroids among Icelandic high school students: A critical test of three perspectives. *Subst Abuse Treat Prev Policy.* 5:32, 2010.

Underwood M. Exploring the social lives of image and performance enhancing drugs: An online ethnography of the ZYZZ fandom of recreational bodybuilders. *Int J Drug Policy.* 39:78, 2017.

Vazquez-Mourelle R. et al. Impact of health authority control measures aimed at reducing the illicit use of anabolic-androgenic steroids. *Eur Addict Res.* 24:28, 2018.

Vitoria Ortiz M. Hormones, politics and sport in the German Democratic Republic (1949-1989). *An R Acad Nac Med.* 128:651, 2011.

Vlad R.A. et al. Doping in sports, a never-ending story? *Adv Pharm Bull.* 8:529, 2018.

Westerman M.E. et al. Heavy testosterone use among bodybuilders: An uncommon cohort of illicit substance users. *Mayo Clin Proc.* 91:175, 2016.

Wichstrom L. Predictors of future anabolic androgenic steroid use. *Med Sci Sports Exerc.* 38:1578, 2006.

Wichstrom L. et al. Use of anabolic-androgenic steroids in adolescence: Winning, looking good or being bad? *J Stud Alcohol.* 62:5, 2001.

Winters S.J. Androgens: Endocrine physiology and pharmacology. *NIDA Res Monogr.* 102:113, 1990.

Woerdeman J. et al. Anabolic androgenic steroids in amateur sports in the Netherlands. *Ned Tijdschr Geneeskd.* 154:A2004, 2010.

Wood R.I. Anabolic steroids: A fatal attraction? *J Neuroendocrinol.* 18:227, 2006.

Wood R.I. et al. Testosterone and sport: Current perspectives. *Horm Behav.* 61:147, 2012.

Wroblewska A.M. Androgenic--anabolic steroids and body dysmorphia in young men. *J Psychosom Res.* 42:225, 1997.

Yesalis C.E. et al. Incidence of the nonmedical use of

anabolic-androgenic steroids. *NIDA Res Monogr.* 102:97, 1990.

Yesalis C.E., et al. Self-reported use of anabolic-androgenic steroids by elite power lifters. *Phys Sportsmed.* 16:91, 1988.

References: Biochemistry of Anabolic Steroids

Aagaard P. Making muscles "stronger": Exercise, nutrition, drugs. *J Musculoskelet Neuronal Interact.* 4:165, 2004.

Abdullaev A.R. The influence of glucocorticoids and anabolic steroids on immunity indices in rheumatism in children of preschool age. *Pediatriia.* 43:50, 1964.

Abzianidze E.N. The reaction of hormones of hypophysis-thyroid gland's endocrinal axis on vibration pathology and on condition of its correction with liquid oxygen and anabolic steroids. *Georgian Med News.* 75, 2007.

Ahima R.S. et al. Regulation of glucocorticoid receptor immunoreactivity in the rat hippocampus by androgenic-anabolic steroids. *Brain Res.* 585:311, 1992.

Aikawa K. et al. Synthesis and biological evaluation of novel selective androgen receptor modulators (SARMS) part III: Discovery of 4-(5-oxopyrrolidine-1-yl)benzonitrile derivative 2f as a clinical candidate. *Bioorg Med Chem.* 25:3330, 2017.

Aikawa K. et al. Synthesis and biological evaluation of novel selective androgen receptor modulators (SARMs). Part I *Bioorg Med Chem.* 23:2568, 2015.

Albanese A.A. Anticatabolic applications of newer anabolic steroids. *Med Times.* 96:871, 1968.

Albanese A.A. Nutritional and metabolic effects of anabolic steroids and corticosteroids. *J Am Med Women's Assoc.* 24:123, 1969.

Albanese A.A. et al. Nutritional and metabolic effects of some newer steroids. Iv. Parenteral anabolic steroids. *N Y State J Med.* 65:2116, 1965.

Alsio J. et al. Impact of nandrolone decanoate on gene expression in endocrine systems related to the adverse effects of anabolic androgenic steroids. *Basic Clin Pharmacol Toxicol.* 105:307, 2009.

Anderson I.A. The metabolic effects of certain anabolic steroids. *Acta Endocrinol Suppl.* 39(Suppl 63):54, 1961.

Appell H.J. et al. Ultrastructural and morphometric investigations on the effects of training and administration of anabolic steroids on the myocardium of guinea pigs. *Int J Sports Med.* 4:268, 1983.

Arazi H. et al. Use of anabolic androgenic steroids produces greater oxidative stress responses to resistance exercise in strength-trained men. *Toxicol Rep.* 4:282, 2017.

Asano M. et al. Synthesis and biological evaluation of novel selective androgen receptor modulators (SARMs). Part II: Optimization of 4-(pyrrolidin-1-yl)benzonitrile derivatives. *Bioorg Med Chem Lett.* 27:1897, 2017.

Barbosa J. et al. Effects of anabolic steroids on haptoglobin, orosomucoid, plasminogen, fibrinogen, transferrin, ceruloplasmin, alpha-1-antitrypsin, beta-glucuronidase and total serum proteins. *J Clin Endocrinol Metab.* 33:388, 1971.

Bartsch W. Anabolic steroids--action on cellular level. *Wien Med Wochenschr.* 143:363, 1993.

Basualto-Alarcon C. et al. Testosterone signals through mTOR and androgen receptor to induce muscle hypertrophy. *Med Sci Sports Exerc.* 45:1712, 2013.

Bathori M. et al. Phytoecdysteroids and anabolic-androgenic steroids--structure and effects on humans. *Curr Med Chem.* 15:75, 2008.

Bayat G. et al. Chronic endurance exercise antagonizes the cardiac UCP2 and UCP3 protein up-regulation induced by nandrolone decanoate. *J Basic Clin Physiol Pharmacol.* 28:609, 2017.

Behrendt H. Effect of anabolic steroids on rat heart muscle cells. I. Intermediate filaments. *Cell Tissue Res.* 180:303, 1977.

Bhasin S. et al. Selective androgen receptor modulators as function promoting therapies. *Curr Opin Clin Nutr Metab Care.* 12:232, 2009.

Bischoff F. et al. The state and distribution of steroid hormones in biologic systems; solubilities of testosterone, progesterone and alpha-estradiol in aqueous salt and protein solution and in serum. *J Biol Chem.* 174:663, 1948.

Bjorkhem-Bergman L. et al. Vitamin D receptor rs2228570 polymorphism is associated with LH levels in men exposed to anabolic androgenic steroids. *BMC Res Notes.* 11:51, 2018.

Boris A. et al. Comparative androgenic, myotrophic and antigonadotrophic properties of some anabolic steroids. *Steroids.* 15:61, 1970.

Brownlee K. et al. Relationship between circulating cortisol and testosterone: Influence of physical exercise. *J Sport Sci Med.* 4:76, 2005.

Bullock G.R. et al. Changes in mitochondrial structure and ribosomal activity in muscle as a consequence of the interaction between a glucocorticoid and some anabolic steroids. *Biochem J.* 115:47P, 1969.

Cadwallader A.B. et al. The androgen receptor and its use in biological assays: Looking toward effect-based testing and its applications. *J Anal Toxicol.* 35:594, 2011.

Camerino B. et al. Structure and effects of anabolic steroids. *Pharmacol Ther B.* 1:233, 1975.

Carteri R.B. et al. Anabolic-androgen steroids effects on bioenergetics responsiveness of synaptic and extra-synaptic mitochondria. *Toxicol Lett.* 307:72, 2019.

Celec P. et al. Effects of anabolic steroids and antioxidant vitamins on ethanol-induced tissue injury. *Life Sci.* 74:419, 2003.

Cheung A.S. et al. Physiological basis behind ergogenic effects of anabolic androgens. *Mol Cell Endocrinol.* 464:14, 2018.

Choi S.M. et al. Comparative safety evaluation of selective androgen receptor modulators and anabolic androgenic steroids. *Expert Opin Drug Saf.* 14:1773, 2015.

Dalbo V.J. et al. Testosterone and trenbolone enanthate increase mature myostatin protein expression despite increasing skeletal muscle hypertrophy and satellite cell number in rodent muscle. *Andrologia.* 49:2017.

Damiao B. et al. Anabolic steroids and their effects of on neuronal density in cortical areas and hippocampus of mice. *Braz J Biol.* 81:537, 2021.

Danhaive P.A. et al. Binding of glucocorticoid antagonists to androgen and glucocorticoid hormone receptors in rat skeletal muscle. *J Steroid Biochem.* 24:481, 1986.

Dayton W.R. et al. Cellular and molecular regulation of muscle growth and development in meat animals. *J Anim Sci.* 86:E217, 2008.

Dayton W.R. et al. Meat science and muscle biology symposium--role of satellite cells in anabolic steroid-induced muscle growth in feedlot steers. *J Anim Sci.* 92:30, 2014.

Delgato, J., et al. Prolonged treatment with the anabolic-androgenic steroid stanozolol increases antioxidant defences in rat skeletal muscle. *J Physiol Biochem. 66: 63-71, 2010.*

Diel P. et al. C2c12 myoblastoma cell differentiation and proliferation is stimulated by androgens and associated with a modulation of myostatin and pax7 expression. *J Mol Endocrinol.* 40:231, 2008.

Dkhil M.A. et al. Epigenetic modifications of gene promoter DNA in the liver of adult female mice masculinized by testosterone. *J Steroid Biochem Mol Biol.* 145:121, 2015.

Donahue J.L. et al. Androgens, anabolic-androgenic steroids, and inhibitors. *Am J Ther.* 7:365, 2000.

Duclos M. et al. Acute and chronic effects of exercise on tissue sensitivity to glucocorticoids. *J Appl Physiol.* 94:869, 2003.

Dumont N.A. et al. Intrinsic and extrinsic mechanisms regulating satellite cell function. *Development.* 142:1572, 2015.

Egner I.M. et al. A cellular memory mechanism aids overload hypertrophy in muscle long after an episodic exposure to anabolic steroids. *J Physiol.* 591:6221, 2013.

Eriksson A. et al. Skeletal muscle morphology in powerlifters with and without anabolic steroids. *Histochem Cell Biol.* 124:167, 2005.

Eriksson A. et al. Hypertrophic muscle fibers with fissures in powerlifters; fiber splitting or defect regeneration? *Histochem Cell Biol.* 126:409, 2006.

Esquivel A. et al. Sulfate metabolites improve retrospectivity after oral testosterone administration. *Drug Test Anal.* 11:392, 2019.

Fiegel G. Drugs interacting with anabolic steroids. *Clin Ter.* 136:415, 1991.

Finardi G. et al. The effects of the new anabolic steroids on sodium and potassium metabolism in man. *Presse Med.* 71:2387, 1963.

Fineschi V. Anabolic androgenic steroids (AAS) as doping agents: Chemical structures, metabolism, cellular responses, physiological and pathological effects. *Mini Rev Med Chem.* 11:359, 2011.

Fontana K. et al. Hepatocyte nuclear phenotype: The cross-talk between anabolic androgenic steroids and exercise in transgenic mice. *Histol Histopathol.* 23:1367, 2008.

Fontana K. et al. Effects of anabolic steroids and high-intensity aerobic exercise on skeletal muscle of transgenic mice. *PLoS One.* 8:e80909, 2013.

Foss G.L. Oral methyl testosterone. *Br Med J.* 2:11, 1939.

Fragkaki A.G. et al. Structural characteristics of anabolic androgenic steroids contributing to binding to the androgen receptor and to their anabolic and androgenic activities. Applied modifications in the steroidal structure. *Steroids.* 74:172, 2009.

Geldof L. et al. In vitro metabolism study of a black market product containing SARM LGD-4033. *Drug Test Anal.* 9:168, 2017.

Germanakis I. et al. Oxidative stress and myocardial dysfunction in young rabbits after short term anabolic steroids administration. *Food Chem Toxicol.* 61:101, 2013.

Ghizoni M.F. et al. The anabolic steroid nandrolone enhances motor and sensory functional recovery in rat median nerve repair with long interpositional nerve grafts. *Neurorehabil Neural Repair.* 27:269, 2013.

Goldman A.L. et al. A reappraisal of testosterone's binding in circulation: Physiological and clinical implications. *Endocr Rev.* 38:302, 2017.

Gongora J. et al. The in vitro metabolism of testosterone to delta 4-androstenedione 3,17 and cis-testosterone by rabbit liver homogenate. *Fed Proc.* 7:42, 1948.

Gribbin H.R. et al. Mode of action and use of anabolic steroids. *Br J Clin Pract.* 30:3, 1976.

Grossman J. et al. Effects of anabolic steroids on albumin metabolism. *J Clin Endocrinol Metab.* 25:698, 1965.

Gustafsson J.A. et al. Studies on steroid receptors in human and rabbit skeletal muscle - clues to the understanding of the mechanism of action of anabolic steroids. *Prog Clin Biol Res.* 142:261, 1984.

Guzman M. et al. Treatment with anabolic steroids increases the activity of the mitochondrial outer carnitine palmitoyltransferase in rat liver and fast-twitch muscle. *Biochem Pharmacol.* 41:833, 1991.

Haak A. et al. Clinical and biochemical aspects of the action of anabolic steroids. *Ned Tijdschr Geneeskd.* 104:2052, 1960.

Hallberg M. Impact of anabolic androgenic steroids on neuropeptide systems. *Mini Rev Med Chem.* 11:399, 2011.

Haupt H.A. Anabolic steroids and growth hormone. *Am J Sports Med.* 21:468, 1993.

He F. et al. Redox mechanism of reactive oxygen species in exercise. *Front Physiol.* 7:486, 2016.

Herbst K.L. et al. Testosterone action on skeletal muscle. *Curr Opin Clin Nutr Metab Care.* 7:271, 2004.

Hickson R.C. et al. Glucocorticoid antagonism by exercise and androgenic-anabolic steroids. *Med Sci Sports Exerc.* 22:331, 1990.

Huffman M.M. et al. The metabolism of testosterone. *Rev Can Biol.* 7:185, 1948.

Illei G. et al. The effect of anabolic steroids on the secretion of pituitary gonadotropins. *Acta Physiol Acad Sci Hung.* 22:189, 1962.

Ishigami R. et al. Studies on drug diabetes. 3. Abnormal carbohydrate metabolism caused by anabolic steroids. *Naika Hokan.* 11:359, 1964.

Janne O.A. Androgen interaction through multiple steroid receptors. *NIDA Res Monogr.* 102:178, 1990.

Jiang Y. mTOR goes to the nucleus. *Cell Cycle.* 9:868, 2010.

Kadi F. Cellular and molecular mechanisms responsible for the action of testosterone on human skeletal muscle. A basis for illegal performance enhancement. *Br J Pharmacol.* 154:522, 2008.

Kadi F. et al. The expression of androgen receptors in human neck and limb muscles: Effects of training and self-administration of androgenic-anabolic steroids. *Histochem Cell Biol.* 113:25, 2000.

Kadi F. et al. Effects of anabolic steroids on the muscle cells of strength-trained athletes. *Med Sci Sports Exerc.* 31:1528, 1999.

Kamanga-Sollo E. et al. IGF-1 mRNA levels in bovine satellite cell cultures: Effects of fusion and anabolic steroid treatment. *J Cell Physiol.* 201:181, 2004.

Kamanga-Sollo E. et al. Roles of IGF-1and the estrogen, androgen and IGF-1 receptors in estradiol-17beta- and trenbolone acetate-stimulated proliferation of cultured bovine satellite cells. *Domest Anim Endocrinol.* 35:88, 2008.

Kicman A.T. Pharmacology of anabolic steroids. *Br J Pharmacol.* 154:502, 2008.

Kicman A.T. et al. Anabolic steroids in sport: Biochemical, clinical and analytical perspectives. *Ann Clin Biochem.* 40:321, 2003.

Kochakian C.D. History, chemistry and pharmacodynamics of anabolic-androgenic steroids. *Wien Med Wochenschr.* 143:359, 1993.

Laurent M.R. et al. Androgens have antiresorptive effects on trabecular disuse osteopenia independent from muscle atrophy. *Bone.* 93:33, 2016.

Lindstrom M. et al. Satellite cell heterogeneity with respect to expression of MYOD, myogenin, DLK1 and c-MET in human skeletal muscle: Application to a cohort of power lifters and sedentary men. *Histochem Cell Biol.* 134:371, 2010.

Lippi G. et al. Biochemistry and physiology of anabolic androgenic steroids doping. *Mini Rev Med Chem.* 11:362, 2011.

Little K. Interaction between catabolic and anabolic steroids. *Curr Ther Res Clin Exp.* 12:658, 1970.

MacDougall J.D. et al. Muscle ultrastructural characteristics of elite powerlifters and bodybuilders. *Eur J Appl Physiol Occup Physiol.* 48:117, 1982.

Magalhães W.S. et al. Human metabolism of the anabolic steroid methasterone: Detection and kinetic excretion of new phase 1 urinary metabolites and investigation of phase II metabolism by GC-MS and UPLC-MS/MS. *J. Braz. Chem. So.* 30:1150, 2019.

Marocolo M. et al. Combined effects of exercise training and high doses of anabolic steroids on cardiac autonomic modulation and ventricular repolarization properties in rats. *Can J Physiol Pharmacol.* 97:1185, 2019.

Matassarin F.W. The use of testosterone propionate in nitrogen retention. *J Kans Med Soc.* 49:287, 1948.

Mehta P.H. et al. Neural mechanisms of the testosterone-aggression relation: The role of orbitofrontal cortex. *J Cogn Neurosci.* 22:2357, 2010.

Mehta P.H. et al. Testosterone and cortisol jointly regulate dominance: Evidence for a dual-hormone hypothesis. *Horm Behav.* 58:898, 2010.

Melcangi R.C. et al. The action of steroid hormones on peripheral myelin proteins: A possible new tool for the rebuilding of myelin? *J Neurocytol.* 29:327, 2000.

Metcalf W. et al. A quantitative expression for nitrogen retention with anabolic steroids. IV. Oxandrolone. *Metabolism.* 14:59, 1965.

Mhaouty-Kodja S. Role of the androgen receptor in the central nervous system. *Mol Cell Endocrinol.* 465:103, 2018.

Molano F. et al. Rat liver lysosomal and mitochondrial activities are modified by anabolic-androgenic steroids. *Med Sci Sports Exerc.* 31:243, 1999.

Mosler S. et al. Modulation of follistatin and myostatin propeptide by anabolic steroids and gender. *Int J Sports Med.* 34:567, 2013.

Muto T. et al. The mechanism of anabolic steroids on the acceleration of the anabolic activity. *Acta Med Biol.* 16:53, 1969.

Narayanan R. et al. Development of selective androgen receptor modulators (SARMs). *Mol Cell Endocrinol.* 465:134, 2018.

Neto W. Effects of strength training and anabolic steroid in the peripheral nerve and skeletal muscle morphology of aged rats. *Front Aging Neurosci.* 9:1, 2017.

Nieschlag E. et al. Mechanisms in endocrinology: Medical consequences of doping with anabolic androgenic steroids: Effects on reproductive functions. *Eur J Endocrinol.* 173:R47, 2015.

Nordstrom A. et al. Higher muscle mass but lower gynoid fat mass in athletes using anabolic androgenic steroids. *J Strength Cond Res.* 26:246, 2012.

Oberlander J.G. et al. The buzz about anabolic androgenic steroids: Electrophysiological effects in excitable tissues. *Neuroendocrinology.* 96:141, 2012.

Ohlsson C. et al. Genetic determinants of serum testosterone concentrations in men. *PLoS Genet.* 7:e1002313, 2011.

Onakomaiya M.M. et al. Mad men, women and steroid cocktails: A review of the impact of sex and other factors on anabolic androgenic steroids effects on affective behaviors. *Psychopharmacology.* 233:549, 2016.

Parssinen M. et al. The effect of supraphysiological doses of anabolic androgenic steroids on collagen metabolism. *Int J Sports Med.* 21:406, 2000.

Penatti C.A. et al. Chronic exposure to anabolic androgenic steroids alters neuronal function in the mammalian forebrain via androgen receptor- and estrogen receptor-mediated mechanisms. *J Neurosci.* 29:12484, 2009.

Pieretti S. et al. Brain nerve growth factor unbalance induced by anabolic androgenic steroids in rats. *Med Sci Sports Exerc.* 45:29, 2013.

Piper T. et al. Studies on the in vivo metabolism of the SARM yk11: Identification and characterization of metabolites potentially useful for doping controls. *Drug Test Anal.* 10:1646, 2018.

Reitzner S.M. et al. Modulation of exercise training related adaptation of body composition and regulatory pathways by anabolic steroids. *J Steroid Biochem Mol Biol.* 190:44, 2019.

Rojas D. et al. Selective androgen receptor modulators: Comparative excretion study of bicalutamide in bovine urine and faeces. *Drug Test Anal.* 9:1017, 2017.

Roman M. et al. Computational assessment of pharmacokinetics and biological effects of some anabolic and androgen steroids. *Pharm Res.* 35:41, 2018.

Ruokonen A. et al. Response of serum testosterone and its precursor steroids, SHBG and CBG to anabolic steroid and testosterone self-administration in man. *J Steroid Biochem.* 23:33, 1985.

Saborido A. et al. Stanozolol treatment decreases the mitochondrial ROS generation and oxidative stress induced by acute exercise in rat skeletal muscle. *J Appl Physiol (1985).* 110:661, 2011.

Saborido A. et al. Effect of anabolic steroids on mitochondria and sarcotubular system of skeletal muscle. *J Appl Physiol (1985).* 70:1038, 1991.

Said R S. et al. Myogenic satellite cells: Biological milieu and possible clinical applications. *Pak J Biol Sci.* 20:1, 2017.

Saito T. et al. Studies on the action mechanisms of anabolic steroids. I. Clinico-pharmacological studies on their effects upon the far advanced pulmonary tuberculous patients. *IRYO.* 20:565, 1966.

Salem N.A. et al. The impact of nandrolone decanoate abuse on experimental animal model: Hormonal and biochemical assessment. *Steroids.* 153:108526, 2019.

Salmons S. Myotrophic effects of anabolic steroids. *Vet Res Commun.* 7:19, 1983.

Satoh K. et al. Morphological effects of an anabolic steroid on muscle fibres of the diaphragm in mice. *J Electron Microsc.* 49:531, 2000.

Schanzer W. Metabolism of anabolic androgenic steroids. *Clin Chem.* 42:1001, 1996.

Schanzer W. et al. Metabolism of anabolic steroids in humans: Synthesis of 6 beta-hydroxy metabolites of 4-chloro-1,2-dehydro-17 alpha-methyltestosterone, fluoxymesterone, and metandienone. *Steroids.* 60:353, 1995.

Schanzer W. et al. 17-epimerization of 17 alpha-methyl anabolic steroids in humans: Metabolism and synthesis of 17 alpha-hydroxy-17 beta-methyl steroids. *Steroids.* 57:537, 1992.

Sculthorpe N. et al. Androgens affect myogenesis in vitro and increase local igf-1 expression. *Med Sci Sports Exerc.* 44:610, 2012.

Seynnes O.R. et al. Effect of androgenic-anabolic steroids and heavy strength training on patellar tendon morphological and mechanical properties. *J Appl Physiol (1985).* 115:84, 2013.

Shahidi N.T. A review of the chemistry, biological action, and clinical applications of anabolic-androgenic steroids. *Clin Ther.* 23:1355, 2001.

Sinha-Hikim I. et al. Effects of testosterone supplementation on skeletal muscle fiber hypertrophy and satellite cells in community-dwelling older men. *J Clin Endocrinol Metab.* 91:3024, 2006.

Sinha-Hikim I. et al. Testosterone-induced muscle hypertrophy is associated with an increase in satellite cell number in healthy, young men. *Am J Physiol Endocrinol Metab.* 285:E197, 2003.

Solomon Z.J. et al. Selective androgen receptor modulators: Current knowledge and clinical applications. *Sex Med Rev.* 7:84, 2019.

Starkov A.A. et al. Regulation of the energy coupling in mitochondria by some steroid and thyroid hormones. *Biochim Biophys Acta.* 1318:173, 1997.

Sun M. et al. Nandrolone attenuates aortic adaptation to exercise in rats. *Cardiovasc Res.* 97:686, 2013.

Takada M. Pharmacological action of anabolic steroids. *Nihon Rinsho.* 52:606, 1994.

Takayama H. et al. Mechanism of action of anabolic steroids. Dynamic observations on protein metabolism by the isotopic method. *Nihon Naibunpi Gakkai Zasshi.* 38:652, 1962.

Tang H. et al. MRI and image quantitation for drug assessment - growth effects of anabolic steroids and precursors. *Conf Proc IEEE Eng Med Biol Soc.* 7:7044, 2005.

Tirassa P. et al. High-dose anabolic androgenic steroids modulate concentrations of nerve growth factor and expression of its low affinity receptor (p75-NGFR) in male rat brain. *J Neurosci Res.* 47:198, 1997.

Toth N. et al. 20-hydroxyecdysone increases fiber size in a muscle-specific fashion in rat. *Phytomedicine.* 15:691, 2008.

Tsika R.W. et al. Effect of anabolic steroids on overloaded and overloaded suspended skeletal muscle. *J Appl Physiol (1985).* 63:2128, 1987.

Tsika R.W. et al. Effect of anabolic steroids on skeletal muscle mass during hindlimb suspension. *J Appl Physiol (1985).* 63:2122, 1987.

van der Vies J. Pharmacokinetics of anabolic steroids. *Wien Med Wochenschr.* 143:366, 1993.

van Wayjen R.G. Metabolic effects of anabolic steroids. *Wien Med Wochenschr.* 143:368, 1993.

Vicencio J.M. et al. Anabolic androgenic steroids and intracellular calcium signaling: A mini review on mechanisms and physiological implications. *Mini Rev Med Chem.* 11:390, 2011.

Weicker H. et al. Influence of training and anabolic steroids on the LDH isozyme pattern of skeletal and heart muscle fibers of guinea pigs. *Int J Sports Med.* 3:90, 1982.

Winters S.J. Androgens: Endocrine physiology and pharmacology. *NIDA Res Monogr.* 102:113, 1990.

Wynn V. The anabolic steroids. *Practitioner.* 200:509, 1968.

Wynn V. Metabolic effects of anabolic steroids. *Br J Sports Med.* 9:60, 1975.

Yu J.G. et al. Effects of long term supplementation of anabolic androgen steroids on human skeletal muscle. *PLoS One.* 9:e105330, 2014.

Zeng F. et al. Androgen interacts with exercise through the mTOR pathway to induce skeletal muscle hypertrophy. *Biol Sport.* 34:313, 2017.

References: Anabolic Steroids and Performance

Alen M. et al. Changes in muscle power production capacity in power athletes self-administering androgenic anabolic steroids. *Duodecim.* 100:1096, 1984.

Alen M. et al. Changes in neuromuscular performance and muscle fiber characteristics of elite power athletes self-administering androgenic and anabolic steroids. *Acta Physiol Scand.* 122:535, 1984.

Alway S.E. et al. Effect of anabolic steroids on new fiber formation and fiber area during stretch-overload. *J Appl Physiol.* 74:832, 1993.

Andrews M.A. et al. Physical effects of anabolic-androgenic steroids in healthy exercising adults: A systematic review and meta-analysis. *Curr Sports Med Rep.* 17:232, 2018.

Ariel G. The effect of anabolic steroid upon skeletal muscle contractile force. *J Sports Med Phys Fitness.* 13:187, 1973.

Ariel G. Prolonged effects of anabolic steroid upon muscular contractile force. *Med Sci Sports.* 6:62, 1974.

Ariel G. et al. Effect of anabolic steroids on reflex components. *J Appl Physiol.* 32:795, 1972.

Bahrke M.S. et al. Weight training. A potential confounding factor in examining the psychological and behavioural effects of anabolic-androgenic steroids. *Sports Med.* 18:309, 1994.

Baume N. et al. Effect of multiple oral doses of androgenic anabolic steroids on endurance performance and serum indices of physical stress in healthy male subjects. *Eur J Appl Physiol.* 98:329, 2006.

Bhasin S. et al. The effects of supraphysiologic doses of testosterone on muscle size and strength in normal men. *N Engl J Med.* 335:1, 1996.

Bhasin S. et al. Testosterone dose-response relationships in healthy young men. *Am J Physiol Endocrinol Metab.* 281:E1172, 2001.

Blazevich A.J. et al. Effect of testosterone administration and weight training on muscle architecture. *Med Sci Sports Exerc.* 33:1688, 2001.

Bochud M. et al. Urinary sex steroid and glucocorticoid hormones are associated with muscle mass and strength in healthy adults. *J Clin Endocrinol Metab.* 104:2195, 2019.

Bouchard, C., et al. Familial aggregation of VO2max response to exercise training: results from the HERITAGE Family Study. J. Appl Physiol. 87:1003-1008, 1999.

Celotti F. et al. Anabolic steroids: A review of their effects on the muscles, of their possible mechanisms of action and of their use in athletics. *J Steroid Biochem Mol Biol.* 43:469, 1992.

Ciopponi T. et al. Anabolic steroids: Update 2002. *Sports Med.* 6:1, 2002.

Conceicao M.S. et al. Muscle fiber hypertrophy and

myonuclei addition: A systematic review and meta-analysis. *Med Sci Sports Exerc.* 50:1385, 2018.

Dalton J.T. et al. The selective androgen receptor modulator GTX024 (enodosarm) improves lean body mass and physical function in healthy elderly men and post-menopausal women: Results of a double-blind, placebo-controlled phase ii trial. *J Cachexia Sarcopenia Muscle.* 2:153, 2011.

Dimauro J. et al. Effects of anabolic steroids and high intensity exercise on rat skeletal muscle fibres and capillarization. A morphometric study. *Eur J Appl Physiol Occup Physiol.* 64:204, 1992.

Edgren R.A. A comparative study of the anabolic and androgenic effects of various steroids. *Acta Endocrinol.* 44:SUPPL87:1, 1963.

Egner I.M. et al. A cellular memory mechanism aids overload hypertrophy in muscle long after an episodic exposure to anabolic steroids. *J Physiol.* 591:6221, 2013.

Elashoff J.D. et al. Effects of anabolic-androgenic steroids on muscular strength. *Ann Intern Med.* 115:387, 1991.

Eriksson A. et al. Skeletal muscle morphology in power-lifters with and without anabolic steroids. *Histochem Cell Biol.* 124:167, 2005.

Fahey T. et al. Sport and exercise physiology: Performance- enhancing substances - anabolic steroids. In. *Encyclopedia of Life Support Systems (EOLSS):* UNESCO; 2015.

Fahey T.D. et al. The effects of an anabolic steroid on the strength, body composition, and endurance of college males when accompanied by a weight training program. *Med Sci Sports.* 5:272, 1973.

Ferry A. et al. Respective effects of anabolic/androgenic steroids and physical exercise on isometric contractile properties of regenerating skeletal muscles in the rat. *Arch Physiol Biochem*. 108:257, 2000.

Foster Z.J. et al. Anabolic-androgenic steroids and testosterone precursors: Ergogenic aids and sport. *Curr Sports Med Rep*. 3:234, 2004.

Franchimont P. et al. Anabolic steroids and physical aptitude. *Rev Med Liege*. 34:163, 1979.

Franke W.W. et al. Hormonal doping and androgenization of athletes: A secret program of the German Democratic Republic government. *Clin Chem*. 43:1262, 1997.

Freed D. et al. Anabolic steroids in athletics. *Br Med J*. 3:761, 1972.

Freed D.L. et al. Anabolic steroids in athelics: Crossover double-blind trial on weightlifters. *Br Med J*. 2:471, 1975.

Fritzsche D. et al. Anabolic steroids (metenolone) improve muscle performance and hemodynamic characteristics in cardiomyoplasty. *Ann Thorac Surg*. 59:961, 1995.

Giorgi A. et al. Muscular strength, body composition and health responses to the use of testosterone enanthate: A double blind study. *J Sci Med Sport*. 2:341, 1999.

Hartgens F. et al. Effects of androgenic-anabolic steroids in athletes. *Sports Med*. 34:513, 2004.

Husak J.F. et al. Steroid use and human performance: Lessons for integrative biologists. *Integr Comp Biol*. 49:354, 2009.

Johnson L.C. et al. Anabolic steroid: Effects on strength development. *Science*. 164:957, 1969.

Johnson L.C. et al. Effect of anabolic steroid treatment on endurance. *Med Sci Sports*. 7:287, 1975.

Johnson N.J. et al. Anabolic steroids and sporting performance. *J Clin Pharm Ther*. 13:171, 1988.

Johnson N.P. Was superman a junky? The fallacy of anabolic steroids. *J S C Med Assoc.* 86:46, 1990.

Kadi F. Adaptation of human skeletal muscle to training and anabolic steroids. *Acta Physiol Scand Suppl.* 646:1, 2000.

Kadi F. et al. Effects of anabolic steroids on the muscle cells of strength-trained athletes. *Med Sci Sports Exerc.* 31:1528, 1999.

Kennedy M.C. et al. Do anabolic-androgenic steroids enhance sporting performance? *Med J Aust.* 166:60, 1997.

Keul J. et al. Anabolic steroids: Damages, effect on performance, and on metabolism. *Med Klin.* 71:497, 1976.

Krause Neto W. et al. Total training load may explain similar strength gains and muscle hypertrophy seen in aged rats submitted to resistance training and anabolic steroids. *Aging Male.* 21:65, 2018.

LaBotz M. et al. Use of performance-enhancing substances. *Pediatrics.* 138:2016.

Lamb D.R. Anabolic steroids in athletics: How well do they work and how dangerous are they? *Am J Sports Med.* 12:31, 1984.

Levandowski R. et al. Anabolic steroids: Performance enhancers? *N J Med.* 88:663, 1991.

Limbird T.J. Anabolic steroids in the training and treatment of athletes. *Compr Ther.* 11:25, 1985.

McKillop G. et al. Acute metabolic effects of exercise in bodybuilders using anabolic steroids. *Br J Sports Med.* 23:186, 1989.

Neto W. Effects of strength training and anabolic steroid in the peripheral nerve and skeletal muscle morphology of aged rats. *Front Aging Neurosci.* 9:1, 2017.

Oberlander J.G. et al. The buzz about anabolic androgenic steroids: Electrophysiological effects in excitable tissues. *Neuroendocrinology.* 96:141, 2012.

Rogerson S. et al. The effect of short-term use of testosterone enanthate on muscular strength and power in healthy young men. *J Strength Cond Res.* 21:354, 2007.

Rogozkin V. Metabolic effects of anabolic steroid on skeletal muscle. *Med Sci Sports.* 11:160, 1979.

Salvador A. et al. Lack of effects of anabolic-androgenic steroids on locomotor activity in intact male mice. *Percept Mot Skills.* 88:319, 1999.

Schroeder E.T. et al. Value of measuring muscle performance to assess changes in lean mass with testosterone and growth hormone supplementation. *Eur J Appl Physiol.* 112:1123, 2012.

Smith D.A. et al. The efficacy of ergogenic agents in athletic competition. Part I: Androgenic-anabolic steroids. *Ann Pharmacother.* 26:520, 1992.

Soe M. et al. The effect of anabolic androgenic steroids on muscle strength, body weight and lean body mass in body-building men. *Ugeskr Laeger.* 151:610, 1989.

Tahmindjis A.J. The use of anabolic steroids by athletes to increase body weight and strength. *Med J Aust.* 1:991, 1976.

Tamaki T. et al. Anabolic steroids increase exercise tolerance. *Am J Physiol Endocrinol Metab.* 280:E973, 2001.

Tapper J. et al. Muscles of the trunk and pelvis are responsive to testosterone administration: Data from testosterone dose-response study in young healthy men. *Andrology.* 6:64, 2018.

Vingren J.L. et al. Post-resistance exercise ethanol ingestion and acute testosterone bioavailability. *Med Sci Sports Exerc.* 45:1825, 2013.

Vitoria Ortiz M. Hormones, politics and sport in the

German Democratic Republic (1949-1989). *An R Acad Nac Med.* 128:651, 2011.

Wang M.Q. et al. Changes in body size of elite high school football players: 1963-1989. *Percept Mot Skills.* 76:379, 1993.

Ward P. The effect of an anabolic steroid on strength and lean body mass. *Med Sci Sports.* 5:277, 1973.

Win-May M. et al. The effect of anabolic steroids on physical fitness. *J Sports Med Phys Fitness.* 15:266, 1975.

Yeater R. et al. Resistance trained athletes using or not using anabolic steroids compared to runners: Effects on cardiorespiratory variables, body composition, and plasma lipids. *Br J Sports Med.* 30:11, 1996.

Yu J.G. et al. Effects of long term supplementation of anabolic androgen steroids on human skeletal muscle. *PLoS One.* 9:e105330, 2014.

References: Anabolic Steroids and Athletes

Al Bishi K.A. et al. Prevalence and awareness of anabolic androgenic steroids (AAS) among gymnasts in the western province of Riyadh, Saudi Arabia. *Electron Physician.* 9:6050, 2017.

Alen M. et al. Changes in neuromuscular performance and muscle fiber characteristics of elite power athletes self-administering androgenic and anabolic steroids. *Acta Physiol Scand.* 122:535, 1984.

Alharbi F.F. et al. Knowledge, attitudes and use of anabolic-androgenic steroids among male gym users: A community based survey in Riyadh, Saudi Arabia. *Saudi Pharm J.* 27:254, 2019.

Allahverdipour H. et al. Vulnerability and the intention to anabolic steroids use among Iranian gym users:

An application of the theory of planned behavior. *Subst Use Misuse.* 47:309, 2012.

Almaiman A.A. et al. Side effects of anabolic steroids used by athletes at Unaizah gyms, Saudi Arabia: A pilot study. *J Sports Med Phys Fitness.* 59:489, 2019.

Bahrke M.S. et al. Abuse of anabolic androgenic steroids and related substances in sport and exercise. *Curr Opin Pharmacol.* 4:614, 2004.

Baume N. et al. Evaluation of longitudinal steroid profiles from male football players in UEFA competitions between 2008 and 2013. *Drug Test Anal.* 8:603, 2016.

Beel A. et al. Current perspectives on anabolic steroids. *Drug Alcohol Rev.* 17:87, 1998.

Bergman R. et al. The use and abuse of anabolic steroids in Olympic-caliber athletes. *Clin Orthop Relat Res.* 169, 1985.

Bierly J.R. Use of anabolic steroids by athletes. Do the risks outweigh the benefits? *Postgrad Med.* 82:67, 1987.

Bowers L.D. et al. A half-century of anabolic steroids in sport. *Steroids.* 74:285, 2009.

Bowers L.D. et al. Anabolic steroids, athletic drug testing, and the Olympic games. *Clin Chem.* 42:999, 1996.

Brooks, et al. *Exercise Physiology: Human Bioenergetics and its Applications.* 2005 (5th edition)

Brown G.A. et al. Testosterone pro-hormone supplements. *Med Sci Sports Exerc.* 38:1451, 2006.

Bruner, R., et al. *Recovery Power: Advanced Nutrition and Training Methods for Competitive Athletes,* 1988.

de Ronde W. Use of androgenic anabolic steroids before and during the Olympic games: Less but has not died out. *Ned Tijdschr Geneeskd.* 152:1820, 2008.

Dodge T. et al. The use of anabolic androgenic steroids and polypharmacy: A review of the literature. *Drug Alcohol Depend.* 114:100, 2011.

Fahey, T.D., et al. *Steroid Alternative Handbook,* San Jose, CA: Sport Science Publications, 1991

Fahey, T.D., et al The effects of intermittent liquid meal feeding on selected hormones and substrates during intense weight training" *Int. J. Sports Nutrition* 3: 67-75, 1993.

Fahey, T.D.,et al. "Body composition and VO2max of exceptional weight-trained athletes." *J. Appl. Physiol.* 39:559-561, 1975

Fahey, T.D., et al. *Specialist in Sports Conditioning.* Carpenteria, CA: ISSA, 2018 4th edition.

Fahey, T.D Predictors of performance in elite discus throwers *Biol. Sport* 19:103-108, 2002

Fahey, T. Pharmacology of bodybuilding. In: Reilly, T. and M. Orme, editors. *The Clinical Pharmacology of Sport and Exercise.* Amsterdam: Elsevier Science B.V., 1997.

Fahey, T.D.,et al. Serum testosterone, body composition, and strength of young adults." *Med. Sci.Sports* 8:31-34, 1976.

Ferner R.E. et al. Anabolic steroids: The power and the glory? *BMJ.* 297:877, 1988.

Fink J. et al. Anabolic-androgenic steroids: Procurement and administration practices of doping athletes. *Phys Sportsmed.* 47:10, 2019.

Fitch K.D. Androgenic-anabolic steroids and the Olympic games. *Asian J Androl.* 10:384, 2008.

Franke W.W. et al. Hormonal doping and androgenization of athletes: A secret program of the German Democratic Republic government. *Clin Chem.* 43:1262, 1997.

Frankle M. et al. Athletes on anabolic-androgenic steroids. *Phys Sportsmed.* 20:75, 1992.

Frankle M.A. et al. Use of androgenic anabolic steroids by athletes. *JAMA.* 252:482, 1984.

Freed D. et al. Anabolic steroids in athletics. *Br Med J.* 3:761, 1972.

Frison E. et al. Exposure to media predicts use of dietary supplements and anabolic-androgenic steroids among Flemish adolescent boys. *Eur J Pediatr.* 172:1387, 2013.

Ganesan K. et al. Anabolic steroids. In. *StatPearls.* Treasure Island (FL)2019.

Geddes J.A. Anabolic steroids and the athlete: Counseling patients about risks and side effects. *Can Fam Physician.* 37:979, 1991.

Gillen Z.M. et al. Performance differences between national football league and high school American football combine participants. *Res Q Exerc Sport.* 90:227, 2019.

Goldberg L. et al. Use of anabolic-androgenic steroids by athletes. *N Engl J Med.* 322:775, 1990.

Gribbin H.R. et al. Mode of action and use of anabolic steroids. *Br J Clin Pract.* 30:3, 1976.

Hall R.C. et al. Abuse of supraphysiologic doses of anabolic steroids. *South Med J.* 98:550, 2005.

Harkness R.A. et al. Effects of large doses of anabolic steroids. *Br J Sports Med.* 9:70, 1975.

Hartgens F. et al. Effects of androgenic-anabolic steroids in athletes. *Sports Med.* 34:513, 2004.

Hervey G.R. Are athletes wrong about anabolic steroids? *Br J Sports Med.* 9:74, 1975.

Hickson R.C. et al. Anabolic steroids and training. *Clin Sports Med.* 5:461, 1986.

Hoffman J.R. et al. Effect of muscle oxygenation during resistance exercise on anabolic hormone response. *Med Sci Sports Exerc.* 35:1929, 2003.

Holden S.C. et al. Anabolic steroids in athletics. *Tex Med.* 86:32, 1990.

Hough D.O. Anabolic steroids and ergogenic aids. *Am Fam Physician.* 41:1157, 1990.

Huhtaniemi I. Anabolic-androgenic steroids--a double-edged sword? *Int J Androl.* 17:57, 1994.

Imhof P. Anabolic steroids and sports. *Schweiz Z Sportmed.* 18:79, 1970.

Jacka B. et al. Health care engagement behaviors of men who use performance- and image-enhancing drugs in Australia. *Subst Abus.* 41:139, 2020.

Jasuja G.K. et al. Patterns of testosterone prescription overuse. *Curr Opin Endocrinol Diabetes Obes.* 24:240, 2017.

Johnson D.A. Use of anabolic steroids by athletes. *JAMA.* 251:1430, 1984.

Kalinski M.I. "State-sponsored" doping: A transition from the former soviet union to present day Russia. *BLDE Univer J Health Sci.* 2:1, 2017.

Lindqvist Bagge A.S. et al. Somatic effects of AAS abuse: A 30-years follow-up study of male former power sports athletes. *J Sci Med Sport.* 20:814, 2017.

MacDougall J.D. et al. Muscle ultrastructural characteristics of elite powerlifters and bodybuilders. *Eur J Appl Physiol Occup Physiol.* 48:117, 1982.

McBride J.A. et al. The availability and acquisition of illicit anabolic androgenic steroids and testosterone preparations on the internet. *Am J Mens Health.* 12:1352, 2018.

McBride J.A. et al. Recovery of spermatogenesis following testosterone replacement therapy or anabolic-androgenic steroid use. *Asian J Androl.* 18:373, 2016.

McDuff D. et al. Recreational and ergogenic substance

use and substance use disorders in elite athletes: A narrative review. *Br J Sports Med.* 53:754, 2019.

Medras M. et al. Use of testosterone and anabolic androgenic steroids in sport. *Endokrynol Pol.* 60:204, 2009.

Mellion M.B. Anabolic steroids in athletics. *Am Fam Physician.* 30:113, 1984.

Moriarty H.J. Anabolic steroids in sport. *N Z Med J.* 110:42, 1997.

Oseid S. How can we prevent and control the use and misuse of anabolic steroids in international sports? *Br J Sports Med.* 11:174, 1977.

Papaloucas M. et al. Pheromones: A new ergogenic aid in sport? *Int J Sports Physiol Perform.* 10:939, 2015.

Payne A.H. Anabolic steroids in athletics (or the rise of the mediocrity). *Br J Sports Med.* 9:83, 1975.

Perls T.T. Growth hormone and anabolic steroids: Athletes are the tip of the iceberg. *Drug Test Anal.* 1:419, 2009.

Pope H.G., Jr. et al. Anabolic-androgenic steroid use among 1,010 college men. *Phys Sportsmed.* 16:75, 1988.

Reyes-Vallejo L. Current use and abuse of anabolic steroids. *Actas Urol Esp.* 2020.

Ritter J.M. Sex, steroids and anabolic androgens in athletics. *Br J Clin Pharmacol.* 74:1, 2012.

Rogol A.D. et al. Clinical review 31: Anabolic-androgenic steroids and athletes: What are the issues? *J Clin Endocrinol Metab.* 74:465, 1992.

Rollo I. A nursing perspective on the misuse of anabolic steroids. *Nurs Times.* 100:30, 2004.

Skarberg K. et al. Multisubstance use as a feature of addiction to anabolic-androgenic steroids. *Eur Addict Res.* 15:99, 2009.

Smit D.L. et al. Baseline characteristics of the Haarlem study: 100 male amateur athletes using anabolic andro-genic steroids. *Scand J Med Sci Sports.* 30:531, 2020.

Stolt A. et al. Qt interval and QT dispersion in en-durance athletes and in power athletes using large doses of anabolic steroids. *Am J Cardiol.* 84:364, 1999.

Strauss R.H. et al. Anabolic steroids in the athlete. *Annu Rev Med.* 42:449, 1991.

VanHelder W.P. et al. Anabolic steroids in sport. *Can J Sport Sci.* 16:248, 1991.

Vitoria Ortiz M. Hormones, politics and sport in the German Democratic Republic (1949-1989). *An R Acad Nac Med.* 128:651, 2011.

Wright J.E. Anabolic steroids and athletics. *Exerc Sport Sci Rev.* 8:149, 1980.

Yu J.G. et al. Potential effects of long term abuse of an-abolic androgen steroids on human skeletal muscle. *J Sports Med Phys Fitness.* 2020.

Zlotsky N.A. Anabolic steroids and athletes. *Conn Med.* 53:241, 1989.

Zoob Carter B.N. et al. The impact of the covid-19 pandemic on male strength athletes who use non-pre-scribed anabolic-androgenic steroids. *Front Psychiatry.* 12:636706, 2021.

References: Anabolic Steroids, Bodybuilding, and Body Composition

Abbate V. et al. Anabolic steroids detected in body-building dietary supplements - a significant risk to public health. *Drug Test Anal.* 7:609, 2015.

Alen M. et al. Physical health and fitness of an elite bodybuilder during 1-year of self-administration of testosterone and anabolic steroids: A case study. *Int J Sports Med.* 6:24, 1985.

Almaiman A.A. Effect of testosterone boosters on body functions: Case report. *Int J Health Sci (Qassim).* 12:86, 2018.

Amaku E.O. A study of the effect of anabolic steroids on nitrogen balance. *West Afr J Pharmacol Drug Res.* 4:1, 1977.

Angoorani H. et al. The misuse of anabolic-androgenic steroids among Iranian recreational male body-builders and their related psycho-socio-demographic factors. *Iran J Public Health.* 44:1662, 2015.

Aparicio V.A. et al. Effects of the dietary amount and source of protein, resistance training and anabolic-androgenic steroids on body weight and lipid profile of rats. *Nutr Hosp.* 28:127, 2013.

Babigian A. et al. Management of gynecomastia due to use of anabolic steroids in bodybuilders. *Plast Reconstr Surg.* 107:240, 2001.

Baldo-Enzi G. et al. Lipid and apoprotein modifications in body builders during and after self-administration of anabolic steroids. *Metabolism.* 39:203, 1990.

Baumann S. et al. Myocardial scar detected by cardiovascular magnetic resonance in a competitive bodybuilder with longstanding abuse of anabolic steroids. *Asian J Sports Med.* 5:e24058, 2014.

Baume N. et al. Research of stimulants and anabolic steroids in dietary supplements. *Scand J Med Sci Sports.* 16:41, 2006.

Bhasin S. et al. The mechanisms of androgen effects on body composition: Mesenchymal pluripotent cell as the target of androgen action. *J Gerontol.* 58A:1103, 2003.

Boehncke E. et al. Influence of anabolic steroids on the n-retention in fattening calves. *Fortschr Tierphysiol Tierernahr.* 18, 1976.

Brand R. et al. Using response-time latencies to measure athletes' doping attitudes: The brief implicit attitude test identifies substance abuse in bodybuilders. *Subst Abus Treat Prev Pol.* 9:36, 2014.

Braseth N.R. et al. Exertional rhabdomyolysis in a body builder abusing anabolic androgenic steroids. *Eur J Emerg Med.* 8:155, 2001.

Calabrese L.H. et al. The effects of anabolic steroids and strength training on the human immune response. *Med Sci Sports Exerc.* 21:386, 1989.

Carvajal R. Contaminated dietary supplements. *N Engl J Med.* 362:274; author reply 274, 2010.

Chasland L.C. et al. Higher circulating androgens and higher physical activity levels are associated with less central adiposity and lower risk of cardiovascular death in older men. *Clin Endocrinol.* 90:375, 2019.

Christou G.A. et al. Acute myocardial infarction in a young bodybuilder taking anabolic androgenic steroids: A case report and critical review of the literature. *Eur J Prev Cardiol.* 23:1785, 2016.

Cohen P.A. American roulette--contaminated dietary supplements. *N Engl J Med.* 361:1523, 2009.

Cordaro F.G. et al. Selling androgenic anabolic steroids by the pound: Identification and analysis of popular websites on the internet. *Scand J Med Sci Sports.* 21:e247, 2011.

Dickerman R.D. et al. Echocardiography in fraternal twin bodybuilders with one abusing anabolic steroids. *Cardiology.* 88:50, 1997.

Dickerman R.D. et al. Sudden cardiac death in a 20-year-old bodybuilder using anabolic steroids. *Cardiology.* 86:172, 1995.

Dickerman R.D. et al. Left ventricular size and function in elite bodybuilders using anabolic steroids. *Clin J Sport Med.* 7:90, 1997.

Ebenbichler C.F. et al. Hyperhomocysteinemia in bodybuilders taking anabolic steroids. *Eur J Intern Med.* 12:43, 2001.

Eriksson A. et al. Skeletal muscle morphology in powerlifters with and without anabolic steroids. *Histochem Cell Biol.* 124:167, 2005.

Fahey T.D. et al. The effects of an anabolic steroid on the strength, body composition, and endurance of college males when accompanied by a weight training program. *Med Sci Sports.* 5:272, 1973.

Favretto D. et al. When color fails: Illicit blue tablets containing anabolic androgen steroids. *J Pharm Biomed Anal.* 83:260, 2013.

Fennessey P.V. et al. Anabolic steroids in body builders: Use, metabolic disposition and physiological effects. *J Pharm Biomed Anal.* 6:999, 1988.

Figueiredo V.C. et al. Cosmetic doping--when anabolic-androgenic steroids are not enough. *Subst Use Misuse.* 49:1163, 2014.

Forbes G.B. The effect of anabolic steroids on lean body mass: The dose response curve. *Metabolism.* 34:571, 1985.

Freed D.L. et al. Anabolic steroids in athletics: Crossover double-blind trial on weightlifters. *Br Med J.* 2:471, 1975.

Garthe I. et al. Athletes and supplements: Prevalence and perspectives. *Int J Sport Nutr Exerc Metab.* 28:126, 2018.

Geyer H. et al. Nutritional supplements cross-contaminated and faked with doping substances. *J Mass Spectrom.* 43:892, 2008.

Goldfield G.S. et al. Body image, disordered eating, and anabolic steroids in male bodybuilders: Current versus former users. *Phys Sportsmed.* 37:111, 2009.

Grogan S. et al. Experiences of anabolic steroid use: In-depth interviews with men and women body builders. *J Health Psychol.* 11:845, 2006.

Hartgens F. et al. Misuse of androgenic-anabolic steroids and human deltoid muscle fibers: Differences between polydrug regimens and single drug administration. *Eur J Appl Physiol.* 86:233, 2002.

Heim J. et al. HDL breakdown in an athlete taking anabolic steroids. *Presse Med.* 25:458, 1996.

Huang G. et al. Circulating biomarkers of testosterone's anabolic effects on fat-free mass. *J Clin Endocrinol Metab.* 2019.

Ilhan E. et al. Acute myocardial infarction and renal infarction in a bodybuilder using anabolic steroids. *Turk Kardiyol Dern Ars.* 38:275, 2010.

Iriart J.A. et al. Body cult and use of anabolic steroids by bodybuilders. *Cad Saude Publica.* 25:773, 2009.

Isaksson B. et al. Body composition during long-term administration of cortisone and anabolic steroids in an asthmatic subject. *Metabolism.* 16:162, 1967.

Juhl S. et al. Concomitant arterial and venous thrombosis in a body builder with severe hyperhomocysteinemia and abuse of anabolic steroids. *Ugeskr Laeger.* 166:3508, 2004.

Kafrouni M.I. et al. Hepatotoxicity associated with dietary supplements containing anabolic steroids. *Clin Gastroenterol Hepatol.* 5:809, 2007.

Kintz P. et al. Testing for anabolic steroids in hair from two bodybuilders. *Forensic Sci Int.* 101:209, 1999.

Kouri E.M. et al. Fat-free mass index in users and

nonusers of anabolic-androgenic steroids. *Clin J Sport Med.* 5:223, 1995.

Lusetti M. et al. Appearance/image- and performance-enhancing drug users: A forensic approach. *Am J Forensic Med Pathol.* 39:325, 2018.

Martello S. et al. Survey of nutritional supplements for selected illegal anabolic steroids and ephedrine using IC-MS/MS and GC-MS methods, respectively. *Food Addit Contam.* 24:258, 2007.

Maughan R. Contamination of supplements: An interview with professor Ron Maughan by Louise M. Burke. *Int J Sport Nutr Exerc Metab.* 14:493, 2004.

Maughan R.J. Contamination of dietary supplements and positive drug tests in sport. *J Sports Sci.* 23:883, 2005.

Maughan R.J. Quality assurance issues in the use of dietary supplements, with special reference to protein supplements. *J Nutr.* 143:1843S, 2013.

Maughan R.J. et al. The use of dietary supplements by athletes. *J Sports Sci.* 25 Suppl 1:S103, 2007.

Maughan R.J. et al. Dietary supplements for athletes: Emerging trends and recurring themes. *J Sports Sci.* 29 Suppl 1:S57, 2011.

Maung A.A. et al. Perioperative nutritional support: Immunonutrition, probiotics, and anabolic steroids. *Surg Clin North Am.* 92:273, 2012.

McKillop G. et al. Acute metabolic effects of exercise in bodybuilders using anabolic steroids. *Br J Sports Med.* 23:186, 1989.

Melnik B. et al. Abuse of anabolic-androgenic steroids and bodybuilding acne: An underestimated health problem. *J Dtsch Dermatol Ges.* 5:110, 2007.

Mitchell L. et al. Correlates of muscle dysmorphia symptomatology in natural bodybuilders: Distinguishing factors in the pursuit of hyper-muscularity. *Body Image.* 22:1, 2017.

Nakhaee M.R. et al. Prevalence of use of anabolic steroids by bodybuilders using three methods in a city of Iran. *Addict Health.* 5:77, 2013.

Nakhaee M.R. et al. Prevalence of use of anabolic steroids by bodybuilders using three methods in a city of Iran. *Addict Health.* 5:77, 2013. https://www.ncbi.nlm.nih.gov/pubmed/24494162

Nasseri A. et al. Effects of resistance exercise and the use of anabolic androgenic steroids on hemodynamic characteristics and muscle damage markers in bodybuilders. *J Sports Med Phys Fitness.* 56:1041, 2016.

National Institute on Drug Abuse. Steroids and other appearance and performance enhancing drugs (APEDs). *https://www.drugabuse.gov.* 2018.

Nordstrom A. et al. Higher muscle mass but lower gynoid fat mass in athletes using anabolic androgenic steroids. *J Strength Cond Res.* 26:246, 2012.

Nottin S. et al. Cardiovascular effects of androgenic anabolic steroids in male bodybuilders determined by tissue doppler imaging. *Am J Cardiol.* 97:912, 2006.

Overbeek G.A. et al. The effect of testosterone propionate on the body weight of monkeys. *Biochem J.* 40:lxvi, 1946.

Parr M.K. et al. High amounts of 17-methylated anabolic-androgenic steroids in effervescent tablets on the dietary supplement market. *Biomed Chromatogr.* 21:164, 2007.

Parr M.K. et al. Analytical strategies for the detection of non-labelled anabolic androgenic steroids in nutritional supplements. *Food Addit Contam.* 21:632, 2004.

Pertusi R. et al. Evaluation of aminotransferase elevations in a bodybuilder using anabolic steroids: Hepatitis or rhabdomyolysis? *J Am Osteopath Assoc.* 101:391, 2001.

Pope H.G., Jr. et al. Anorexia nervosa and "reverse anorexia" among 108 male bodybuilders. *Compr Psychiatry.* 34:406, 1993.

Reitzner S.M. et al. Modulation of exercise training related adaptation of body composition and regulatory pathways by anabolic steroids. *J Steroid Biochem Mol Biol.* 190:44, 2019.

Rosca A.E. et al. Impact of chronic administration of anabolic androgenic steroids and taurine on blood pressure in rats. *Braz J Med Biol Res.* 49:e5116, 2016.

Santos A.M. et al. Illicit use and abuse of anabolic-androgenic steroids among Brazilian bodybuilders. *Subst Use Misuse.* 46:742, 2011.

Sepehri G. et al. Frequency of anabolic steroids abuse in bodybuilder athletes in Kerman City. *Addict Health.* 1:25, 2009.

Siekierzynska-Czarnecka A. et al. Death caused by pulmonary embolism in a body builder taking anabolic steroids (metanabol). *Wiad Lek.* 43:972, 1990.

Striegel H. et al. Contaminated nutritional supplements--legal protection for elite athletes who tested positive: A case report from Germany. *J Sports Sci.* 23:723, 2005.

Tapper J. et al. Muscles of the trunk and pelvis are responsive to testosterone administration: Data from testosterone dose-response study in young healthy men. *Andrology.* 6:64, 2018.

Tsarouhas K. et al. Use of nutritional supplements contaminated with banned doping substances by recreational adolescent athletes in Athens, Greece. *Food Chem Toxicol.* 115:447, 2018.

Underwood M. Exploring the social lives of image and

performance enhancing drugs: An online ethnography of the ZYZZ fandom of recreational bodybuilders. *Int J Drug Policy*. 39:78, 2017.

van der Merwe P.J. et al. Unintentional doping through the use of contaminated nutritional supplements. *S Afr Med J*. 95:510, 2005.

Van Poucke C. et al. Determination of anabolic steroids in dietary supplements by liquid chromatography-tandem mass spectrometry. *Anal Chim Acta*. 586:35, 2007.

Wang M.Q. et al. Desire for weight gain and potential risks of adolescent males using anabolic steroids. *Percept Mot Skills*. 78:267, 1994.

Westerman M.E. et al. Heavy testosterone use among bodybuilders: An uncommon cohort of illicit substance users. *Mayo Clin Proc*. 91:175, 2016.

Woodward C. et al. Hepatocellular carcinoma in body builders; an emerging rare but serious complication of androgenic anabolic steroid use. *Ann Hepatobiliary Pancreat Surg*. 23:174, 2019.

References: Anabolic Steroids and Females

al Shareef S. et al. Anabolic steroid use disorder. In. *Statpearls*. Treasure Island (FL)2019.

American College of Obstetrics and Gynecology. ACOG committee opinion no. 484: Performance enhancing anabolic steroid abuse in women. *Obstet Gynecol*. 117:1016, 2011.

Arndt H.J. Data on hormone-related voice disorders in women. *Arch Ohren Nasen Kehlkopfheilkd*. 182:659, 1963.

Arndt H.J. Voice damages in women due to androgenic

and anabolic hormones. *Dtsch Med Wochenschr.* 88:2336, 1963.

Bahrke M.S. et al. Abuse of anabolic androgenic steroids and related substances in sport and exercise. *Curr Opin Pharmacol.* 4:614, 2004.

Bakker K. et al. Liver lesions due to long-term use of anabolic steroids and oral contraceptives. *Ned Tijdschr Geneeskd.* 120:2214, 1976.

Balasch J. Sex steroids and bone: Current perspectives. *Hum Reprod Update.* 9:207, 2003.

Bensoussan Y. et al. Case report: The long-term effects of anabolic steroids on the female voice over a 20-year period. *Clin Case Rep.* 7:1067, 2019.

Berning J.M. et al. Anabolic androgenic steroids: Use and perceived use in nonathlete college students. *J Am Coll Health.* 56:499, 2008.

Bird H.A. et al. A controlled trial of nandrolone de-canoate in the treatment of rheumatoid arthritis in postmenopausal women. *Ann Rheum Dis.* 46:237, 1987.

Birkenhager J.C. Estrogens, anabolic steroids and postmenopausal osteoporosis: What are the facts? *Ned Tijdschr Geneeskd.* 135:973, 1991.

Birzniece V. et al. Sex steroids and the GH axis: Implications for the management of hypopituitarism. *Best Pract Res Clin Endocrinol Metab.* 31:59, 2017.

Black E.F. The use of testosterone propionate in gynaecology. *Can Med Assoc J.* 47:124, 1942.

Bolch O.H., Jr. et al. Induction of premature menstruation with catatoxic steroids. *Am J Obstet Gynecol.* 111:1107, 1971.

Bolch O.H., Jr. et al. Induction of premature menstruation with anabolic steroids. *Am J Obstet Gynecol.* 117:121, 1973.

Borjesson A. et al. Recruitment to doping and help-seeking behavior of eight female AAS users. *Subst Abuse Treat Prev Policy.* 11:11, 2016.

Bourg R. Secretory activity of the mammary glands; sequellae of massive testosterone doses in women following castration. *Ann Endocrinol (Paris).* 11:254, 1950.

Brasil G.A. et al. Nandrolone decanoate induces cardiac and renal remodeling in female rats, without modification in physiological parameters: The role of ANP system. *Life Sci.* 137:65, 2015.

Brenner P.F. et al. A study of the abortifacient effect of oxymetholone in early gestation. *Contraception.* 11:669, 1975.

Brooke-Wavell K. et al. The influence of physical activity on the response of bone mineral density to 5 years tibolone. *Maturitas.* 35:229, 2000.

Buisson C. et al. Metabolic and isotopic signature of short-term DHEA administration in women: Comparison with findings in men. *Drug Test Anal.* 10:1744, 2018.

Caliman I.F. et al. Long-term treatment with nandrolone decanoate impairs mesenteric vascular relaxation in both sedentary and exercised female rats. *Steroids.* 120:7, 2017.

Chantal Y. et al. Exploring the social image of anabolic steroids users through motivation, sportspersonship orientations and aggression. *Scand J Med Sci Sports.* 19:228, 2009.

Choi P.Y. et al. Violence toward women and illicit androgenic-anabolic steroid use. *Ann Clin Psychiatry.* 6:21, 1994.

Clark A.S. et al. Chronic administration of anabolic steroids disrupts pubertal onset and estrous cyclicity in rats. *Biol Reprod.* 68:465, 2003.

Compston J.E. Sex steroids and bone. *Physiol Rev.* 81:419, 2001.

Coomber R. et al. The supply of steroids and other performance and image enhancing drugs (PIEDs) in one English city: Fakes, counterfeits, supplier trust, common beliefs and access. *Perf Enhanc Health.* 3:135, 2014.

Cox D.W. et al. Perturbations of the human menstrual cycle by oxymetholone. *Am J Obstet Gynecol.* 121:121, 1975.

Damste P.H. Virilization of the voice due to the use of anabolic steroids. *Ned Tijdschr Geneeskd.* 107:891, 1963.

Derman R.J. Effects of sex steroids on women's health: Implications for practitioners. *Am J Med.* 98:137S, 1995.

Dickey R.P. et al. Drugs that affect the breast and lactation. *Clin Obstet Gynecol.* 18:95, 1975.

Diloksambandh V. Anabolic steroids and female reproductive organs. *J Med Assoc Thai.* 61 Suppl 3:31, 1978.

Diniz D. et al. The illegal market for gender-related drugs as portrayed in the Brazilian news media: The case of misoprostol and women. *Cad Saude Publica.* 27:94, 2011.

Eklund E. et al. Serum androgen profile and physical performance in women olympic athletes. *Br J Sports Med.* 51:1301, 2017.

Eliakim A. et al. A case study of virilizing adrenal tumor in an adolescent female elite tennis player--insight into the use of anabolic steroids in young athletes. *J Strength Cond Res.* 25:46, 2011.

Elliot D.L. et al. Definition and outcome of a curriculum to prevent disordered eating and body-shaping drug use. *J Sch Health.* 76:67, 2006.

Fahey, T.D. et al. The effects of prolonged, intense exercise on estradiol, progesterone, LH and FSH concentrations during mid-menstrual cycle." *Biol. Sport.* 14: 175-183, 1997.

Farooqi V. et al. Anabolic steroids for rehabilitation after hip fracture in older people. *Cochrane Database Syst Rev.* CD008887, 2014.

Field A.E. et al. Exposure to the mass media, body shape concerns, and use of supplements to improve weight and shape among male and female adolescents. *Pediatrics.* 116:e214, 2005.

Franke W.W. et al. Hormonal doping and androgenization of athletes: A secret program of the German Democratic Republic government. *Clin Chem.* 43:1262, 1997.

Garg R.K. et al. High density lipoprotein. *J Assoc Physicians India.* 39:269, 1991.

Gennari C. et al. Effects of nandrolone decanoate therapy on bone mass and calcium metabolism in women with established post-menopausal osteoporosis: A double-blind placebo-controlled study. *Maturitas.* 11:187, 1989.

Gentil P. et al. Nutrition, pharmacological and training strategies adopted by six bodybuilders: Case report and critical review. *Eur J Transl Myol.* 27:6247, 2017.

Giannitrapani L. et al. Sex hormones and risk of liver tumor. *Ann N Y Acad Sci.* 1089:228, 2006.

Giltay E.J. et al. Effects of sex steroids on plasma total homocysteine levels: A study in transsexual males and females. *J Clin Endocrinol Metab.* 83:550, 1998.

Glueck C.J. Nonpharmacologic and pharmacologic alteration of high-density lipoprotein cholesterol: Therapeutic approaches to prevention of atherosclerosis. *Am Heart J.* 110:1107, 1985.

Goldfield G.S. Body image, disordered eating and anabolic steroid use in female bodybuilders. *Eat Disord.* 17:200, 2009.

Grogan S. et al. Experiences of anabolic steroid use: In-depth interviews with men and women body builders. *J Health Psychol.* 11:845, 2006.

Gruber A.J. et al. Compulsive weightlifting and anabolic drug abuse among women rape victims. *Compr Psychiatry.* 40:273, 1999.

Gruber A.J. et al. Psychiatric and medical effects of anabolic-androgenic steroid use in women. *Psychother Psychosom.* 69:19, 2000.

Hahner S. et al. Dehydroepiandrosterone to enhance physical performance: Myth and reality. *Endocrinol Metab Clin North Am.* 39:127, 2010.

Handelsman D.J. et al. Circulating testosterone as the hormonal basis of sex differences in athletic performance. *Endocr Rev.* 39:803, 2018.

Hassager C. et al. The carboxy-terminal propeptide of type I procollagen in serum as a marker of bone formation: The effect of nandrolone decanoate and female sex hormones. *Metabolism.* 40:205, 1991.

Hassager C. et al. Collagen synthesis in post-menopausal women during therapy with anabolic steroid or female sex hormones. *Metabolism.* 39:1167, 1990.

Hedstrom M. et al. Positive effects of anabolic steroids, vitamin d and calcium on muscle mass, bone mineral density and clinical function after a hip fracture. A randomised study of 63 women. *J Bone Joint Surg Br.* 84:497, 2002.

Hermans E.J. et al. Effects of exogenous testosterone on the ventral striatal bold response during reward anticipation in healthy women. *Neuroimage.* 52:277, 2010.

Hickson R.C. et al. Anabolic steroids and training. *Clin Sports Med.* 5:461, 1986.

Hildebrandt T. et al. Development and validation of the appearance and performance enhancing drug use schedule. *Addict Behav.* 36:949, 2011.

Honour J.W. Steroid abuse in female athletes. *Curr Opin Obstet Gynecol.* 9:181, 1997.

Huang G. et al. Do anabolic-androgenic steroids have performance-enhancing effects in female athletes? *Mol Cell Endocrinol.* 464:56, 2018.

Ip E.J. et al. Women and anabolic steroids: An analysis of a dozen users. *Clin J Sport Med.* 20:475, 2010.

Ishak K.G. Hepatic lesions caused by anabolic and contraceptive steroids. *Semin Liver Dis.* 1:116, 1981.

Janssen J.A. Impact of physical exercise on endocrine aging. *Front Horm Res.* 47:68, 2016.

Jones O.S. Use of testosterone in the female. *Med Times.* 78:568, 1950.

Kanayama G. et al. Anabolic steroid abuse among teenage girls: An illusory problem? *Drug Alcohol Depend.* 88:156, 2007.

Kanayama G. et al. Over-the-counter drug use in gymnasiums: An underrecognized substance abuse problem? *Psychother Psychosom.* 70:137, 2001.

Kanayama G. et al. Illicit anabolic-androgenic steroid use. *Horm Behav.* 58:111, 2010.

Kibble M.W. et al. Adverse effects of anabolic steroids in athletes. *Clin Pharm.* 6:686, 1987.

Kicman A.T. Pharmacology of anabolic steroids. *Br J Pharmacol.* 154:502, 2008.

Laurell C.B. et al. A comparison of plasma protein changes induced by danazol, pregnancy, and estrogens. *J Clin Endocrinol Metab.* 49:719, 1979.

Luci M. et al. Dehydroepiandrosterone [DHEA(s)]: Anabolic hormone? *Recenti Prog Med.* 101:333, 2010.

Maravelias C. et al. Adverse effects of anabolic steroids in athletes. A constant threat. *Toxicol Lett.* 158:167, 2005.

Martinez-Patino M.J. et al. The unfinished race: 30 years of gender verification in sport. *Lancet.* 388:541, 2016.

Moffatt R.J. et al. Effects of anabolic steroids on lipoprotein profiles of female weight lifters. *Phys Sportsmed.* 18:106, 1990.

Molero Y. et al. Illicit drug use among gym-goers: A cross-sectional study of gym-goers in Sweden. *Sports Med Open.* 3:31, 2017.

Mosler S. et al. Modulation of follistatin and myostatin propeptide by anabolic steroids and gender. *Int J Sports Med.* 34:567, 2013.

Mostert C.H. et al. Gender differences in licit and illicit substance use reported by incoming freshman college students. *Tenn Med.* 101:34, 2008.

Mullen J.E. et al. Urinary steroid profile in females - the impact of menstrual cycle and emergency contraceptives. *Drug Test Anal.* 9:1034, 2017.

Muller A. Anabolic drugs and the feminine voice. *Pract Otorhinolaryngol (Basel).* 26:91, 1964.

Nagata J.M. et al. Predictors of muscularity-oriented disordered eating behaviors in U.S. Young adults: A prospective cohort study. *Int J Eat Disord.* 52:1380, 2019.

Need A.G. et al. Anabolic steroids in postmenopausal osteoporosis. *Wien Med Wochenschr.* 143:392, 1993.

Need A.G. et al. Effects of nandrolone decanoate on forearm mineral density and calcium metabolism in osteoporotic postmenopausal women. *Calcif Tissue Int.* 41:7, 1987.

Nieschlag E. et al. Mechanisms in endocrinology: Medical consequences of doping with anabolic androgenic steroids: Effects on reproductive functions. *Eur J Endocrinol.* 173:R47, 2015.

Onakomaiya M.M. et al. Mad men, women and steroid cocktails: A review of the impact of sex and other factors on anabolic androgenic steroids effects on affective behaviors. *Psychopharmacology.* 233:549, 2016.

Penatti C.A. et al. Effects of chronic exposure to an anabolic androgenic steroid cocktail on alpha5-receptor-mediated gabaergic transmission and neural signaling in the forebrain of female mice. *Neuroscience.* 161:526, 2009.

Pereira E. et al. Prevalence and profile of users and non-users of anabolic steroids among resistance training practitioners. *BMC Public Health.* 19:1650, 2019.

Perello J. Virilization of the female larynx. *Acta Otorinolaryngol Iber Am.* 15:139, 1964.

Perez-Laso C. et al. Effects of adult female rat androgenization on brain morphology and metabolomic profile. *Cereb Cortex.* 28:2846, 2018.

Pollanen E. et al. Differential influence of peripheral and systemic sex steroids on skeletal muscle quality in pre- and postmenopausal women. *Aging Cell.* 10:650, 2011.

Pope H.G., Jr. et al. Muscle dysmorphia. An underrecognized form of body dysmorphic disorder. *Psychosomatics.* 38:548, 1997.

Quaglio G. et al. Anabolic steroids: Dependence and complications of chronic use. *Intern Emerg Med.* 4:289, 2009.

Rachon D. et al. Prevalence and risk factors of anabolic-androgenic steroids (AAS) abuse among adolescents and young adults in Poland. *Soz Praventivmed.* 51:392, 2006.

Raschka C. et al. Recreational athletes and doping--a survey in 11 gyms in the area of Frankfurt/Main. *MMW Fortschr Med.* 155 Suppl 2:41, 2013.

Salinas Vert I. et al. Defects of adrenal steroidogenesis in patients with hirsutism. *Med Clin (Barc).* 110:171, 1998.

Salinger S.L. Proliferative effect of testosterone propionate on human vaginal epithelium. *Acta Endocrinol.* 4:265, 1950.

Schols A.M. et al. Physiologic effects of nutritional support and anabolic steroids in patients with chronic obstructive pulmonary disease. A placebo-controlled randomized trial. *Am J Respir Crit Care Med.* 152:1268, 1995.

Shahidi N.T. A review of the chemistry, biological action, and clinical applications of anabolic-androgenic steroids. *Clin Ther.* 23:1355, 2001.

Shapiro J. et al. Testosterone and other anabolic steroids as cardiovascular drugs. *Am J Ther.* 6:167, 1999.

Sirianni R. et al. Nandrolone and stanozolol upregulate aromatase expression and further increase IGF-1-dependent effects on MCF-7 breast cancer cell proliferation. *Mol Cell Endocrinol.* 363:100, 2012.

Skarberg K. et al. The development of multiple drug use among anabolic-androgenic steroid users: Six subjective case reports. *Subst Abuse Treat Prev Policy.* 3:24, 2008.

Stenman U.H. et al. Gonadotropins in doping: Pharmacological basis and detection of illicit use. *Br J Pharmacol.* 154:569, 2008.

Stergiopoulos K. et al. Anabolic steroids, acute myocardial infarction and polycythemia: A case report and review of the literature. *Vasc Health Risk Manag.* 4:1475, 2008.

Strauss R.H. et al. Anabolic steroid use and perceived effects in ten weight-trained women athletes. *JAMA.* 253:2871, 1985.

Talaat M. et al. Histologic and histochemical study of effects of anabolic steroids on the female larynx. *Ann Otol Rhinol Laryngol.* 96:468, 1987.

Tapper J. et al. The effects of testosterone administration on muscle areas of the trunk and pelvic floor in hysterectomized women with low testosterone levels: Proof-of-concept study. *Menopause.* 26:1405, 2019.

Taylor W. Risk factors associated with the use of sex hormones. *Anticancer Res.* 7:943, 1987.

Thiblin I. et al. Sudden unexpected death in a female fitness athlete, with a possible connection to the use of anabolic androgenic steroids (AAS) and ephedrine. *Forensic Sci Int.* 184:e7, 2009.

Tripathi A. et al. Iatrogenic dependence of anabolic-androgenic steroid in an Indian non-athletic woman. *BMJ Case Rep.* 2014:2014.

Van Eenoo P. et al. Endogenous origin of norandrosterone in female urine: Indirect evidence for the production of 19-norsteroids as by-products in the conversion from androgen to estrogen. *J Steroid Biochem Mol Biol.* 78:351, 2001.

Verheyden K. et al. Excretion of endogenous boldione in human urine: Influence of phytosterol consumption. *J Steroid Biochem Mol Biol.* 117:8, 2009.

Vingren J.L. et al. Effect of resistance exercise on muscle steroidogenesis. *J Appl Physiol (1985).* 105:1754, 2008.

Vorona E. et al. Adverse effects of doping with anabolic androgenic steroids in competitive athletics, recreational sports and bodybuilding. *Minerva Endocrinol.* 43:476, 2018.

Walker C.J. et al. Doping in sport--1. Excretion of 19-norandrosterone by healthy women, including those using contraceptives containing norethisterone. *Steroids.* 74:329, 2009.

Whetzel C.A. et al. Measuring DHEA-s in saliva: Time of day differences and positive correlations between two different types of collection methods. *BMC Res Notes.* 3:204, 2010.

Wollina U. et al. Side-effects of topical androgenic and anabolic substances and steroids. A short review. *Acta Dermatovenerol Alp Pannonica Adriat.* 16:117, 2007.

Wood R.I. et al. Testosterone and sport: Current perspectives. *Horm Behav.* 61:147, 2012.

Wu F.C. Endocrine aspects of anabolic steroids. *Clin Chem.* 43:1289, 1997.

Yesalis C.E. et al. Anabolic-androgenic steroids and related substances. *Curr Sports Med Rep.* 1:246, 2002.

Yilmaz B. et al. Endocrinology of hirsutism: From androgens to androgen excess disorders. *Front Horm Res.* 53:108, 2019.

Zahm S.H. et al. The epidemiology of soft tissue sarcoma. *Semin Oncol.* 24:504, 1997.

References: Anabolic Steroids and Aging

Advisory Panel on Testosterone Replacement in Men. Report of National Institute on Aging Advisory Panel on Testosterone Replacement in Men. *J Clin Endocrinol Metab.* 86:4611, 2001.

Afiadata A. et al. Testosterone replacement therapy:

Who to evaluate, what to use, how to follow, and who is at risk? *Hosp Pract.* 42:69, 2014.

Ahlering T.E. et al. Testosterone replacement therapy reduces biochemical recurrence after radical prostatectomy. *BJU Int.* 2020.

Ahmed T. et al. Is testosterone replacement safe in men with cardiovascular disease? *Cureus.* 12:e7324, 2020.

Aleman-Mateo H. et al. Association between insulin resistance and low relative appendicular skeletal muscle mass: Evidence from a cohort study in community-dwelling older men and women participants. *J Gerontol A Biol Sci Med Sci.* 69:871, 2014.

Alexandersen P. et al. The aging male: Testosterone deficiency and testosterone replacement. An up-date. *Atherosclerosis.* 173:157, 2004.

Allan C.A. et al. Age-related changes in testosterone and the role of replacement therapy in older men. *Clin Endocrinol.* 60:653, 2004.

Almehmadi Y. et al. Testosterone replacement therapy improves the health-related quality of life of men diagnosed with late-onset hypogonadism. *Arab J Urol.* 14:31, 2016.

Angelova P. et al. Testosterone replacement therapy improves erythrocyte membrane lipid composition in hypogonadal men. *Aging Male.* 15:173, 2012.

As P. et al. Benefits and consequences of testosterone replacement therapy: A review. *Eur Endocrinol.* 9:59, 2013.

American Society of Andrology.. Testosterone replacement therapy for male aging: ASA position statement. *J Androl.* 27:133, 2006.

Baillargeon J. et al. Testosterone replacement therapy and hospitalization rates in men with

COPD. *Chron Respir Dis.* 16:1479972318793004, 2019.

Bain J. Andropause. Testosterone replacement therapy for aging men. *Can Fam Physician.* 47:91, 2001.

Barbonetti A. et al. Testosterone replacement therapy. *Andrology.* 2020.

Barqawi A. et al. Testosterone replacement therapy and the risk of prostate cancer. Is there a link? *Int J Impot Res.* 18:323, 2006.

Basaria S. et al. Effects of testosterone replacement in men with opioid-induced androgen deficiency: A randomized controlled trial. *Pain.* 156:280, 2015.

Bassil N. et al. The benefits and risks of testosterone replacement therapy: A review. *Ther Clin Risk Manag.* 5:427, 2009.

Batrinos M.L. Testosterone and aggressive behavior in man. *Int J Endocrinol Metab.* 10:563, 2012.

Bhasin S. et al. Issues in testosterone replacement in older men. *J Clin Endocrinol Metab.* 83:3435, 1998.

Bhasin S. et al. Testosterone therapy in men with hypogonadism: An endocrine society clinical practice guideline. *J Clin Endocrinol Metab.* 103:1715, 2018.

Bhasin S. et al. Effect of testosterone replacement on measures of mobility in older men with mobility limitation and low testosterone concentrations: Secondary analyses of the testosterone trials. *Lancet Diabetes Endocrinol.* 6:879, 2018.

Bhasin S. et al. The effects of supraphysiologic doses of testosterone on muscle size and strength in normal men. *N Engl J Med.* 335:1, 1996.

Boden W.E. et al. Testosterone concentrations and risk of cardiovascular events in androgen-deficient men with atherosclerotic cardiovascular disease. *Am Heart J.* 224:65, 2020.

Borst S.E. et al. Testosterone replacement therapy for older men. *Clin Interv Aging.* 2:561, 2007.

Brand T.C. et al. Testosterone replacement therapy and prostate cancer: A word of caution. *Curr Urol Rep.* 8:185, 2007.

Busnelli A. et al. 'Forever young'-testosterone replacement therapy: A blockbuster drug despite flabby evidence and broken promises. *Hum Reprod.* 32:719, 2017.

Catakoglu A.B. et al. Testosterone replacement therapy and cardiovascular events. *Turk Kardiyol Dern Ars.* 45:664, 2017.

Celik O. et al. Testosterone replacement therapy: Should it be performed in erectile dysfunction? *Nephrourol Mon.* 5:858, 2013.

Chahla E.J. et al. Testosterone replacement therapy and cardiovascular risk factors modification. *Aging Male.* 14:83, 2011.

Cheng Y. et al. Factors associated with the initiation of testosterone replacement therapy in men from the 45 and up study. *Aust J Gen Pract.* 47:698, 2018.

Cho N.H. et al. Letter: Association of thigh muscle mass with insulin resistance and incident type 2 diabetes mellitus in Japanese Americans (Diabetes Metab J 2018;42:488-95). *Diabetes Metab J.* 43:123, 2019.

Cole A.P. et al. Impact of testosterone replacement therapy on thromboembolism, heart disease and obstructive sleep apnoea in men. *BJU Int.* 121:811, 2018.

Collet T.H. et al. Endogenous testosterone levels and the risk of incident cardiovascular events in elderly men: The MROS prospective study. *J Endocr Soc.* 4:bvaa038, 2020.

Corona G. et al. Testosterone therapy: What we have learned from trials. *J Sex Med.* 17:447, 2020.

Corona G.G. et al. Testosterone replacement therapy

and cardiovascular risk: A review. *World J Mens Health.* 33:130, 2015.

Crossland H. et al. The impact of immobilisation and inflammation on the regulation of muscle mass and insulin resistance: Different routes to similar end-points. *J Physiol.* 597:1259, 2019.

Cruz-Topete D. et al. Uncovering sex-specific mechanisms of action of testosterone and redox balance. *Redox Biol.* 31:101490, 2020.

Cui Y. et al. The effect of testosterone replacement therapy on prostate cancer: A systematic review and meta-analysis. *Prostate Cancer Prostatic Dis.* 17:132, 2014.

Cunningham G.R. Testosterone replacement therapy for late-onset hypogonadism. *Nat Clin Pract Urol.* 3:260, 2006.

Cunningham G.R. Andropause or male menopause? Rationale for testosterone replacement therapy in older men with low testosterone levels. *Endocr Pract.* 19:847, 2013.

Dean J.D. et al. The international society for sexual medicine's process of care for the assessment and management of testosterone deficiency in adult men. *J Sex Med.* 12:1660, 2015.

Dimitriadis F. et al. Effect of testosterone replacement treatment on constitutional and sexual symptoms in type 2 diabetic men: Need for rules. *Asian J Androl.* 17:217, 2015.

Dimopoulou C. et al. EMAS position statement: Testosterone replacement therapy in the aging male. *Maturitas.* 84:94, 2016.

Dontas A.S. et al. Long-term effects of anabolic steroids on renal functions in the aged subject. *J Gerontol.* 22:268, 1967.

Efesoy O. et al. The effect of testosterone replacement

therapy on penile hemodynamics in hypogonadal men with erectile dysfunction, having veno-occlusive dysfunction. *Am J Mens Health*. 12:634, 2018.

Farooqi V. et al. Anabolic steroids for rehabilitation after hip fracture in older people. *Cochrane Database Syst Rev*. CD008887, 2014.

Fillo J. et al. The effect of long term testosterone replacement therapy on bone mineral density. *Bratisl Lek Listy*. 120:291, 2019.

Francomano D. et al. Cardiovascular effect of testosterone replacement therapy in aging male. *Acta Biomed*. 81 Suppl 1:101, 2010.

Gagliano-Juca T. et al. Trials of testosterone replacement reporting cardiovascular adverse events. *Asian J Androl*. 20:131, 2018.

Gagliano-Juca T. et al. Effects of testosterone replacement on electrocardiographic parameters in men: Findings from two randomized trials. *J Clin Endocrinol Metab*. 102:1478, 2017.

Gagliano-Juca T. et al. Differential effects of testosterone on peripheral neutrophils, monocytes and platelets in men: Findings from two trials. *Andrology*. 2020.

Gharahdaghi N. et al. Testosterone therapy induces molecular programming augmenting physiological adaptations to resistance exercise in older men. *J Cachexia Sarcopenia Muscle*. 10:1276, 2019.

Groti K. et al. The impact of testosterone replacement therapy on glycemic control, vascular function, and components of the metabolic syndrome in obese hypogonadal men with type 2 diabetes. *Aging Male*. 21:158, 2018.

Guo C. et al. Efficacy and safety of testosterone replacement therapy in men with hypogonadism: A meta-analysis study of placebo-controlled trials. *Exp Ther Med.* 11:853, 2016.

Guo W. et al. Testosterone plus low-intensity physical training in late life improves functional performance, skeletal muscle mitochondrial biogenesis, and mitochondrial quality control in male mice. *PLoS One.* 7:e51180, 2012.

Guzzoni V. et al. Tendon remodeling in response to resistance training, anabolic androgenic steroids and aging. *Cells.* 7:2018.

Gysel T. et al. Association between insulin resistance, lean mass and muscle torque/force in proximal versus distal body parts in healthy young men. *J Musculoskelet Neuronal Interact.* 14:41, 2014.

Hackett G. Metabolic effects of testosterone therapy in men with type 2 diabetes and metabolic syndrome. *Sex Med Rev.* 2019.

Hackett G. et al. Serum testosterone, testosterone replacement therapy and all-cause mortality in men with type 2 diabetes: Retrospective consideration of the impact of PDE5 inhibitors and statins. *Int J Clin Pract.* 70:244, 2016.

Han S.J. et al. Association of thigh muscle mass with insulin resistance and incident type 2 diabetes mellitus in Japanese Americans. *Diabetes Metab J.* 42:488, 2018.

Haring R. et al. No evidence found for an association between trial characteristics and treatment effects in randomized trials of testosterone therapy in men: A meta-epidemiological study. *J Clin Epidemiol.* 122:12, 2020.

Hassan J. et al. Testosterone deficiency syndrome: Benefits, risks, and realities associated with testosterone replacement therapy. *Can J Urol.* 23:20, 2016.

Heo J.E. et al. Association between the thigh muscle

and insulin resistance according to body mass index in middle-aged Korean adults. *Diabetes Metab J.* 2020.

Hirasawa Y. et al. Evaluation of skeletal muscle mass indices, assessed by bioelectrical impedance, as indicators of insulin resistance in patients with type 2 diabetes. *J Phys Ther Sci.* 31:190, 2019.

Hosoi T. et al. Effect of testosterone replacement therapy on sarcopenia: Case report of an older man with late-onset hypogonadism. *Geriatr Gerontol Int.* 20:85, 2020.

Huang G. et al. Effects of testosterone replacement on metabolic and inflammatory markers in men with opioid-induced androgen deficiency. *Clin Endocrinol (Oxf).* 85:232, 2016.

Huang G. et al. Effects of testosterone replacement on pain catastrophizing and sleep quality in men with opioid-induced androgen deficiency. *Pain Med.* 18:1070, 2017.

Jaeger E.C.B. et al. Testosterone replacement causes dose-dependent improvements in spatial memory among aged male rats. *Psychoneuroendocrinology.* 113:104550, 2020.

Jayasena C.N. et al. A systematic review of randomized controlled trials investigating the efficacy and safety of testosterone therapy for female sexual dysfunction in postmenopausal women. *Clin Endocrinol.* 90:391, 2019.

Jeong S.M. et al. Effect of testosterone replacement treatment in testosterone deficiency syndrome patients with metabolic syndrome. *Korean J Urol.* 52:566, 2011.

Jones S.D., Jr. et al. Erythrocytosis and polycythemia secondary to testosterone replacement therapy in the aging male. *Sex Med Rev.* 3:101, 2015.

Jones T.H. et al. Randomized controlled trials - mechanistic studies of testosterone and the cardiovascular system. *Asian J Androl.* 20:120, 2018.

Jung H.J. et al. Effect of testosterone replacement therapy on cognitive performance and depression in men with testosterone deficiency syndrome. *World J Mens Health.* 34:194, 2016.

Junjie W. et al. Testosterone replacement therapy has limited effect on increasing bone mass density in older men: A meta-analysis. *Curr Pharm Des.* 25:73, 2019.

Kalra S. et al. Testosterone replacement in male hypogonadism. *Clin Pharmacol.* 2:149, 2010.

Kaplan A.L. et al. Testosterone replacement therapy following the diagnosis of prostate cancer: Outcomes and utilization trends. *J Sex Med.* 11:1063, 2014.

Kato Y. et al. The five-year effects of testosterone replacement therapy on lipid profile and glucose tolerance among hypogonadal men in japan: A case control study. *Aging Male.* 1, 2019.

Kawanabe S. et al. Association of the muscle/fat mass ratio with insulin resistance in gestational diabetes mellitus. *Endocr J.* 66:75, 2019.

Kempegowda P. et al. Long-term testosterone undecanoate replacement therapy: Impact of ethnicity. *Clin Endocrinol.* 92:428, 2020.

Kohn T.P. et al. Effects of testosterone replacement therapy on lower urinary tract symptoms: A systematic review and meta-analysis. *Eur Urol.* 69:1083, 2016.

Kovac J.R. et al. A positive role for anabolic androgenic steroids: Preventing metabolic syndrome and type 2 diabetes mellitus. *Fertil Steril.* 102:e5, 2014.

Kwong J.C.C. et al. Testosterone deficiency: A review and comparison of current guidelines. *J Sex Med.* 16:812, 2019.

Lang P.O. et al. Testosterone replacement therapy in

reversing "andropause": What is the proof-of-principle? *Rejuvenation Res.* 15:453, 2012.

Lee S.W. et al. Appendicular skeletal muscle mass and insulin resistance in an elderly Korean population: The Korean social life, health and aging project-health examination cohort. *Diabetes Metab J.* 39:37, 2015.

Legros J.J. et al. Oral testosterone replacement in symptomatic late-onset hypogonadism: Effects on rating scales and general safety in a randomized, placebo-controlled study. *Eur J Endocrinol.* 160:821, 2009.

Lenfant L. et al. Testosterone replacement therapy (TRT) and prostate cancer: An updated systematic review with a focus on previous or active localized prostate cancer. *Urol Oncol.* 2020.

Leung K.M. et al. Update on testosterone replacement therapy in hypogonadal men. *Curr Urol Rep.* 16:57, 2015.

Lim D. et al. Can testosterone replacement decrease the memory problem of old age? *Med Hypotheses.* 60:893, 2003.

Linderman J.K. et al. Effect of special operations training on testosterone, lean body mass, and strength and the potential for therapeutic testosterone replacement: A review of the literature. *J Spec Oper Med.* 20:94, 2020.

Lindqvist Bagge A.S. et al. Somatic effects of AAS abuse: A 30-years follow-up study of male former power sports athletes. *J Sci Med Sport.* 20:814, 2017.

Loo S.Y. et al. Cardiovascular and cerebrovascular safety of testosterone replacement therapy among aging men with low testosterone levels: A cohort study. *Am J Med.* 2019.

Mangolim A.S. et al. Effectiveness of testosterone

therapy in obese men with low testosterone levels, for losing weight, controlling obesity complications, and preventing cardiovascular events: Protocol of a systematic review of randomized controlled trials. *Medicine.* 97:e0482, 2018.

Mascarenhas A. et al. Factors that may be influencing the rise in prescription testosterone replacement therapy in adult men: A qualitative study. *Aging Male.* 19:90, 2016.

Matsumoto A.M. Testosterone replacement in men with age-related low testosterone: What did we learn from the testosterone trials? *Curr Opin Endocr Metab Res.* 6:34, 2019.

McClintock T.R. et al. Testosterone replacement therapy is associated with an increased risk of urolithiasis. *World J Urol.* 37:2737, 2019.

McCullough A. Alternatives to testosterone replacement: Testosterone restoration. *Asian J Androl.* 17:201, 2015.

McGill J.J. et al. Androgen deficiency in older men: Indications, advantages, and pitfalls of testosterone replacement therapy. *Cleve Clin J Med.* 79:797, 2012.

Millar A.C. et al. Predicting low testosterone in aging men: A systematic review. *CMAJ.* 188:E321, 2016.

Moon D.G. et al. The ideal goal of testosterone replacement therapy: Maintaining testosterone levels or managing symptoms? *J Clin Med.* 8:2019.

Moon S.S. Low skeletal muscle mass is associated with insulin resistance, diabetes, and metabolic syndrome in the Korean population: The Korea National Health and Nutrition Examination Survey (KNHANES) 2009-2010. *Endocr J.* 61:61, 2014.

Nakano K. et al. Testosterone replacement therapy for

late-onset hypogonadism after radical prostatectomy: A case report. *Hinyokika Kiyo.* 60:397, 2014.

Nam S.Y. et al. Low-dose growth hormone treatment combined with diet restriction decreases insulin resistance by reducing visceral fat and increasing muscle mass in obese type 2 diabetic patients. *Int J Obes Relat Metab Disord.* 25:1101, 2001.

Nam Y.S. et al. Testosterone replacement, muscle strength, and physical function. *World J Mens Health.* 36:110, 2018.

Nian Y. et al. Testosterone replacement therapy improves health-related quality of life for patients with late-onset hypogonadism: A meta-analysis of randomized controlled trials. *Andrologia.* 49:2017.

Nightingale T.E. et al. Body composition changes with testosterone replacement therapy following spinal cord injury and aging: A mini review. *J Spinal Cord Med.* 41:624, 2018.

Ohlsson C. et al. High serum testosterone is associated with reduced risk of cardiovascular events in elderly men. The MROS (osteoporotic fractures in men) study in Sweden. *J Am Coll Cardiol.* 58:1674, 2011.

Ohlsson C. et al. Genetic determinants of serum testosterone concentrations in men. *PLoS Genet.* 7:e1002313, 2011.

Okada K. et al. Improved lower urinary tract symptoms associated with testosterone replacement therapy in Japanese men with late-onset hypogonadism. *Am J Mens Health.* 12:1403, 2018.

Paduch D.A. et al. Testosterone replacement in androgen-deficient men with ejaculatory dysfunction: A randomized controlled trial. *J Clin Endocrinol Metab.* 100:2956, 2015.

Pantalone K.M. et al. Testosterone replacement

therapy and the risk of adverse cardiovascular outcomes and mortality. *Basic Clin Androl.* 29:5, 2019.

Park H.S. et al. Determinants of bone mass and insulin resistance in Korean postmenopausal women: Muscle area, strength, or composition? *Yonsei Med J.* 60:742, 2019.

Patrick Selph J. et al. Testosterone replacement therapy in men with prostate cancer: What is the evidence? *Sex Med Rev.* 1:135, 2013.

Perry P.J. et al. Bioavailable testosterone as a correlate of cognition, psychological status, quality of life, and sexual function in aging males: Implications for testosterone replacement therapy. *Ann Clin Psychiatry.* 13:75, 2001.

Pintana H. et al. Testosterone replacement attenuates cognitive decline in testosterone-deprived lean rats, but not in obese rats, by mitigating brain oxidative stress. *Age.* 37:84, 2015.

Ponce O.J. et al. The efficacy and adverse events of testosterone replacement therapy in hypogonadal men: A systematic review and meta-analysis of randomized, placebo-controlled trials. *J Clin Endocrinol Metab.* 2018.

Ponce O.J. et al. The efficacy and adverse events of testosterone replacement therapy in hypogonadal men: A systematic review and meta-analysis of randomized, placebo-controlled trials. *J Clin Endocrinol Metab.* 2018.

Pongkan W. et al. Roles of testosterone replacement in cardiac ischemia-reperfusion injury. *J Cardiovasc Pharmacol Ther.* 21:27, 2016.

Ramachandran S. et al. Testosterone replacement therapy: Pre-treatment sex hormone-binding globulin levels and age may identify clinical subgroups. *Andrology.* 2020.

Retzler J. et al. Preferences for the administration of

testosterone gel: Evidence from a discrete choice experiment. *Patient Prefer Adherence.* 13:657, 2019.

Saad F. et al. Effects of long-term testosterone replacement therapy, with a temporary intermission, on glycemic control of nine hypogonadal men with type 1 diabetes mellitus - a series of case reports. *Aging Male.* 18:164, 2015.

Salman M. et al. Early weight loss predicts the reduction of obesity in men with erectile dysfunction and hypogonadism undergoing long-term testosterone replacement therapy. *Aging Male.* 20:45, 2017.

Sansone A. et al. Testosterone replacement therapy: The emperor's new clothes. *Rejuvenation Res.* 20:9, 2017.

Santella C. et al. Testosterone replacement therapy and the risk of prostate cancer in men with late-onset hypogonadism. *Am J Epidemiol.* 2019.

Sattler F.R. et al. Testosterone and growth hormone improve body composition and muscle performance in older men. *J Clin Endocrinol Metab.* 94:1991, 2009.

Seko T. et al. Lower limb muscle mass is associated with insulin resistance more than lower limb muscle strength in non-diabetic older adults. *Geriatr Gerontol Int.* 19:1254, 2019.

Shaikh K. et al. Biomarkers and noncalcified coronary artery plaque progression in older men treated with testosterone. *J Clin Endocrinol Metab.* 105:2020.

Shigehara K. et al. Effect of testosterone replacement therapy on sexual function and glycemic control among hypogonadal men with type 2 diabetes mellitus. *Int J Impot Res.* 31:25, 2019.

Shigehara K. et al. Effects of testosterone replacement therapy on nocturia and quality of life in men with hypogonadism: A subanalysis of a previous prospective randomized controlled study in japan. *Aging Male.* 18:169, 2015.

Shigehara K. et al. Effects of testosterone replacement therapy on hypogonadal men with osteopenia or osteoporosis: A subanalysis of a prospective randomized controlled study in Japan (earth study). *Aging Male.* 20:139, 2017.

Shin Y.S. et al. The optimal indication for testosterone replacement therapy in late onset hypogonadism. *J Clin Med.* 8:2019.

Sloan J.P. et al. A pilot study of anabolic steroids in elderly patients with hip fractures. *J Am Geriatr Soc.* 40:1105, 1992.

Snyder P.J. et al. Effects of testosterone treatment in older men. *N Engl J Med.* 374:611, 2016.

Snyder P.J. et al. Lessons from the testosterone trials. *Endocr Rev.* 39:369, 2018.

Snyder P.J. et al. The testosterone trials: Seven coordinated trials of testosterone treatment in elderly men. *Clin Trials.* 11:362, 2014.

Spitzer M. et al. Risks and benefits of testosterone therapy in older men. *Nat Rev Endocrinol.* 9:414, 2013.

Srikanthan P. et al. Relative muscle mass is inversely associated with insulin resistance and pre-diabetes. Findings from the third national health and nutrition examination survey. *J Clin Endocrinol Metab.* 96:2898, 2011.

Storer T.W. et al. Effects of testosterone supplementation for 3 years on muscle performance and physical function in older men. *J Clin Endocrinol Metab.* 102:583, 2017.

Storer T.W. et al. Testosterone attenuates age-related fall in aerobic function in mobility limited older men with low testosterone. *J Clin Endocrinol Metab.* 101:2562, 2016.

Storer T.W. et al. Changes in muscle mass, muscle strength, and power but not physical function are related to testosterone dose in healthy older men. *J Am Geriatr Soc.* 56:1991, 2008.

Strollo F. et al. Low-intermediate dose testosterone replacement therapy by different pharmaceutical preparations improves frailty score in elderly hypogonadal hyperglycaemic patients. *Aging Male.* 16:33, 2013.

Sumii K. et al. Prospective assessment of health-related quality of life in men with late-onset hypogonadism who received testosterone replacement therapy. *Andrologia.* 48:198, 2016.

Surampudi P.N. et al. Hypogonadism in the aging male diagnosis, potential benefits, and risks of testosterone replacement therapy. *Int J Endocrinol.* 2012:625434, 2012.

Tan S. et al. Effects of testosterone supplementation on separate cognitive domains in cognitively healthy older men: A meta-analysis of current randomized clinical trials. *Am J Geriatr Psychiatry.* 27:1232, 2019.

Tao J. et al. Testosterone supplementation in patients with chronic heart failure: A meta-analysis of randomized controlled trials. *Front Endocrinol (Lausanne).* 11:110, 2020.

Traustadottir T. et al. Long-term testosterone supplementation in older men attenuates age-related decline in aerobic capacity. *J Clin Endocrinol Metab.* 103:2861, 2018.

Tsametis C.P. et al. Testosterone replacement therapy: For whom, when and how? *Metabolism.* 86:69, 2018.

Volpato S. et al. The benefit and risk of testosterone

replacement therapy in older men: Effects on lipid metabolism. *Acta Biomed.* 81 Suppl 1:95, 2010.

Volpi R. et al. Extra-prostatic complications of testosterone replacement therapy. *J Endocrinol Invest.* 28:75, 2005.

Wald M. et al. Testosterone replacement therapy for older men. *J Androl.* 27:126, 2006.

Wallis C.J. et al. Survival and cardiovascular events in men treated with testosterone replacement therapy: An intention-to-treat observational cohort study. *Lancet Diabetes Endocrinol.* 4:498, 2016.

Walther A. et al. Testosterone and dehydroepiandrosterone treatment in ageing men: Are we all set? *World J Mens Health.* 2019.

Wang C. et al. Validity and clinically meaningful changes in the psychosexual daily questionnaire and derogatis interview for sexual function assessment: Results from the testosterone trials. *J Sex Med.* 15:997, 2018.

Washington T.A. et al. Lactate dehydrogenase regulation in aged skeletal muscle: Regulation by anabolic steroids and functional overload. *Exp Gerontol.* 57:66, 2014.

Yabluchanskiy A. et al. Is testosterone replacement therapy in older men effective and safe? *Drugs Aging.* 36:981, 2019.

Yassin A. et al. Effects of testosterone replacement therapy withdrawal and re-treatment in hypogonadal elderly men upon obesity, voiding function and prostate safety parameters. *Aging Male.* 19:64, 2016.

Yeap B.B. et al. Epidemiological and mendelian randomization studies of dihydrotestosterone and estradiol and leukocyte telomere length in men. *J Clin Endocrinol Metab.* 101:1299, 2016.

Yeap B.B. et al. Testosterone treatment in older men: Clinical implications and unresolved questions from the testosterone trials. *Lancet Diabetes Endocrinol.* 6:659, 2018.

Zhou T. et al. Effects of testosterone supplementation on body composition in HIV patients: A meta-analysis of double-blinded randomized controlled trials. *Curr Med Sci.* 38:191, 2018.

Zitzmann M. Testosterone replacement treatment in older people with and without co-morbidities. *Internist.* 61:549, 2020.

References: Anabolic Steroids and Children

Bierich J.R. Anabolic steroids and growth. *Minerva Med.* 62:2572, 1971.

Bierich J.R. Effects and side effects of anabolic steroids in children. *Acta Endocrinol Suppl.* 39(Suppl 63):89, 1961.

Blashill A.J. et al. Anabolic-androgenic steroids and condom use: Potential mechanisms in adolescent males. *J Sex Res.* 51:690, 2014.

Blashill A.J. et al. Sexual orientation and anabolic-androgenic steroids in U.S. Adolescent boys. *Pediatrics.* 133:469, 2014.

Buckley W.E. et al. Estimated prevalence of anabolic steroid use among male high school seniors. *JAMA.* 260:3441, 1988.

Canlorbe P. et al. Effect of 2 anabolic steroids on "essential" delayed growth. *Ann Pediatr.* 16:582, 1969.

Chaudhuri R.K. Anabolic steroids and growth promotion. *Indian J Pediatr.* 31:313, 1964.

Clark A.S. et al. Chronic administration of anabolic

steroids disrupts pubertal onset and estrous cyclicity in rats. *Biol Reprod.* 68:465, 2003.

Colombini G. Anabolic steroids in pediatrics. *Pediatria (Napoli).* 70:993, 1962.

Cunningham R.L. et al. Pubertal exposure to anabolic androgenic steroids increases spine densities on neurons in the limbic system of male rats. *Neuroscience.* 150:609, 2007.

Damasceno E.F. et al. Branch retinal vein occlusion and anabolic steroids abuse in young bodybuilders. *Acta Ophthalmol.* 87:580, 2009.

Deamer W.C. Stimulation of growth in boys by sublingual testosterone therapy. *Am J Dis Child.* 75:850, 1948.

Denham B.E. Anabolic-androgenic steroids and adolescents: Recent developments. *J Addict Nurs.* 23:167, 2012.

Dodge T. et al. Influence of parent-adolescent communication about anabolic steroids on adolescent athletes' willingness to try performance-enhancing substances. *Subst Use Misuse.* 50:1307, 2015.

DuRant R.H. et al. Use of multiple drugs among adolescents who use anabolic steroids. *N Engl J Med.* 328:922, 1993.

Ercoli A. et al. Steroidal ethers: Effect of some anabolic steroids on the growth curve, body composition and weight of various organs in male castrated rats. *Boll Soc Ital Biol Sper.* 39:2090, 1963.

Escamilla R.F. Treatment of preadolescent eunuchoidism with testosterone linguets. *Am Pract Dig Treat.* 3:425, 1949.

Fahey, T.D., et al. "Pubertal stage differences in hormonal and hematological responses to maximal exercise in males." *J. Appl. Physiol.* 46: 823-827, 1979.

Fruchart G. Hypodermic insertions of testosterone in

hypogenitalism in adolescents. *J Sci Med Lille.* 68:150, 1950.

Fujii T. et al. Effects of some anabolic steroids on the growth in male and female rats. *Endocrinol Jpn.* 9:93, 1962.

Galletti F. et al. Steroidal ethers: Effect of some anabolic steroids on the growth curve and weight of various organs in intact adult rats. *Boll Soc Ital Biol Sper.* 39:2095, 1963.

Ganson K.T. et al. Exploring anabolic-androgenic steroid use and teen dating violence among adolescent males. *Subst Use Misuse.* 54:779, 2019.

Gautier E. et al. Anabolic steroids in anuria in the child. *Minerva Med.* 52:366, 1961.

Gebhardt A. et al. The effect of anabolic steroids on mandibular growth. *Am J Orthod Dentofacial Orthop.* 123:435, 2003.

Goldberg L. et al. Effects of a multidimensional anabolic steroid prevention intervention. The adolescents training and learning to avoid steroids (Atlas) program. *JAMA.* 276:1555, 1996.

Goth E. Management of retarded growth with anabolic steroids. *Ther Hung.* 12:140, 1964.

Griffiths S. et al. Pornography use in sexual minority males: Associations with body dissatisfaction, eating disorder symptoms, thoughts about using anabolic steroids and quality of life. *Aust N Z J Psychiatry.* 52:339, 2018.

Groughs W. et al. The effect of hormones and anabolic steroids on growth and development. I. Growth hormone, thyroid hormone, glucocorticoids, androgenic hormones of the adrenal glands and gonads. *Ned Tijdschr Geneeskd.* 108:1797, 1964.

Gupta S. Anabolic steroids in childhood malnutrition. *J*

Indian Med Assoc. 48:111, 1967.

Gustafsson G. et al. Acquired aplastic anaemia in children treated with corticosteroids and anabolic steroids. *Scand J Haematol.* 26:195, 1981.

Halliburton A.E. et al. Health beliefs as a key determinant of intent to use anabolic-androgenic steroids (AAS) among high-school football players: Implications for prevention. *Int J Adolesc Youth.* 23:269, 2018.

Hansen H.G. On the use of anabolic steroids in children. *Monatsschr Kinderheilkd.* 110:236, 1962.

Harding F.E. Sublingual methyl testosterone for boyhood emotional, physical, and genital immaturity. *J Pediatr.* 32:351, 1948.

Hoffman J.R. et al. Nutritional supplementation and anabolic steroid use in adolescents. *Med Sci Sports Exerc.* 40:15, 2008.

Johnston J.A. Factors influencing retention of nitrogen and calcium in period of growth; effect of methyl testosterone. *Am J Dis Child.* 74:52, 1947.

Jones R.W. et al. The effects of anabolic steroids on growth, body composition, and metabolism in boys with chronic renal failure on regular hemodialysis. *J Pediatr.* 97:559, 1980.

Kageyama A. Water intake and output in newborn infants--effect of anabolic steroids. *Nihon Sanka Fujinka Gakkai Zasshi.* 18:165, 1966.

Kerr J.M. et al. Anabolic-androgenic steroids: Use and abuse in pediatric patients. *Pediatr Clin North Am.* 54:771, 2007.

Kindlundh A.M. et al. Adolescent use of anabolic-androgenic steroids and relations to self-reports of social, personality and health aspects. *Eur J Public Health.* 11:322, 2001.

Kindlundh A.M. et al. Factors associated with adolescent use of doping agents: Anabolic-androgenic steroids. *Addiction*. 94:543, 1999.

Kokkevi A. et al. Daily exercise and anabolic steroids use in adolescents: A cross-national European study. *Subst Use Misuse*. 43:2053, 2008.

Lane J.R. et al. The influence of endogenous and exogenous sex hormones in adolescents with attention to oral contraceptives and anabolic steroids. *J Adolesc Health*. 15:630, 1994.

Linsk J.A. Testosterone therapy in children; a review of the literature. *Arch Pediatr*. 67:371, 1950.

Lumia A.R. et al. Impact of anabolic androgenic steroids on adolescent males. *Physiol Behav*. 100:199, 2010.

Mattila V.M. et al. Use of dietary supplements and anabolic-androgenic steroids among Finnish adolescents in 1991-2005. *Eur J Public Health*. 20:306, 2010.

Melloni R.H., Jr. et al. Adolescent exposure to anabolic/androgenic steroids and the neurobiology of offensive aggression: A hypothalamic neural model based on findings in pubertal Syrian hamsters. *Horm Behav*. 58:177, 2010.

Metzl J.D. Anabolic steroids and the pediatric community. *Pediatrics*. 116:1542, 2005.

Middleman A.B. et al. High-risk behaviors among high school students in Massachusetts who use anabolic steroids. *Pediatrics*. 96:268, 1995.

Mitchell G.L. Report to the commissioner of baseball of an independent investigation into the illegal use of steroids and other performance enhancing substances by players in major league baseball. 2007.

Modlinski R. et al. The effect of anabolic steroids on the gastrointestinal system, kidneys, and adrenal glands. *Curr Sports Med Rep*. 5:104, 2006.

Mohd Mutalip S.S. et al. Pubertal anabolic androgenic steroid exposure in male rats affects levels of gonadal steroids, mating frequency, and pregnancy outcome. *J Basic Clin Physiol Pharmacol.* 30:29, 2018.

Moore D.C. et al. Studies of anabolic steroids: V. Effect of prolonged oxandrolone administration on growth in children and adolescents with uncomplicated short stature. *Pediatrics.* 58:412, 1976.

Moore D.C. et al. Studies of anabolic steroids. VI. Effect of prolonged administration of oxandrolone on growth in children and adolescents with gonadal dysgenesis. *J Pediatr.* 90:462, 1977.

Nagata J.M. et al. Association between legal performance-enhancing substances and use of anabolic-androgenic steroids in young adults. *JAMA Pediatr.* 174:992, 2020.

Nicholls A.R. et al. Children's first experience of taking anabolic-androgenic steroids can occur before their 10th birthday: A systematic review identifying 9 factors that predicted doping among young people. *Front Psychol.* 8:1015, 2017.

Nilsson S. et al. Attitudes and behaviors with regards to androgenic anabolic steroids among male adolescents in a county of Sweden. *Subst Use Misuse.* 40:1, 2005.

Nilsson S. et al. Attitudes and behaviors with regards to androgenic anabolic steroids among male adolescents in a county of Sweden. *Subst Use Misuse.* 39:1183, 2004.

Nilsson S. et al. The prevalence of the use of androgenic anabolic steroids by adolescents in a county of Sweden. *Eur J Public Health.* 11:195, 2001.

Nilsson S. et al. Trends in the misuse of androgenic anabolic steroids among boys 16-17 years old in a primary health care area in Sweden. *Scand J Prim Health Care.* 19:181, 2001.

Nyda M.J. et al. The effect on the linear growth, weight gain, and histologic pattern of the testes of young rats by large doses of DOCA, lipoadrenal cortex, thyroid, thyroxine, testosterone propionate and physiologic doses of testosterone propionate. *J Clin Endocrinol Metab.* 10:818, 1950.

Prader A. The influence of anabolic steroids on growth. *Acta Endocrinol Suppl.* 39(Suppl 63):78, 1961.

Rachon D. et al. Prevalence and risk factors of ana-bolic-androgenic steroids (AAS) abuse among adoles-cents and young adults in Poland. *Soz Praventivmed.* 51:392, 2006.

Ray C.G. et al. Studies of anabolic steroids. 3. The ef-fect of oxandrolone on height and skeletal maturation in mongoloid children. *Am J Dis Child.* 110:618, 1965.

Ray C.G. et al. Studies of anabolic steroids. II. The ef-fect of oxandrolone on height and skeletal maturation in mongoloid children (a preliminary report). *Am J Dis Child.* 106:375, 1963.

Ricci L.A. et al. Adolescent anabolic/androgenic steroids: Aggression and anxiety during exposure pre-dict behavioral responding during withdrawal in Syrian hamsters (*mesocricetus auratus*). *Horm Behav.* 64:770, 2013.

Rogol A.D. Can anabolic steroids or human growth hormone affect the growth and maturation of adoles-cent athletes? *Pediatr Exerc Sci.* 26:423, 2014.

Rogol A.D. et al. Anabolic-androgenic steroids and the adolescent. *Pediatr Ann.* 21:175, 1992.

Rogol A.D. et al. Anabolic-androgenic steroids pro-foundly affect growth at puberty in boys. *NIDA Res Monogr.* 102:187, 1990.

Sadowska-Krepa E. et al. High-dose testosterone enanthate supplementation boosts oxidative stress, but exerts little effect on the antioxidant barrier in sedentary adolescent male rat liver. *Pharmacol Rep.* 69:673, 2017.

Sandvik M.R. et al. Anabolic-androgenic steroid use and correlates in Norwegian adolescents. *Eur J Sport Sci.* 18:903, 2018.

Stilger V.G. et al. Anabolic-androgenic steroid use among high school football players. *J Community Health.* 24:131, 1999.

Terney R. et al. The use of anabolic steroids in high school students. *Am J Dis Child.* 144:99, 1990.

Thevis M. et al. Determination of the prevalence of anabolic steroids, stimulants, and selected drugs subject to doping controls among elite sport students using analytical chemistry. *J Sports Sci.* 26:1059, 2008.

Thompson P.D. et al. Use of anabolic steroids among adolescents. *N Engl J Med.* 329:888, 1993.

Thorlindsson T. et al. Sport and use of anabolic androgenic steroids among Icelandic high school students: A critical test of three perspectives. *Subst Abuse Treat Prev Policy.* 5:32, 2010.

van de Pijpekamp G.H. Use of anabolic steroids in children. *Paediatr Indones.* 4:Suppl:185, 1964.

Wang M.Q. et al. Desire for weight gain and potential risks of adolescent males using anabolic steroids. *Percept Mot Skills.* 78:267, 1994.

Wichstrom L. et al. Use of anabolic-androgenic steroids in adolescence: Winning, looking good or being bad? *J Stud Alcohol.* 62:5, 2001.

Windsor R. et al. Prevalence of anabolic steroids use by male and female adolescents. *Med Sci Sports Exerc.* 21:494, 1989.

Yesalis C.E. et al. Self-reported use of anabolic-androgenic steroids by elite power lifters. *Phys Sportsmed.* 16:91, 1988. https://www.ncbi.nlm.nih.gov/pubmed/27404754

References: Anabolic Steroids and Sexual Physiology

Alibegovic A. Testicular morphology in hypogonadotropic hypogonadism after the abuse of anabolic steroids. *Forensic Sci Med Pathol.* 14:564, 2018.

Armstrong J.M. et al. Impact of anabolic androgenic steroids on sexual function. *Transl Androl Urol.* 7:483, 2018

Behre H.M. et al. Rationale, design and methods of the esprit study: Energy, sexual desire and body proportions with Androgel, testosterone 1% gel therapy, in hypogonadal men. *Aging Male.* 11:101, 2008.

Birzniece V. et al. Sex steroids and the GH axis: Implications for the management of hypopituitarism. *Best Pract Res Clin Endocrinol Metab.* 31:59, 2017.

Christou M.A. et al. Effects of anabolic androgenic steroids on the reproductive system of athletes and recreational users: A systematic review and meta-analysis. *Sports Med.* 47:1869, 2017.

Clark A.S. et al. Sex- and age-specific effects of anabolic androgenic steroids on reproductive behaviors and on gabaergic transmission in neuroendocrine control regions. *Brain Res.* 1126:122, 2006.

Cordaro F.G. et al. Selling androgenic anabolic steroids by the pound: Identification and analysis of popular websites on the internet. *Scand J Med Sci Sports.* 21:e247, 2011.

Cruz M. et al. [anabolic steroids and pathology of sex development]. *Munch Med Wochenschr.* 113:949, 1971.

de Luis D.A. et al. Anabolic steroids and gynecomastia. Review of the literature. *An Med Interna.* 18:489, 2001.

de Souza G.L. et al. Anabolic steroids and male infertility: A comprehensive review. *BJU Int.* 108:1860, 2011.

Diamandis E.P. A replacement for the testosterone "sex gap". *Clin Chem Lab Med.* 54:e61, 2016.

Drakeley A. et al. Duration of azoospermia following anabolic steroids. *Fertil Steril.* 81:226, 2004.

Drobnis E.Z. et al. Exogenous androgens and male reproduction. *Adv Exp Med Biol.* 1034:25, 2017.

El Osta R. et al. Anabolic steroids abuse and male infertility. *Basic Clin Androl.* 26:2, 2016.

Feinberg M.J. et al. The effect of anabolic-androgenic steroids on sexual behavior and reproductive tissues in male rats. *Physiol Behav.* 62:23, 1997.

Fernandez J.D. et al. Metabolic effects of hormone therapy in transgender patients. *Endocr Pract.* 22:383, 2016.

Ferrari W. et al. [action of anabolic steroids on the development of the genital system in the rabbit. VI Anabolic and androgenic activity of 13 beta-ethyl-17 beta-hydroxy-17 alpha-ethyl-4-gonen-3-one (norboletone) in the rat]. *Boll Soc Ital Biol Sper.* 44:1310, 1968.

Friedl K.E. et al. Self-treatment of gynecomastia in bodybuilders who use anabolic steroids. *Phys Sportsmed.* 17:67, 1989.

Giannico O. Treatment of sexual impotence with associated testosterone and vitamin E. *Clin Nuova Rass Prog Med Int.* 10:231, 1950.

Goldsmith E.D. et al. Interference with testosterone-induced growth of the seminal vesicles and coagulating glands in male mice by a folic acid antagonist. *Nature.* 164:62, 1949.

Heller C.G. et al. Improvement in spermatogenesis following depression of human testis with testosterone. *Fertil Steril.* 1:415, 1950.

Heller C.G. et al. The effect of testosterone administration upon the human testis. *J Clin Endocrinol Metab.* 10:816, 1950.

Hengevoss J. et al. Combined effects of androgen anabolic steroids and physical activity on the hypothalamic-pituitary-gonadal axis. *J Steroid Biochem Mol Biol.* 150:86, 2015.

Illei G. et al. The effect of anabolic steroids on the secretion of pituitary gonadotropins. *Acta Physiol Acad Sci Hung.* 22:189, 1962.

Ip E.J. et al. The Castro study: Unsafe sexual behaviors and illicit drug use among gay and bisexual men who use anabolic steroids. *Am J Addict.* 28:101, 2019.

Jones I.C. The action of testosterone on the adrenal cortex of the hypophysectomized, prepuberally castrated male mouse. *Endocrinology.* 44:427, 1949.

Kanayama G. et al. Prolonged hypogonadism in males following withdrawal from anabolic-androgenic steroids: An under-recognized problem. *Addiction.* 110:823, 2015.

Karila T. et al. Concomitant abuse of anabolic androgenic steroids and human chorionic gonadotrophin impairs spermatogenesis in power athletes. *Int J Sports Med.* 25:257, 2004.

Kim J.Y. et al. Anabolic-androgenic steroids and appetitive sexual behavior in male rats. *Horm Behav.* 66:585, 2014.

Knuth U.A. et al. Anabolic steroids and semen parameters in bodybuilders. *Fertil Steril.* 52:1041, 1989.

Lykhonosov M.P. et al. The medical aspect of using anabolic androgenic steroids in males attending gyms of Saint-Petersburg. *Probl Endokrinol.* 65:19, 2019.

Lykhonosov M.P. et al. Peculiarity of recovery of the hypothalamic-pituitary-gonadal (HPG) axis, in men after using androgenic anabolic steroids]. *Probl Endokrinol.* 66:104, 2020.

Martikainen H. et al. Testicular responsiveness to human chorionic gonadotrophin during transient hypogonadotrophic hypogonadism induced by androgenic/anabolic steroids in power athletes. *J Steroid Biochem.* 25:109, 1986.

McBride J.A. et al. The availability and acquisition of illicit anabolic androgenic steroids and testosterone preparations on the internet. *Am J Mens Health.* 12:1352, 2018.

McBride J.A. et al. Recovery of spermatogenesis following testosterone replacement therapy or anabolic-androgenic steroid use. *Asian J Androl.* 18:373, 2016.

Miner J.N. et al. An orally active selective androgen receptor modulator is efficacious on bone, muscle, and sex function with reduced impact on prostate. *Endocrinology.* 148:363, 2007.

Morgentaler, A. Strategies for testosterone therapy in men with metastatic prostate cancer in clinical practice: Introducing modified bipolar androgen therapy. *Andro Clin Res Ther.* 1: http://online.liebertpub.com/doi/10.1089/andro.2020.0009, 2021.

Naraghi M.A. et al. The effects of swimming exercise and supraphysiological doses of nandrolone decanoate on the testis in adult male rats: A transmission electron microscope study. *Folia Morphol.* 69:138, 2010.

Nieschlag E. et al. Mechanisms in endocrinology: Medical consequences of doping with anabolic androgenic steroids: Effects on reproductive functions. *Eur J Endocrinol.* 173:R47, 2015.

Onakomaiya M.M. et al. Mad men, women and steroid cocktails: A review of the impact of sex and other factors on anabolic androgenic steroids effects on affective behaviors. *Psychopharmacology.* 233:549, 2016.

Pena J.E. et al. Reversible azoospermia: Anabolic steroids may profoundly affect human immunodeficiency virus-seropositive men undergoing assisted reproduction. *Obstet Gynecol.* 101:1073, 2003.

Penatti C.A. et al. Chronic exposure to anabolic androgenic steroids alters activity and synaptic function in neuroendocrine control regions of the female mouse. *Neuropharmacology.* 61:653, 2011.

Pundir J. et al. Anabolic steroids and male subfertility. *J Obstet Gynaecol.* 28:810, 2008.

Rahnema C.D. et al. Anabolic steroid-induced hypogonadism: Diagnosis and treatment. *Fertil Steril.* 101:1271, 2014.

Rasmussen J.J. et al. Former abusers of anabolic androgenic steroids exhibit decreased testosterone levels and hypogonadal symptoms years after cessation: A case-control study. *PLoS One.* 11:e0161208, 2016.

Roselli C.E. The effect of anabolic-androgenic steroids on aromatase activity and androgen receptor binding in the rat preoptic area. *Brain Res.* 792:271, 1998.

Salerno M. et al. Anabolic androgenic steroids and carcinogenicity focusing on Leydig cell: A literature review. *Oncotarget.* 9:19415, 2018.

Semet M. et al. The impact of drugs on male fertility: A review. *Andrology.* 5:640, 2017.

Smit D.L. et al. Outpatient clinic for users of anabolic androgenic steroids: An overview. *Neth J Med.* 76:167, 2018.

Sorensen M.B. et al. Azoospermia in 2 body-builders after taking anabolic steroids. *Ugeskr Laeger.* 157:1044, 1995.

Torres-Calleja J. et al. Effect of androgenic anabolic steroids on semen parameters and hormone levels in bodybuilders. *Fertil Steril.* 74:1055, 2000.

Turner J.E. et al. Effect of prolonged administration of anabolic and androgenic steroids on reproductive function in the mare. *J Reprod Fertil Suppl.* 32:213, 1982.

Vargas R.A. et al. The prostate after administration of anabolic androgenic steroids: A morphometrical study in rats. *Int Braz J Urol.* 39:675, 2013.

References: Anabolic Steroids and the Cardiovascular System

Alen M. et al. Serum lipids in power athletes self-administering testosterone and anabolic steroids. *Int J Sports Med.* 6:139, 1985.

Alhadad A. et al. Pulmonary embolism associated with protein c deficiency and abuse of anabolic-androgen steroids. *Clin Appl Thromb Hemost.* 16:228, 2010.

Angell P. et al. Anabolic steroids and cardiovascular risk. *Sports Med.* 42:119, 2012.

Angell P.J. et al. Anabolic steroid use and longitudinal, radial, and circumferential cardiac motion. *Med Sci Sports Exerc.* 44:583, 2012.

Baggish A.L. et al. Cardiovascular toxicity of illicit anabolic-androgenic steroid use. *Circulation.* 135:1991, 2017.

Baggish A.L. et al. Long-term anabolic-androgenic steroid use is associated with left ventricular dysfunction. *Circ Heart Fail.* 3:472, 2010.

Bowman S. Anabolic steroids and infarction. *BMJ.* 300:750, 1990.

Bigi M.A.B. et al. Aortopathic effect of androgenic anabolic steroids. *J Echocardiogr.* 19:113, 2021.

Campbell R.S. et al. Studies on the influence of anabolic steroids on experimental atheroma: Androstanolone. *J Endocrinol.* 20:246, 1960.

Campbell S.E. et al. Pathologic remodeling of the myocardium in a weightlifter taking anabolic steroids. *Blood Press.* 2:213, 1993.

Carbone A. et al. Cardiac damage in athlete's heart: When the "supernormal" heart fails! *World J Cardiol.* 9:470, 2017.

Christou G.A. et al. Acute myocardial infarction in a young bodybuilder taking anabolic androgenic steroids: A case report and critical review of the literature. *Eur J Prev Cardiol.* 23:1785, 2016.

Cohen J.C. et al. Altered serum lipoprotein profiles in male and female power lifters ingesting anabolic steroids. *Phys Sportsmed.* 14:131, 1986.

Cohen J.C. et al. Insulin resistance and diminished glucose tolerance in powerlifters ingesting anabolic steroids. *J Clin Endocrinol Metab.* 64:960, 1987.

Cohen J.C. et al. Hypercholesterolemia in male power lifters using anabolic-androgenic steroids. *Phys Sportsmed.* 16:49, 1988.

Cohen L.I. et al. Lipoprotein (a) and cholesterol in body builders using anabolic androgenic steroids. *Med Sci Sports Exerc.* 28:176, 1996.

D'Andrea A. et al. Anabolic-androgenic steroids and athlete's heart: When big is not beautiful! *Int J Cardiol.* 203:486, 2016.

D'Andrea A. et al. Correction to: Left atrial myocardial dysfunction after chronic abuse of anabolic androgenic steroids: A speckle tracking echocardiography analysis. *Int J Cardiovasc Imaging.* 34:1561, 2018.

D'Andrea A. et al. Left atrial myocardial dysfunction after chronic abuse of anabolic androgenic steroids: A speckle tracking echocardiography analysis. *Int J Cardiovasc Imaging.* 34:1549, 2018.

Dickerman R.D. et al. Cardiovascular complications and anabolic steroids. *Eur Heart J.* 17:1912, 1996.

Dickerman R.D. et al. Echocardiography in fraternal twin bodybuilders with one abusing anabolic steroids. *Cardiology.* 88:50, 1997.

Dickerman R.D. et al. Sudden cardiac death in a 20-year-old bodybuilder using anabolic steroids. *Cardiology.* 86:172, 1995.

Do Carmo E.C. et al. Anabolic steroid associated to physical training induces deleterious cardiac effects. *Med Sci Sports Exerc.* 43:1836, 2011.

Dubinskii A.A. et al. Effect of anabolic steroids on the rabbits with cholesterol atherosclerosis. *Biull Eksp Biol Med.* 93:23, 1982.

Ebenbichler C.F. et al. Hyperhomocysteinemia in bodybuilders taking anabolic steroids. *Eur J Intern Med.* 12:43, 2001.

Edvardsson B. Hypertensive encephalopathy associated with anabolic-androgenic steroids used for bodybuilding. *Acta Neurol Belg.* 115:457, 2015.

Far H.R. et al. Cardiac hypertrophy in deceased users of anabolic androgenic steroids: An investigation of autopsy findings. *Cardiovasc Pathol.* 21:312, 2012.

Farzam K. Anabolic-androgenic steroids and cardiometabolic derangements. Cureus. 13:e12492, 2021.

Fiegel G. et al. Catamnestic results following therapy of heart patients with anabolic steroids. *Med Klin.* 61:1870, 1966.

Fineschi V. et al. Anabolic steroid abuse and cardiac sudden death: A pathologic study. *Arch Pathol Lab Med.* 125:253, 2001.

Fisher M. et al. Myocardial infarction with extensive intracoronary thrombus induced by anabolic steroids. *Br J Clin Pract.* 50:222, 1996.

Frohlich J. et al. Lipid profile of body builders with and without self-administration of anabolic steroids. *Eur J Appl Physiol Occup Physiol.* 59:98, 1989.

Garevik N. et al. Long term perturbation of endocrine parameters and cholesterol metabolism after discontinued abuse of anabolic androgenic steroids. *J Steroid Biochem Mol Biol.* 127:295, 2011.

Garner O. et al. Cardiomyopathy induced by anabolic-androgenic steroid abuse. *BMJ Case Rep.* 2018:2018.

Gheshlaghi F. et al. Cardiovascular manifestations of anabolic steroids in association with demographic variables in body building athletes. *J Res Med Sci.* 20:165, 2015.

Glazer G. Atherogenic effects of anabolic steroids on serum lipid levels. A literature review. *Arch Intern Med.* 151:1925, 1991.

Goldstein D.R. et al. Clenbuterol and anabolic steroids: A previously unreported cause of myocardial infarction with normal coronary arteriograms. *South Med J.* 91:780, 1998.

Golestani R. et al. Adverse cardiovascular effects of anabolic steroids: Pathophysiology imaging. *Eur J Clin Invest.* 42:795, 2012.

Goncalves R.V. et al. Trans-fatty acids aggravate anabolic steroid-induced metabolic disturbances and differential gene expression in muscle, pancreas and adipose tissue. *Life Sci.* 232:116603, 2019.

Ha E.T. et al. Non-ischemic cardiomyopathy secondary

to left ventricular hypertrophy due to long-term ana-bolic-androgenic steroid use in a former Olympic athlete. *Cureus.* 10:e3313, 2018.

Hackett G. Metabolic effects of testosterone therapy in men with type 2 diabetes and metabolic syndrome. *Sex Med Rev.* 2019.

Hajimoradi B. et al. Echocardiographic findings in power athletes abusing anabolic androgenic steroids. *Asian J Sports Med.* 4:10, 2013.

Halvorsen S. et al. Acute myocardial infarction in a young man who had been using androgenic anabolic steroids. *Tidsskr Nor Laegeforen.* 124:170, 2004.

Han H.C. et al. Steroid-induced cardiomyopathy. *Med J Aust.* 203:226, 2015.

Hartgens F. et al. Prospective echocardiographic assessment of androgenic-anabolic steroids effects on cardiac structure and function in strength athletes. *Int J Sports Med.* 24:344, 2003.

Hartgens F. et al. Body composition, cardiovascular risk factors and liver function in long-term androgenic-anabolic steroids using bodybuilders three months after drug withdrawal. *Int J Sports Med.* 17:429, 1996.

Hartgens F. et al. Effects of androgenic-anabolic steroids on apolipoproteins and lipoprotein (a). *Br J Sports Med.* 38:253, 2004.

Hassan N.A. et al. Doping and effects of anabolic androgenic steroids on the heart: Histological, ultrastructural, and echocardiographic assessment in strength athletes. *Hum Exp Toxicol.* 28:273, 2009.

Heim J. et al. HDL breakdown in an athlete taking anabolic steroids. *Presse Med.* 25:458, 1996.

Hernandez-Guerra A.I. et al. Sudden cardiac death in anabolic androgenic steroids abuse: Case report and literature review. *Forensic Sci Res.* 4:267, 2019.

Herschman Z. Cardiac effects of anabolic steroids. *Anesthesiology.* 72:772, 1990.

Hourigan L.A. et al. Intracoronary stenting for acute myocardial infarction (AMI) in a 24-year-old man using anabolic androgenic steroids. *Aust N Z J Med.* 28:838, 1998.

Huie M.J. An acute myocardial infarction occurring in an anabolic steroid user. *Med Sci Sports Exerc.* 26:408, 1994.

Ilhan E. et al. Acute myocardial infarction and renal infarction in a bodybuilder using anabolic steroids. *Turk Kardiyol Dern Ars.* 38:275, 2010.

Ilic I. et al. The impact of anabolic androgenic steroids abuse and type of training on left ventricular remodeling and function in competitive athletes. *Vojnosanit Pregl.* 71:383, 2014.

Joukar S. et al. Heart reaction to nandrolone decanoate plus two different intensities of endurance exercise: Electrocardiography and stereological approach. *Addict Health.* 10:180, 2018.

Kanayama G. et al. Ruptured tendons in anabolic-androgenic steroid users: A cross-sectional cohort study. *Am J Sports Med.* 43:2638, 2015.

Karhunen M.K. et al. Anabolic steroids alter the haemodynamic effects of endurance training and deconditioning in rats. *Acta Physiol Scand.* 133:297, 1988.

Kasikcioglu E. Anabolic-androgenic steroids: A bad tenor for cardiovascular orchestra (myocardial infarction with intracoronary thrombus induced by anabolic steroids). *Anadolu Kardiyol Derg.* 5:148, 2005.

Kasikcioglu E. et al. Aortic elastic properties in athletes using anabolic-androgenic steroids. *Int J Cardiol.* 114:132, 2007.

Kasikcioglu E. et al. Androgenic anabolic steroids also

impair right ventricular function. *Int J Cardiol.* 134:123, 2009.

Kennedy C. Myocardial infarction in association with misuse of anabolic steroids. *Ulster Med J.* 62:174, 1993.

Kennedy M.C. et al. Myocardial infarction and cerebral haemorrhage in a young body builder taking anabolic steroids. *Aust N Z J Med.* 23:713, 1993.

Kim C. et al. Testosterone and cardiac mass and function in men with type 1 diabetes in the epidemiology of diabetes interventions and complications study. *Clin Endocrinol.* 84:693, 2016.

Kindermann W. Cardiovascular side effects of anabolic-androgenic steroids. *Herz.* 31:566, 2006.

Hartgens, F., et al.. Prospective echocardiographic assessment of androgenic-anabolic steroids effects on cardiac structure and function in strength athletes. Int j sports med 2003; 24: 344 - 351. *Int J Sports Med.* 25:241, 2004.

Kloner R.A. et al. Testosterone and cardiovascular disease. *J Am Coll Cardiol.* 67:545, 2016.

Kouri E.M. et al. Changes in lipoprotein-lipid levels in normal men following administration of increasing doses of testosterone cypionate. *Clin J Sport Med.* 6:152, 1996.

Labib M. et al. The adverse effects of anabolic steroids on serum lipids. *Ann Clin Biochem.* 33 (Pt 3):263, 1996.

Lajarin F. et al. Evolution of serum lipids in two male bodybuilders using anabolic steroids. *Clin Chem.* 42:970, 1996.

Lane H.A. et al. Impaired vasoreactivity in bodybuilders using androgenic anabolic steroids. *Eur J Clin Invest.* 36:483, 2006.

Liu J.D. et al. Anabolic-androgenic steroids and cardiovascular risk. *Chin Med J (Engl).* 132:2229, 2019.

Lorimer D.A. et al. Cardiac dysfunction in athletes receiving anabolic steroids. *DICP.* 24:1060, 1990.

Madea B. et al. Long-term cardiovascular effects of anabolic steroids. *Lancet.* 352:33, 1998.

Marocolo M. et al. Combined effects of exercise training and high doses of anabolic steroids on cardiac autonomic modulation and ventricular repolarization properties in rats. *Can J Physiol Pharmacol.* 97:1185, 2019.

McCullough D. et al. How the love of muscle can break a heart: Impact of anabolic androgenic steroids on skeletal muscle hypertrophy, metabolic and cardiovascular health. *Rev Endocr Metab Disord.* 22:389, 2021.

McKillop G. et al. Increased left ventricular mass in a bodybuilder using anabolic steroids. *Br J Sports Med.* 20:151, 1986.

McNutt R.A. et al. Acute myocardial infarction in a 22-year-old world class weight lifter using anabolic steroids. *Am J Cardiol.* 62:164, 1988.

Medei E. et al. Chronic treatment with anabolic steroids induces ventricular repolarization disturbances: Cellular, ionic and molecular mechanism. *J Mol Cell Cardiol.* 49:165, 2010.

Melchert R.B. et al. The effect of anabolic-androgenic steroids on primary myocardial cell cultures. *Med Sci Sports Exerc.* 24:206, 1992.

Melchert R.B. et al. Cardiovascular effects of androgenic-anabolic steroids. *Med Sci Sports Exerc.* 27:1252, 1995.

Moffatt R.J. et al. Effects of anabolic steroids on lipoprotein profiles of female weight lifters. *Phys Sportsmed.* 18:106, 1990.

Mohler E.R., 3rd et al. The effect of testosterone on

cardiovascular biomarkers in the testosterone trials. *J Clin Endocrinol Metab.* 103:681, 2018.

Montisci M. et al. Anabolic androgenic steroids abuse and cardiac death in athletes: Morphological and toxicological findings in four fatal cases. *Forensic Sci Int.* 217:e13, 2012.

Montisci R. et al. Early myocardial dysfunction after chronic use of anabolic androgenic steroids: Combined pulsed-wave tissue doppler imaging and ultrasonic integrated backscatter cyclic variations analysis. *J Am Soc Echocardiogr.* 23:516, 2010.

Morgentaler A. Defending testosterone, debunking the myths. *Medscape.* June 4, 2015:2015.

Nascimento J.H. et al. Cardiac effects of anabolic steroids: Hypertrophy, ischemia and electrical remodelling as potential triggers of sudden death. *Mini Rev Med Chem.* 11:425, 2011.

Nieminen M.S. et al. Serious cardiovascular side effects of large doses of anabolic steroids in weight lifters. *Eur Heart J.* 17:1576, 1996.

Nottin S. et al. Cardiovascular effects of androgenic anabolic steroids in male bodybuilders determined by tissue doppler imaging. *Am J Cardiol.* 97:912, 2006.

Palatini P. et al. Cardiovascular effects of anabolic steroids in weight-trained subjects. *J Clin Pharmacol.* 36:1132, 1996.

Parker M.W. et al. Anabolic-androgenic steroids: Worse for the heart than we knew? *Circ Heart Fail.* 3:470, 2010.

Payne J.R. et al. Cardiac effects of anabolic steroids. *Heart.* 90:473, 2004.

Pencina K.M. et al. Endogenous circulating testosterone and sex hormone-binding globulin levels and measures of myocardial structure and function: The Framingham Heart Study. *Andrology.* 7:307, 2019.

Peoples K. et al. Hyperhomocysteinemia-induced myocardial infarction in a young male using anabolic steroids. *Am J Emerg Med.* 32:948 e1, 2014.

Polito M.V. et al. Androgenic-anabolic steroids: The new insidious killer leading to heart failure. *Minerva Cardioangiol.* 65:663, 2017.

Pope H.G., Jr. et al. The lifetime prevalence of anabolic-androgenic steroid use and dependence in Americans: Current best estimates. *Am J Addict.* 23:371, 2014.

Rasmussen J.J. et al. Cardiac systolic dysfunction in past illicit users of anabolic androgenic steroids. *Am Heart J.* 203:49, 2018.

Rasmussen J.J. et al. Insulin sensitivity in relation to fat distribution and plasma adipocytokines among abusers of anabolic androgenic steroids. *Clin Endocrinol.* 87:249, 2017.

Rockhold R.W. Cardiovascular toxicity of anabolic steroids. *Annu Rev Pharmacol Toxicol.* 33:497, 1993.

Rosca A.E. et al. Lipid profile changes induced by chronic administration of anabolic androgenic steroids and taurine in rats. *Medicina.* 55:2019.

Rothman R.D. et al. Anabolic androgenic steroid induced myocardial toxicity: An evolving problem in an ageing population. *BMJ Case Rep.* 2011:2011.

Salzano A. et al. Hormonal replacement therapy in heart failure: Focus on growth hormone and testosterone. *Heart Fail Clin.* 15:377, 2019.

Santora L.J. et al. Coronary calcification in body builders using anabolic steroids. *Prev Cardiol.* 9:198, 2006.

Schollert P.V. et al. Dilated cardiomyopathy in a user of anabolic steroids. *Ugeskr Laeger.* 155:1217, 1993.

Schwingel P.A. et al. The influence of concomitant use of alcohol, tobacco, cocaine, and anabolic steroids on lipid profiles of Brazilian recreational bodybuilders. *Subst Use Misuse.* 49:1115, 2014.

Seara F.A.C. et al. Cardiac electrical and contractile disorders promoted by anabolic steroid overdose are associated with late autonomic imbalance and impaired ca(2+) handling. *Steroids.* 148:1, 2019.

Shaikh K. et al. Biomarkers and noncalcified coronary artery plaque progression in older men treated with testosterone. *J Clin Endocrinol Metab.* 105:2020.

Shamloul R.M. et al. Anabolic steroids abuse-induced cardiomyopathy and ischaemic stroke in a young male patient. *BMJ Case Rep.* 2014:2014.

Shapiro J. et al. Testosterone and other anabolic steroids as cardiovascular drugs. *Am J Ther.* 6:167, 1999.

Sivalokanathan S. et al. The cardiac effects of performance-enhancing medications: Caffeine vs. Anabolic androgenic steroids. *Diagnostics.* 11:2021.

Tabor J. et al. Examining the effects of anabolic-androgenic steroids on repetitive mild traumatic brain injury (RMTBI) outcomes in adolescent rats. *Brain Sci.* 10:2020.

Stolt A. et al. Qt interval and QT dispersion in endurance athletes and in power athletes using large doses of anabolic steroids. *Am J Cardiol.* 84:364, 1999.

Sullivan M.L. et al. Atrial fibrillation and anabolic steroids. *J Emerg Med.* 17:851, 1999.

Sullivan M.L. et al. The cardiac toxicity of anabolic steroids. *Prog Cardiovasc Dis.* 41:1, 1998.

Tagarakis C.V. et al. Anabolic steroids impair the exercise-induced growth of the cardiac capillary bed. *Int J Sports Med.* 21:412, 2000.

Takala T.E. et al. Effects of training and anabolic

steroids on collagen synthesis in dog heart. *Eur J Appl Physiol Occup Physiol.* 62:1, 1991.

Thiblin I. et al. Anabolic steroids and cardiovascular risk: A national population-based cohort study. *Drug Alcohol Depend.* 152:87, 2015.

Thompson P.D. et al. Left ventricular function is not impaired in weight-lifters who use anabolic steroids. *J Am Coll Cardiol.* 19:278, 1992.

Tostes R.C. et al. Reactive oxygen species: Players in the cardiovascular effects of testosterone. *Am J Physiol Regul Integr Comp Physiol.* 310:R1, 2016.

Vaskinn A. et al. Theory of mind in users of anabolic androgenic steroids. *Psychopharmacology* 237:3191, 2020.

Yu J.G. et al. Potential effects of long-term abuse of anabolic androgen steroids on human skeletal muscle. *J Sports Med Phys Fitness.* 60:1040, 2020.

Weicker H. et al. Influence of training and anabolic steroids on the LDH isozyme pattern of skeletal and heart muscle fibers of guinea pigs. *Int J Sports Med.* 3:90, 1982.

Welder A.A. et al. Cardiotoxic effects of cocaine and anabolic-androgenic steroids in the athlete. *J Pharmacol Toxicol Methods.* 29:61, 1993.

White M. et al. Anabolic androgenic steroid use as a cause of fulminant heart failure. *Can J Cardiol.* 34:1369 e1, 2018.

Wysoczanski M. et al. Acute myocardial infarction in a young man using anabolic steroids. *Angiology.* 59:376, 2008.

References: Anabolic Steroids, Psychology, and the Brain

Agis-Balboa R.C. et al. Enhanced fear responses in mice treated with anabolic androgenic steroids. *Neuroreport.* 20:617, 2009.

Altschule M.D. et al. The use of testosterone in the treatment of depressions. *N Engl J Med.* 239:1036, 1948.

Amaral J.M.X. et al. Effective treatment and prevention of attempted suicide, anxiety, and aggressiveness with fluoxetine, despite proven use of androgenic anabolic steroids. *Drug Test Anal.* 13:197, 2021.

Annitto W.J. et al. Anabolic steroids and acute schizophrenic episode. *J Clin Psychiatry.* 41:143, 1980.

Arvary D. et al. Anabolic-androgenic steroids as a gateway to opioid dependence. *N Engl J Med.* 342:1532, 2000.

Bahrke M.S. et al. Psychological and behavioural effects of endogenous testosterone levels and anabolic-androgenic steroids among males. A review. *Sports Med.* 10:303, 1990.

Bahrke M.S. et al. Psychological and behavioural effects of endogenous testosterone and anabolic-androgenic steroids. An update. *Sports Med.* 22:367, 1996.

Bates G. et al. A systematic review investigating the behaviour change strategies in interventions to prevent misuse of anabolic steroids. *J Health Psychol.* 1359105317737607, 2017.

Bates G. et al. Treatments for people who use anabolic androgenic steroids: A scoping review. *Harm Reduct J.* 16:75, 2019.

Bjork T. et al. Eating disorders and anabolic androgenic steroids in males--similarities and differences in self-image and psychiatric symptoms. *Subst Abuse Treat Prev Policy.* 8:30, 2013.

Bjornebekk A. et al. Structural brain imaging of long-term anabolic-androgenic steroid users and non-using weightlifters. *Biol Psychiatry.* 82:294, 2017.

Bond A.J. et al. Assessment of attentional bias and mood in users and non-users of anabolic-androgenic steroids. *Drug Alcohol Depend.* 37:241, 1995.

Brand R. et al. Using response-time latencies to measure athletes' doping attitudes: The brief implicit attitude test identifies substance abuse in bodybuilders. *Subst Abuse Treat Prev Policy.* 9:36, 2014.

Breuer M.E. et al. Aggression in male rats receiving anabolic androgenic steroids: Effects of social and environmental provocation. *Horm Behav.* 40:409, 2001.

Bronson F.H. Effects of prolonged exposure to anabolic steroids on the behavior of male and female mice. *Pharmacol Biochem Behav.* 53:329, 1996.

Bronson F.H. et al. Effect of anabolic steroids on behavior and physiological characteristics of female mice. *Physiol Behav.* 59:49, 1996.

Brower K.J. Withdrawal from anabolic steroids. *Curr Ther Endocrinol Metab.* 5:291, 1994.

Brower K.J. Withdrawal from anabolic steroids. *Curr Ther Endocrinol Metab.* 6:338, 1997.

Brower K.J. et al. Anabolic androgenic steroids and suicide. *Am J Psychiatry.* 146:1075, 1989.

Brower K.J. et al. Evidence for physical and psychological dependence on anabolic androgenic steroids in eight weight lifters. *Am J Psychiatry.* 147:510, 1990.

Chantal Y. et al. Examining a negative halo effect to anabolic steroids users through perceived achievement goals, sportspersonship orientations, and aggressive tendencies. *Scand J Psychol.* 54:173, 2013.

Chantal Y. et al. Exploring the social image of anabolic steroids users through motivation, sportspersonship orientations and aggression. *Scand J Med Sci Sports.* 19:228, 2009.

Chicco A.J. et al. "Roid-rage" at the cellular level: Abolition of endogenous cardioprotection by anabolic steroids reveals new links between the RAAS and cardiac KATP channels : Editorial to: "At1 and aldosterone receptors blockade prevents the chronic effect of nandrolone on the exercise-induced cardioprotection in perfused rat heart subjected to ischemia and reperfusion" by S.R. Marques-Neto et al. *Cardiovasc Drugs Ther.* 28:113, 2014.

Choi P.Y. et al. Violence toward women and illicit androgenic-anabolic steroid use. *Ann Clin Psychiatry.* 6:21, 1994.

Clark A.S. et al. Anabolic-androgenic steroids and aggression in castrated male rats. *Physiol Behav.* 56:1107, 1994.

Clark A.S. et al. Behavioral and physiological responses to anabolic-androgenic steroids. *Neurosci Biobehav Rev.* 27:413, 2003.

Clark A.S. et al. Anabolic-androgenic steroids and brain reward. *Pharmacol Biochem Behav.* 53:741, 1996.

Cooper C.J. et al. Psychiatric disturbances in users of anabolic steroids. *S Afr Med J.* 84:509, 1994.

Cooper C.J. et al. A high prevalence of abnormal personality traits in chronic users of anabolic-androgenic steroids. *Br J Sports Med.* 30:246, 1996.

Cooper S.E. et al. Testosterone enhances risk tolerance without altering motor impulsivity in male rats. *Psychoneuroendocrinology.* 40:201, 2014.

Corrigan B. Anabolic steroids and the mind. *Med J Aust.* 165:222, 1996.

Cunningham R.L. et al. Factors influencing aggression

toward females by male rats exposed to anabolic androgenic steroids during puberty. *Horm Behav.* 51:135, 2007.

Daly R.C. Anabolic steroids, brain and behaviour. *Ir Med J.* 94:102, 2001.

Dunn M. Commentary on Lundholm et al. (2015): What came first, the steroids or the violence? *Addiction.* 110:109, 2015.

Ellingrod V.L. et al. The effects of anabolic steroids on driving performance as assessed by the Iowa driver simulator. *Am J Drug Alcohol Abuse.* 23:623, 1997.

Frahm K.A. et al. Effects of anabolic androgenic steroids and social subjugation on behavior and neurochemistry in male rats. *Pharmacol Biochem Behav.* 97:416, 2011.

Gettler L.T. et al. Are testosterone levels and depression risk linked based on partnering and parenting? Evidence from a large population-representative study of u.S. Men and women. *Soc Sci Med.* 163:157, 2016.

Gonzalez-Marti I. et al. Muscle dysmorphia: Detection of the use-abuse of anabolic androgenic steroids in a Spanish sample. *Adicciones.* 30:243, 2018.

Griffiths S. et al. Pornography use in sexual minority males: Associations with body dissatisfaction, eating disorder symptoms, thoughts about using anabolic steroids and quality of life. *Aust N Z J Psychiatry.* 52:339, 2018.

Griffiths S. et al. The contribution of social media to body dissatisfaction, eating disorder symptoms, and anabolic steroid use among sexual minority men. *Cyberpsychol Behav Soc Netw.* 21:149, 2018.

Gronbladh A. et al. The neurobiology and addiction potential of anabolic androgenic steroids and the effects of growth hormone. *Brain Res Bull.* 126:127, 2016.

Gruber A.J. et al. Compulsive weightlifting and anabolic drug abuse among women rape victims. *Compr Psychiatry.* 40:273, 1999.

Gruber A.J. et al. Psychiatric and medical effects of anabolic-androgenic steroid use in women. *Psychother Psychosom.* 69:19, 2000.

Hallberg M. et al. Anabolic-androgenic steroids affect the content of substance p and substance p(1-7) in the rat brain. *Peptides.* 21:845, 2000.

Hallgren M. et al. Anti-social behaviors associated with anabolic-androgenic steroid use among male adolescents. *Eur Addict Res.* 21:321, 2015.

Hauger L.E. et al. Structural brain characteristics of anabolic-androgenic steroid dependence in men. *Addiction.* 114:1405, 2019.

Hauger L.E. et al. Structural brain characteristics of anabolic-androgenic steroid dependence in men. *Addiction.* 114:1405, 2019.

Henderson L.P. et al. Anabolic androgenic steroids and forebrain gabaergic transmission. *Neuroscience.* 138:793, 2006.

Hildebrandt T. et al. Defining the construct of synthetic androgen intoxication: An application of general brain arousal. *Front Psychol.* 9:390, 2018.

Ip E.J. et al. Polypharmacy, infectious diseases, sexual behavior, and psychophysical health among anabolic steroid-using homosexual and heterosexual gym patrons in san Francisco's Castro district. *Subst Use Misuse.* 52:959, 2017.

Iriart J.A. et al. Body cult and use of anabolic steroids by bodybuilders. *Cad Saude Publica.* 25:773, 2009.

Isaacson R.L. Non-linear effects in the retention of an avoidance task induced by anabolic steroids. *Eur J Pharmacol.* 405:177, 2000.

Isacsson G. Do anabolic steroids induce violence? *Lakartidningen.* 92:2083, 1995.

Isacsson G. et al. Can anabolic steroids cause personality changes? *Nord Med.* 108:180, 1993.

Isacsson G. et al. Anabolic steroids and violent crime--an epidemiological study at a jail in Stockholm, Sweden. *Compr Psychiatry.* 39:203, 1998.

Jacka B. et al. Health care engagement behaviors of men who use performance- and image-enhancing drugs in Australia. *Subst Abus.* 41:139, 2020.

Jasuja G.K. et al. Patterns of testosterone prescription overuse. *Curr Opin Endocrinol Diabetes Obes.* 24:240, 2017.

Johansson P. et al. Anabolic androgenic steroids affects alcohol intake, defensive behaviors and brain opioid peptides in the rat. *Pharmacol Biochem Behav.* 67:271, 2000.

Johansson P. et al. Anabolic androgenic steroids increase beta-endorphin levels in the ventral tegmental area in the male rat brain. *Neurosci Res.* 27:185, 1997.

Joksimovic J. et al. Exercise attenuates anabolic steroids-induced anxiety via hippocampal NPY and mc4 receptor in rats. *Front Neurosci.* 13:172, 2019.

Jorge-Rivera J.C. et al. Anabolic steroids induce region- and subunit-specific rapid modulation of GABA(a) receptor-mediated currents in the rat forebrain. *J Neurophysiol.* 83:3299, 2000.

Kanayama G. et al. Body image and attitudes toward male roles in anabolic-androgenic steroid users. *Am J Psychiatry.* 163:697, 2006.

Kanayama G. et al. Anabolic-androgenic steroid dependence: An emerging disorder. *Addiction.* 104:1966, 2009.

Kanayama G. et al. Treatment of anabolic-androgenic

steroid dependence: Emerging evidence and its implications. *Drug Alcohol Depend.* 109:6, 2010.

Kanayama G. et al. Past anabolic-androgenic steroid
use among men admitted for substance abuse treatment: An underrecognized problem? *J Clin Psychiatry.*
64:156, 2003.

Kanayama G. et al. Features of men with anabolic-androgenic steroid dependence: A comparison with non-
dependent AAS users and with AAS nonusers. *Drug
Alcohol Depend.* 102:130, 2009.

Kanayama G. et al. Cognitive deficits in long-term anabolic-androgenic steroid users. *Drug Alcohol Depend.*
130:208, 2013.

Kanayama G. et al. Associations of anabolic-androgenic steroid use with other behavioral disorders: An
analysis using directed acyclic graphs. *Psychol Med.*
48:2601, 2018.

Katz D.L. et al. Anabolic-androgenic steroid-induced
mental status changes. *NIDA Res Monogr.* 102:215,
1990.

Kaufman M.J. et al. Brain and cognition abnormalities
in long-term anabolic-androgenic steroid users. *Drug
Alcohol Depend.* 152:47, 2015.

Khoodoruth M.A.S. et al. Anabolic steroids-induced
delirium: A case report. *Medicine.* 99: e21639, 2020.

Kindlundh A.M. et al. Adolescent use of anabolic-androgenic steroids and relations to self-reports of social,
personality and health aspects. *Eur J Public Health.*
11:322, 2001.

Klotz F. et al. Criminality among individuals testing
positive for the presence of anabolic androgenic
steroids. *Arch Gen Psychiatry.* 63:1274, 2006.

Klotz F. et al. Violent crime and substance abuse: A
medico-legal comparison between deceased users of

anabolic androgenic steroids and abusers of illicit drugs. *Forensic Sci Int.* 173:57, 2007.

Kouri E.M. et al. Use of anabolic-androgenic steroids: We are talking prevalence rates. *JAMA.* 271:347, 1994.

Lindqvist Bagge A.S. et al. Somatic effects of AAS abuse: A 30-years follow-up study of male former power sports athletes. *J Sci Med Sport.* 20:814, 2017.

Lood Y. et al. Anabolic androgenic steroids in police cases in Sweden 1999-2009. *Forensic Sci Int.* 219:199, 2012.

Lumia A.R. et al. Impact of anabolic androgenic steroids on adolescent males. *Physiol Behav.* 100:199, 2010.

Lundholm L. et al. Anabolic androgenic steroids and violent offending: Confounding by polysubstance abuse among 10,365 general population men. *Addiction.* 110:100, 2015.

Lundholm L. et al. Use of anabolic androgenic steroids in substance abusers arrested for crime. *Drug Alcohol Depend.* 111:222, 2010.

McGinnis M.Y. Anabolic androgenic steroids and aggression: Studies using animal models. *Ann N Y Acad Sci.* 1036:399, 2004.

McGinnis M.Y. et al. Physical provocation potentiates aggression in male rats receiving anabolic androgenic steroids. *Horm Behav.* 41:101, 2002.

McGinnis M.Y. et al. Effects of withdrawal from anabolic androgenic steroids on aggression in adult male rats. *Physiol Behav.* 75:541, 2002.

McIntyre K.L. et al. Anabolic androgenic steroids induce age-, sex-, and dose-dependent changes in GABA(a) receptor subunit MRNAS in the mouse forebrain. *Neuropharmacology.* 43:634, 2002.

Medras M. et al. The central effects of androgenic-anabolic steroid use. *J Addict Med.* 12:184, 2018.

Medras M. et al. [treatment strategies of withdrawal from long-term use of anabolic-androgenic steroids]. *Pol Merkur Lekarski.* 11:535, 2001.

Menard C.S. et al. Up-regulation of androgen receptor immunoreactivity in the rat brain by androgenic-anabolic steroids. *Brain Res.* 622:226, 1993.

Menard C.S. et al. Androgenic-anabolic steroids modify beta-endorphin immunoreactivity in the rat brain. *Brain Res.* 669:255, 1995.

Milhorn H.T., Jr. Anabolic steroids: Another form of drug abuse. *J Miss State Med Assoc.* 32:293, 1991.

Mills J.D. et al. Anabolic steroids and head injury. *Neurosurgery.* 70:205, 2012.

Morrison T.R. et al. Vasopressin differentially modulates aggression and anxiety in adolescent hamsters administered anabolic steroids. *Horm Behav.* 86:55, 2016.

Morton R. et al. Psychiatric effects of anabolic steroids after burn injuries. *Psychosomatics.* 41:66, 2000.

Murray S.B. et al. Anabolic steroid use and body image psychopathology in men: Delineating between appearance- versus performance-driven motivations. *Drug Alcohol Depend.* 165:198, 2016.

Nagata J.M. et al. Predictors of muscularity-oriented disordered eating behaviors in u.S. Young adults: A prospective cohort study. *Int J Eat Disord.* 2019.

Negus S.S. et al. Lack of evidence for opioid tolerance or dependence in rhesus monkeys following high-dose anabolic-androgenic steroid administration. *Psychoneuroendocrinology.* 26:789, 2001.

Novaes Gomes F.G. et al. The beneficial effects of strength exercise on hippocampal cell proliferation and apoptotic signaling is impaired by anabolic androgenic steroids. *Psychoneuroendocrinology.* 50:106, 2014.

Nyberg F. et al. Interactions between opioids and anabolic androgenic steroids: Implications for the development of addictive behavior. *Int Rev Neurobiol.* 102:189, 2012.

Oberlander J.G. et al. Estrous cycle variations in GABA(a) receptor phosphorylation enable rapid modulation by anabolic androgenic steroids in the medial preoptic area. *Neuroscience.* 226:397, 2012.

Pagonis T.A. et al. Psychiatric side effects induced by supraphysiological doses of combinations of anabolic steroids correlate to the severity of abuse. *Eur Psychiatry.* 21:551, 2006.

Pagonis T.A. et al. Psychiatric and hostility factors related to use of anabolic steroids in monozygotic twins. *Eur Psychiatry.* 21:563, 2006.

Petersson A. et al. Convulsions in users of anabolic androgenic steroids: Possible explanations. *J Clin Psychopharmacol.* 27:723, 2007.

Piacentino D. et al. Anabolic-androgenic steroid use and psychopathology in athletes. a systematic review. *Curr Neuropharm.* 11:101, 2015.

Pibiri F. et al. Neurosteroids regulate mouse aggression induced by anabolic androgenic steroids. *Neuroreport.* 17:1537, 2006.

Pope H.G., Jr. et al. Review article: Anabolic-androgenic steroids, violence, and crime: Two cases and literature review. *Am J Addict.* 2021.

Pope H.G., Jr. et al. Muscle dysmorphia. An underrecognized form of body dysmorphic disorder. *Psychosomatics.* 38:548, 1997.

Pope H.G. et al. Risk factors for illicit anabolic-androgenic steroid use in male weightlifters: A cross-sectional cohort study. *Biol Psychiatry.* 71:254, 2012.

Pope H.G. et al. Anabolic steroid users' attitudes towards physicians. *Addiction.* 99:1189, 2004.

Pope H.G., Jr. et al. Affective and psychotic symptoms associated with anabolic steroid use. *Am J Psychiatry.* 145:487, 1988.

Pope H.G., Jr. et al. Homicide and near-homicide by anabolic steroid users. *J Clin Psychiatry.* 51:28, 1990.

Pope H.G., Jr. et al. Psychiatric and medical effects of anabolic-androgenic steroid use. A controlled study of 160 athletes. *Arch Gen Psychiatry.* 51:375, 1994.

Pope H.G., Jr. et al. Anorexia nervosa and "reverse anorexia" among 108 male bodybuilders. *Compr Psychiatry.* 34:406, 1993.

Pope H.G. et al. A diagnostic interview module for anabolic-androgenic steroid dependence: Preliminary evidence of reliability and validity. *Exp Clin Psychopharmacol.* 18:203, 2010.

Pope H.G., Jr. et al. Body image disorders and abuse of anabolic-androgenic steroids among men. *JAMA.* 317:23, 2017.

Rejeski W.J. et al. Anabolic steroids and aggressive behavior in cynomolgus monkeys. *J Behav Med.* 11:95, 1988.

Rejeski W.J. et al. Anabolic-androgenic steroids: Effects on social behavior and baseline heart rate. *Health Psychol.* 9:774, 1990.

Ricci L.A. et al. Adolescent anabolic/androgenic steroids: Aggression and anxiety during exposure predict behavioral responding during withdrawal in Syrian hamsters (*mesocricetus auratus*). *Horm Behav.* 64:770, 2013.

Rohman L. The relationship between anabolic androgenic steroids and muscle dysmorphia: A review. *Eat Disord.* 17:187, 2009.

Salas-Ramirez K.Y. et al. Anabolic androgenic steroids

differentially affect social behaviors in adolescent and adult male syrian hamsters. *Horm Behav.* 53:378, 2008.

Salas-Ramirez K.Y. et al. Anabolic steroids have long-lasting effects on male social behaviors. *Behav Brain Res.* 208:328, 2010.

Sandvik M.R. et al. Anabolic-androgenic steroid use and correlates in Norwegian adolescents. *Eur J Sport Sci.* 18:903, 2018.

Seitz J. et al. White matter abnormalities in long-term anabolic-androgenic steroid users: A pilot study. *Psychiatry Res Neuroimaging.* 260:1, 2017.

Skarberg K. et al. Is there an association between the use of anabolic-androgenic steroids and criminality? *Eur Addict Res.* 16:213, 2010.

Tarlo L. et al. Anabolic steroids in chronic schizophrenia. *Br J Psychiatry.* 110:287, 1964.

Thiblin I. et al. Anabolic androgenic steroids and violence. *Acta Psychiatr Scand Suppl.* 125, 2002.

Thiblin I. et al. Anabolic androgenic steroids and suicide. *Ann Clin Psychiatry.* 11:223, 1999.

Tricker R. et al. The effects of supraphysiological doses of testosterone on angry behavior in healthy eugonadal men--a clinical research center study. *J Clin Endocrinol Metab.* 81:3754, 1996.

Uzych L. Anabolic-androgenic steroids and psychiatric-related effects: A review. *Can J Psychiatry.* 37:23, 1992.

Wallin K.G. et al. Anabolic-androgenic steroids and decision making: Probability and effort discounting in male rats. *Psychoneuroendocrinology.* 57:84, 2015.

Wallin K.G. et al. Anabolic-androgenic steroids impair set-shifting and reversal learning in male rats. *Eur Neuropsychopharmacol.* 25:583, 2015.

Wesson D.W. et al. Stacking anabolic androgenic steroids (AAS) during puberty in rats: A neuroendocrine and behavioral assessment. *Pharmacol Biochem Behav.* 83:410, 2006.

Westlye L.T. et al. Brain connectivity aberrations in anabolic-androgenic steroid users. *Neuroimage Clin.* 13:62, 2017.

Wood R.I. et al. 'Roid rage in rats? Testosterone effects on aggressive motivation, impulsivity and tyrosine hydroxylase. *Physiol Behav.* 110-111:6, 2013.

Wroblewska A.M. Androgenic--anabolic steroids and body dysmorphia in young men. *J Psychosom Res.* 42:225, 1997.

Yesalis C.E. Use of steroids for self-enhancement: An epidemiologic/societal perspective. *AIDS Read.* 11:157, 2001.

Yesalis C.E. Use of steroids for self-enhancement: An epidemiologic/societal perspective. *AIDS Read.* 11:157, 2001.

Yesalis C.E. et al. Indications of psychological dependence among anabolic-androgenic steroid abusers. *NIDA Res Monogr.* 102:196, 1990.

References: Vascular Effects of Anabolic Steroids

Alaraj A.M. et al. Spontaneous subdural haematoma in anabolic steroids dependent weightlifters: Reports of two cases and review of literature. *Acta Neurochir.* 147:85, 2005.

Alves M.J. et al. Abnormal neurovascular control in anabolic androgenic steroids users. *Med Sci Sports Exerc.* 42:865, 2010.

Ansell J.E. et al. Coagulation abnormalities associated with the use of anabolic steroids. *Am Heart J.* 125:367, 1993.

Argalious M.Y. et al. Association of testosterone replacement therapy and the incidence of a composite of postoperative in-hospital mortality and cardiovascular events in men undergoing cardiac surgery. *Anesth Analg.* 130:890, 2020.

Brennan R. et al. "Blood letting"-self-phlebotomy in injecting anabolic-androgenic steroids within performance and image enhancing drug (pied) culture. *Int J Drug Policy.* 55:47, 2018.

Chang S. et al. Anabolic androgenic steroid abuse: The effects on thrombosis risk, coagulation, and fibrinolysis. *Semin Thromb Hemost.* 44:734, 2018.

Choe H. et al. Inherited antithrombin deficiency and anabolic steroids: A risky combination. *Blood Coagul Fibrinolysis.* 27:717, 2016.

D'Ascenzo S. et al. Detrimental effects of anabolic steroids on human endothelial cells. *Toxicol Lett.* 169:129, 2007.

Duarte L. et al. The erythropoietic effects of anabolic steroids. *Proc Soc Exp Biol Med.* 125:1030, 1967.

Ebenbichler C.F. et al. Flow-mediated, endothelium-dependent vasodilatation is impaired in male body builders taking anabolic-androgenic steroids. *Atherosclerosis.* 158:483, 2001.

Falkenberg M. et al. Peripheral arterial thrombosis in two young men using anabolic steroids. *Eur J Vasc Endovasc Surg.* 13:223, 1997.

Faludi G. et al. Anabolic steroids in muscular, neurologic and hematologic disorders. *J Am Med Womens Assoc.* 23:346, 1968.

Ferenchick G.S. et al. Anabolic-androgenic steroid abuse in weightlifters: Evidence for activation of the hemostatic system. *Am J Hematol.* 49:282, 1995.

Frankle M.A. et al. Anabolic androgenic steroids and a

stroke in an athlete: Case report. *Arch Phys Med Rehabil.* 69:632, 1988.

Gagliano-Juca T. et al. Differential effects of testosterone on peripheral neutrophils, monocytes and platelets in men: Findings from two trials. *Andrology.* 8:1324-1331, 2020.

Glueck C.J. et al. Testosterone therapy, thrombophilia, venous thromboembolism, and thrombotic events. *J Clin Med.* 8: 2018.

Grace F. et al. Blood pressure and rate pressure product response in males using high-dose anabolic androgenic steroids (AAS). *J Sci Med Sport.* 6:307, 2003.

Green D.J. et al. Anabolic steroids and vascular responses. *Lancet.* 342:863, 1993.

Gunes Y. et al. Myocardial infarction with intracoronary thrombus induced by anabolic steroids. *Anadolu Kardiyol Derg.* 4:357, 2004.

Harston G.W. et al. Lacunar infarction associated with anabolic steroids and polycythemia: A case report. *Case Rep Neurol.* 6:34, 2014.

Hashmi A. et al. Superior sagittal venous sinus thrombosis in a patient with illicit testosterone use. *Cureus.* 11:e5491, 2019.

Hassan A.F. et al. Effect of exercise training and anabolic androgenic steroids on hemodynamics, glycogen content, angiogenesis and apoptosis of cardiac muscle in adult male rats. *Int J Health Sci (Qassim).* 7:47, 2013.

Hernandez-Guerra A.I. et al. Sudden cardiac death in anabolic androgenic steroids abuse: Case report and literature review. *Forensic Sci Res.* 4:267, 2019.

Hinterberger W. et al. Anabolic steroids and blood cell production. *Wien Med Wochenschr.* 143:380, 1993.

Houghton D.E. et al. Testosterone therapy and venous

thromboembolism: A systematic review and meta-analysis. *Thromb Res.* 172:94, 2018.

Howard C.W. et al. Anabolic steroids and anticoagulants. *Br Med J.* 1:1659, 1977.

Janjic M.M. et al. Anabolic-androgenic steroids induce apoptosis and NOS_2 (nitric-oxide synthase $_2$) in adult rat Leydig cells following in vivo exposure. *Reprod Toxicol.* 34:686, 2012.

Juhl S. et al. Concomitant arterial and venous thrombosis in a body builder with severe hyperhomocysteinemia and abuse of anabolic steroids. *Ugeskr Laeger.* 166:3508, 2004.

Junior J. et al. Androgenic-anabolic steroids inhibited post-exercise hypotension: A case control study. *Braz J Phys Ther.* 22:77, 2018.

Karhunen M.K. et al. Anabolic steroids alter the haemodynamic effects of endurance training and deconditioning in rats. *Acta Physiol Scand.* 133:297, 1988.

Lepori M. et al. The popliteal-artery entrapment syndrome in a patient using anabolic steroids. *N Engl J Med.* 346:1254, 2002.

Li H. et al. Association between use of exogenous testosterone therapy and risk of venous thrombotic events among exogenous testosterone treated and untreated men with hypogonadism. *J Urol.* 195:1065, 2016.

Liljeqvist S. et al. Pulmonary embolism associated with the use of anabolic steroids. *Eur J Intern Med.* 19:214, 2008.

Low M.S. et al. Anabolic androgenic steroids, an easily forgotten cause of polycythaemia and cerebral infarction. *Intern Med J.* 46:497, 2016.

Lowe G.D. Anabolic steroids and fibrinolysis. *Wien Med Wochenschr.* 143:383, 1993.

McCulloch N.A. et al. Multiple arterial thromboses associated with anabolic androgenic steroids. *Clin J Sport Med.* 24:153, 2014.

Nasseri A. et al. Effects of resistance exercise and the use of anabolic androgenic steroids on hemodynamic characteristics and muscle damage markers in bodybuilders. *J Sports Med Phys Fitness.* 56:1041, 2016.

Porello R.A. et al. Neurovascular response during exercise and mental stress in anabolic steroid users. *Med Sci Sports Exerc.* 50:596, 2018.

Ramasamy R. et al. Association between testosterone supplementation therapy and thrombotic events in elderly men. *Urology.* 86:283, 2015.

Rasmussen J.J. et al. Increased blood pressure and aortic stiffness among abusers of anabolic androgenic steroids: Potential effect of suppressed natriuretic peptides in plasma? *J Hypertens.* 36:277, 2018.

Riebe D. et al. The blood pressure response to exercise in anabolic steroid users. *Med Sci Sports Exerc.* 24:633, 1992.

Rocha F.L. et al. Anabolic steroids induce cardiac renin-angiotensin system and impair the beneficial effects of aerobic training in rats. *Am J Physiol Heart Circ Physiol.* 293:H3575, 2007.

Rosca A.E. et al. Influence of chronic administration of anabolic androgenic steroids and taurine on haemostasis profile in rats: A thrombelastographic study. *Blood Coagul Fibrinolysis.* 24:256, 2013.

Rosca A.E. et al. Impact of chronic administration of anabolic androgenic steroids and taurine on blood pressure in rats. *Braz J Med Biol Res.* 49:e5116, 2016.

Schumacher J. et al. Large hepatic hematoma and intraabdominal hemorrhage associated with abuse of anabolic steroids. *N Engl J Med.* 340:1123, 1999.

Shimada Y. et al. Cerebral infarction in a young man using high-dose anabolic steroids. *J Stroke Cerebrovasc Dis.* 21:906 e9, 2012.

Shores M.M. Testosterone treatment and cardiovascular events in prescription database studies. *Asian J Androl.* 20:138, 2018.

Stergiopoulos K. et al. Anabolic steroids, acute myocardial infarction and polycythemia: A case report and review of the literature. *Vasc Health Risk Manag.* 4:1475, 2008.

Tsatsakis A. et al. A mechanistic and pathophysiological approach for stroke associated with drugs of abuse. *J Clin Med.* 8:2019.

References: Anabolic Steroids and Cancer

Abbasnezhad A. et al. The effects of anabolic-androgenic steroids on DNA damage in bodybuilders' blood lymphocytes. Biomarkers. 1, 2021.

Arakawa K. Clinical studies on the effect of anabolic steroids in the therapy of cervix cancer. 1. Effect on protein metabolism in extensive pannysterectomy. *Nihon Naibunpi Gakkai Zasshi.* 43:795, 1967.

Basile J.R. et al. Supraphysiological doses of performance enhancing anabolic-androgenic steroids exert direct toxic effects on neuron-like cells. *Front Cell Neurosci.* 7:69, 2013.

Becker C. et al. Changes in the MIKRNA profile under the influence of anabolic steroids in bovine liver. *Analyst.* 136:1204, 2011.

Bronson F.H. et al. Exposure to anabolic-androgenic steroids shortens life span of male mice. *Med Sci Sports Exerc.* 29:615, 1997.

Cazorla-Saravia P. et al. Is it the creatine or the anabolic androgenic steroids? Need for assessing the steroids role in testicular cancer. *Br J Cancer.* 113:1638, 2015.

Chan Y.X. et al. Lower circulating androgens are associated with overall cancer risk and prostate cancer risk in men aged 25-84 years from the Busselton health study. *Horm Cancer.* 9:391, 2018.

Creagh T.M. et al. Hepatic tumours induced by anabolic steroids in an athlete. *J Clin Pathol.* 41:441, 1988.

Daneshmend T.K. et al. Hepatic angiosarcoma associated with androgenic-anabolic steroids. *Lancet.* 2:1249, 1979.

Debruyne F.M. et al. Testosterone treatment is not associated with increased risk of prostate cancer or worsening of lower urinary tract symptoms: Prostate health outcomes in the registry of hypogonadism in men. *BJU Int.* 119:216, 2017.

Edis A.J. et al. Anabolic steroids and colonic cancer. *Med J Aust.* 142:426, 1985.

Eisenberg M.L. Testosterone replacement therapy and prostate cancer incidence. *World J Mens Health.* 33:125, 2015.

Eliakim A. et al. A case study of virilizing adrenal tumor in an adolescent female elite tennis player--insight into the use of anabolic steroids in young athletes. *J Strength Cond Res.* 25:46, z~.

Falk H. et al. Hepatic angiosarcoma associated with androgenic-anabolic steroids. *Lancet.* 2:1120, 1979.

Frey H. Liver cancer following use of anabolic steroids? *Tidsskr Nor Laegeforen.* 93:2499, 1973.

Garcia-Horton A. et al. Anabolic steroids in myelodysplastic syndromes: A systematic review. *Leuk Res.* 94:106370, 2020.

Goldman B. Liver carcinoma in an athlete taking anabolic steroids. *J Am Osteopath Assoc.* 85:56, 1985.

Hickson R.C. et al. Adverse effects of anabolic steroids. *Med Toxicol Adverse Drug Exp.* 4:254, 1989.

Hupperets P. et al. A retrospective study of the effect of anabolic steroids on the dyshaematopoietic syndrome (preleukaemic syndrome). *Neth J Med.* 26:181, 1983.

Ishak K.G. Hepatic neoplasms associated with contraceptive and anabolic steroids. *Recent Results Cancer Res.* 66:73, 1979.

Ishak K.G. Hepatic lesions caused by anabolic and contraceptive steroids. *Semin Liver Dis.* 1:116, 1981.

Johnson F.L. The association of oral androgenic-anabolic steroids and life-threatening disease. *Med Sci Sports.* 7:284, 1975.

Lovisetto P. et al. Features of liver damage caused by 17-alpha-alkyl-substituted anabolic steroids. *Minerva Med.* 70:769, 1979.

Modlinski R. et al. The effect of anabolic steroids on the gastrointestinal system, kidneys, and adrenal glands. *Curr Sports Med Rep.* 5:104, 2006.

Rawbone R.G. et al. Anabolic steroids and bone marrow toxicity during therapy with methotrexate. *Br J Cancer.* 26:395, 1972.

Rigberg S.V. et al. Potential roles of androgens and the anabolic steroids in the treatment of cancer - a review. *J Med.* 6:271, 1975.

Salerno M. et al. Anabolic androgenic steroids and carcinogenicity focusing on Leydig cell: A literature review. *Oncotarget.* 9:19415, 2018.

Schultzel M.M. et al. Bilateral deltoid myositis ossificans in a weightlifter using anabolic steroids. *Orthopedics.* 37:e844, 2014.

Soe K.L. et al. Liver pathology associated with the use of anabolic-androgenic steroids. *Liver.* 12:73, 1992.
Soe K.L. et al. Liver pathology associated with anabolic androgenic steroids. *Ugeskr Laeger.* 156:2585, 1994.
Souza L.D. et al. Micronucleus as biomarkers of cancer risk in anabolic androgenic steroids users. *Hum Exp Toxicol.* 36:302, 2017.
Stang-Voss C. et al. Structural alterations of liver parenchyma induced by anabolic steroids. *Int J Sports Med.* 2:101, 1981.
Syed S.P. et al. Anabolic steroids causing growth of benign tumors: Androgen receptor in angiolipomas. *J Am Acad Dermatol.* 57:899, 2007.
Tentori L. et al. Doping with growth hormone/IGF-1, anabolic steroids or erythropoietin: Is there a cancer risk? *Pharmacol Res.* 55:359, 2007.

References: Anabolic Steroids and Disease

Adachi M. et al. Effect of anabolic steroids on osteoporosis. *Clin Calcium.* 18:1451, 2008.
Adair F.E. Testosterone in the treatment of breast carcinoma. *Med Clin North Am.* 32:18, 1948.
Adair F.E. et al. The use of testosterone propionate in the treatment of advanced carcinoma of the breast. *Ann Surg.* 123:1023, 1946.
Adami S. et al. Anabolic steroids in corticosteroid-induced osteoporosis. *Wien Med Wochenschr.* 143:395, 1993.
Albarosa U. et al. On the anabolic effects of synthetic steroids in the repair of fractures. *Riforma Med.* 78:1034, 1964.
Algeri R. et al. High doses of anabolic steroids in col-

lateral therapy of malignant neoplasms. Results with 19-norandrostenolone undecylate. *Clin Ter.* 85:505, 1978.

Amadei A. Effect of testosterone propionate on the healing process of fractures; experimental investigation. *Folia Endocrinol Mens Incretologia Incretoterapia.* 3:697, 1950.

Aparicio V.A. et al. Effects of the dietary amount and source of protein, resistance training and anabolic-androgenic steroids on body weight and lipid profile of rats. *Nutr Hosp.* 28:127, 2013.

Badalian L.O. et al. Treatment problems using anabolic steroids in progressive muscular dystrophy. *Klin Med.* 62:23, 1984.

Beatty D.C. et al. The combination of anabolic steroids and corticosteroids in the treatment of rheumatoid arthritis. *Proc R Soc Med.* 57:671, 1964.

Beiner J.M. et al. The effect of anabolic steroids and corticosteroids on healing of muscle contusion injury. *Am J Sports Med.* 27:2, 1999.

Berger J.R. et al. Effect of anabolic steroids on HIV-related wasting myopathy. *South Med J.* 86:865, 1993.

Brennan R. et al. "Blood letting"-self-phlebotomy in injecting anabolic-androgenic steroids within performance and image enhancing drug culture. *Int J Drug Policy.* 55:47, 2018.

Brodsky I. The role of androgens and anabolic steroids in the treatment of cancer. *Semin Drug Treat.* 3:15, 1973.

Caccialanza P. et al. Anabolic steroids in the cicatrization of experimental cutaneous wounds in man. *Minerva Med.* 52:372, 1961.

Calabrese L.H. et al. The effects of anabolic steroids and strength training on the human immune response. *Med Sci Sports Exerc.* 21:386, 1989.

Chan Y.X. et al. Lower circulating androgens are associated with overall cancer risk and prostate cancer risk in men aged 25-84 years from the Busselton Health Study. *Horm Cancer.* 9:391, 2018.

Chatterjee K. Neuralgic amyotrophy treated with anabolic steroids. *J Indian Med Assoc.* 42:385, 1964.

Chen J.F. et al. Androgens and androgen receptor actions on bone health and disease: From androgen deficiency to androgen therapy. *Cells.* 8:2019.

Choi S.M. et al. Comparative safety evaluation of selective androgen receptor modulators and anabolic androgenic steroids. *Expert Opin Drug Saf.* 14:1773, 2015.

Creutzberg E.C. et al. A role for anabolic steroids in the rehabilitation of patients with COPD? A double-blind, placebo-controlled, randomized trial. *Chest.* 124:1733, 2003.

Dmitriev V.B. et al. Role of anabolic steroids in the treatment of gunshot fractures. *Voen Med Zh.* 6:28, 1973.

Dobs A.S. Is there a role for androgenic anabolic steroids in medical practice? *JAMA.* 281:1326, 1999.

Dos Santos M.R. et al. Effect of exercise training and testosterone replacement on skeletal muscle wasting in patients with heart failure with testosterone deficiency. *Mayo Clin Proc.* 91:575, 2016.

Endoh M. et al. Prophylactic treatment of hereditary angioneurotic edema with anabolic steroids. *Tokai J Exp Clin Med.* 5:59, 1980.

Falqueto H. et al. Can conditions of skeletal muscle loss be improved by combining exercise with anabolic-androgenic steroids? A systematic review and meta-analysis of testosterone-based interventions. *Rev Endocr Metab Disord.* 22:161, 2021.

Farooqi V. et al. Anabolic steroids for rehabilitation

after hip fracture in older people. *Sao Paulo Med J.* 134:467, 2016.

Farooqi V. et al. Anabolic steroids for rehabilitation after hip fracture in older people. *Cochrane Database Syst Rev.* CD008887, 2014.

Ferreira I.M. et al. The influence of 6 months of oral anabolic steroids on body mass and respiratory muscles in undernourished COPD patients. *Chest.* 114:19, 1998.

Fillo J. et al. The effect of long term testosterone replacement therapy on bone mineral density. *Bratisl Lek Listy.* 120:291, 2019.

Fiore C.E. et al. The effects of muscle-building exercise on forearm bone mineral content and osteoblast activity in drug-free and anabolic steroids self-administering young men. *Bone Miner.* 13:77, 1991.

Fruehan A.E. et al. Current status of anabolic steroids. *JAMA.* 184:527, 1963.

Gagliano-Juca T. et al. Testosterone replacement therapy and cardiovascular risk. *Nat Rev Cardiol.* 2019.

Gale R.P. Aplastic anaemia treated with anabolic steroids. *Br J Haematol.* 43:483, 1979.

Garcia-Esperon C. et al. Ingestion of anabolic steroids and ischaemic stroke. A clinical case report and review of the literature. *Rev Neurol.* 56:327, 2013.

Gerber C. et al. Anabolic steroids reduce muscle degeneration associated with rotator cuff tendon release in sheep. *Am J Sports Med.* 43:2393, 2015.

Gerber C. et al. Anabolic steroids reduce muscle damage caused by rotator cuff tendon release in an experimental study in rabbits. *J Bone Joint Surg Am.* 93:2189, 2011.

Gerber C. et al. Rotator cuff muscles lose responsiveness to anabolic steroids after tendon tear and musculotendinous retraction: An experimental study in sheep. *Am J Sports Med.* 40:2454, 2012.

Ghizoni M.F. et al. The anabolic steroid nandrolone enhances motor and sensory functional recovery in rat median nerve repair with long interpositional nerve grafts. *Neurorehabil Neural Repair.* 27:269, 2013.

Gullett N.P. et al. Update on clinical trials of growth factors and anabolic steroids in cachexia and wasting. *Am J Clin Nutr.* 91:1143S, 2010.

Gunes A.T. et al. Hormones: Androgens, antiandrogens, anabolic steroids, estrogens--unapproved uses or indications. *Clin Dermatol.* 18:55, 2000.

Guzzoni V. et al. Tendon remodeling in response to resistance training, anabolic androgenic steroids and aging. *Cells.* 7:2018.

Haeger K. Hydrogenated ergotamine alkaloids and anabolic steroids in the treatment of leg ulcers. *Lakartidningen.* 63:641, 1966.

Haeger K. Effects of anabolic steroids in the long-term treatment of ischaemic leg ulcers. *Zentralbl Phlebol.* 7:248, 1968.

Haeusler G. et al. Growth hormone in combination with anabolic steroids in patients with turner syndrome: Effect on bone maturation and final height. *Acta Paediatr.* 85:1408, 1996.

Hakansson A. et al. Anabolic androgenic steroids in the general population: User characteristics and associations with substance use. *Eur Addict Res.* 18:83, 2012.

Hausmann D.F. et al. Anabolic steroids in polytrauma patients. Influence on renal nitrogen and amino acid losses: A double-blind study. *JPEN J Parenter Enteral Nutr.* 14:111, 1990.

Hedstrom M. et al. Positive effects of anabolic steroids, vitamin d and calcium on muscle mass, bone mineral density and clinical function after a hip fracture. A randomised study of 63 women. *J Bone Joint Surg Br.* 84:497, 2002.

Hohmann E. et al. Anabolic steroids after total knee arthroplasty. A double blinded prospective pilot study. *J Orthop Surg Res.* 5:93, 2010.

Hughes T.K. et al. Modulation of immune responses by anabolic androgenic steroids. *Int J Immunopharmacol.* 17:857, 1995.

Hulsbaek S. et al. Feasibility and preliminary effect of anabolic steroids in addition to strength training and nutritional supplement in rehabilitation of patients with hip fracture: A randomized controlled pilot trial (HIP-SAP1 trial). *BMC Geriatr.* 21:323, 2021.

Hulsbaek S. et al. Preliminary effect and feasibility of physiotherapy with strength training and protein-rich nutritional supplement in combination with anabolic steroids in cross-continuum rehabilitation of patients with hip fracture: Protocol for a blinded randomized controlled pilot trial (HIP-SAP1 trial). *Trials.* 20:763, 2019.

Iashchenko B.P. et al. Anabolic steroids in the overall treatment of pulmonary tuberculosis in the middle-aged and elderly. *Probl Tuberk.* 26, 1980.

Ip E.J. et al. Women and anabolic steroids: An analysis of a dozen users. *Clin J Sport Med.* 20:475, 2010.

Ip E.J. et al. The anabolic 500 survey: Characteristics of male users versus nonusers of anabolic-androgenic steroids for strength training. *Pharmacotherapy.* 31:757, 2011.

Isaacs J. et al. The use of anabolic steroids as a strategy in reversing denervation atrophy after delayed nerve repair. *Hand.* 6:142, 2011.

Ishihara H. et al. Acceleration of regeneration of mucosa in small intestine damaged by ionizing radiation using anabolic steroids. *Radiat Res.* 175:367, 2011.

Johns K. et al. Anabolic steroids for the treatment of weight loss in HIV-infected individuals. *Cochrane Database Syst Rev.* CD005483, 2005.

Jones I.A. et al. Anabolic steroids and tendons: A review of their mechanical, structural, and biologic effects. *J Orthop Res.* 36:2830, 2018.

Joss E.E. Anabolic steroids in girls with Turner's syndrome. *Acta Paediatr Scand Suppl.* 343:38, 1988.

Karpakka J.A. et al. The effects of anabolic steroids on collagen synthesis in rat skeletal muscle and tendon. A preliminary report. *Am J Sports Med.* 20:262, 1992.

Kim C.S. et al. The effect of anabolic steroids on ameliorating the adverse effects of chronic corticosteroids on intestinal anastomotic healing in rabbits. *Surg Gynecol Obstet.* 176:73, 1993.

Kovac J.R. et al. A positive role for anabolic androgenic steroids: Preventing metabolic syndrome and type 2 diabetes mellitus. *Fertil Steril.* 102:e5, 2014.

Laurent M.R. et al. Age-related bone loss and sarcopenia in men. *Maturitas.* 122:51, 2019.

Marcocci C. et al. Fluoride and anabolic steroids in the treatment of glucocorticoid-induced osteoporosis. *Front Horm Res.* 30:165, 2002.

Metcalfe D. et al. Anabolic steroids in patients undergoing total knee arthroplasty. *BMJ Open.* 2:2012.

Morton R. et al. Psychiatric effects of anabolic steroids after burn injuries. *Psychosomatics.* 41:66, 2000.

Mulligan K. et al. Anabolic treatment with GH, IGF-1, or anabolic steroids in patients with HIV-associated wasting. *Int J Cardiol.* 85:151, 2002.

Naing C. et al. Anabolic steroids for treating pressure ulcers. *Cochrane Database Syst Rev.* 6:CD011375, 2017.

Need A.G. et al. Anabolic steroids in postmenopausal osteoporosis. *Wien Med Wochenschr.* 143:392, 1993.

Ohlsson C. et al. High serum testosterone is associated with reduced risk of cardiovascular events in elderly men. The MROS (osteoporotic fractures in men) study in Sweden. *J Am Coll Cardiol.* 58:1674, 2011.

Pagonis T.A. et al. Multivitamins and phospholipids complex protects the hepatic cells from androgenic-anabolic-steroids-induced toxicity. *Clin Toxicol.* 46:57, 2008.

Pan L. et al. Effects of anabolic steroids on chronic obstructive pulmonary disease: A meta-analysis of randomised controlled trials. *PLoS One.* 9:e84855, 2014.

Rigberg S.V. et al. Potential roles of androgens and the anabolic steroids in the treatment of cancer - a review. *J Med.* 6:271, 1975.

Salcido R. Anabolic steroids for pressure ulcers revisited. *Adv Skin Wound Care.* 18:344, 2005.

Santos J.D.B. et al. Food-drug interaction: Anabolic steroids aggravate hepatic lipotoxicity and nonalcoholic fatty liver disease induced by trans fatty acids. *Food Chem Toxicol.* 116:360, 2018.

Schols A.M. et al. Physiologic effects of nutritional support and anabolic steroids in patients with chronic obstructive pulmonary disease. A placebo-controlled randomized trial. *Am J Respir Crit Care Med.* 152:1268, 1995.

Serra C. et al. Testosterone improves the regeneration of old and young mouse skeletal muscle. *J Gerontol A Biol Sci Med Sci.* 68:17, 2013.

Seynnes O.R. et al. Effect of androgenic-anabolic steroids and heavy strength training on patellar tendon morphological and mechanical properties. *J Appl Physiol (1985).* 115:84, 2013.

Sharma S. et al. Anabolic steroids in COPD: A review and preliminary results of a randomized trial. *Chron Respir Dis.* 5:169, 2008.

Sun L. et al. Anabolic steroids reduce spinal cord injury-related bone loss in rats associated with increased wnt signaling. *J Spinal Cord Med.* 36:616, 2013.

Tabor J. et al. Neuroendocrine whiplash: Slamming the breaks on anabolic-androgenic steroids following repetitive mild traumatic brain injury in rats may worsen outcomes. *Front Neurol.* 10:481, 2019.

Tainter M.L. et al. Use of anabolic steroids in rehabilitation. *J Am Osteopath Assoc.* 62:796, 1963.

Upadhyaya S.K. et al. Anabolic androgenic steroids in delayed diagnosis of tuberculosis. *J Pharmacol Pharmacother.* 3:345, 2012.

Urtado C.B. et al. Resistance training associated with the administration of anabolic-androgenic steroids improves insulin sensitivity in ovariectomized rats. *Diabetes Metab Syndr Obes.* 4:385, 2011.

Varriale P. et al. Acute myocardial infarction associated with anabolic steroids in a young HIV-infected patient. *Pharmacotherapy.* 19:881, 1999.

Velema M.S. et al. Should androgenic anabolic steroids be considered in the treatment regime of selected chronic obstructive pulmonary disease patients? *Curr Opin Pulm Med.* 18:118, 2012.

Vergel N. Building your body to survive: The use of anabolic steroids for HIV therapy. *Posit Aware.* 9:37, 1998.

Walton. Anabolic steroids and muscular dystrophy. *Neurology.* 42:1435, 1992.

Woerdeman J. et al. Therapeutic effects of anabolic androgenic steroids on chronic diseases associated with muscle wasting. *Expert Opin Investig Drugs.* 20:87, 2011.

References: Miscellaneous Side-effects of Anabolic Steroids

Abelenda M. et al. Brown adipose tissue thermogenesis in testosterone-treated rats. *Acta Endocrinol.* 126:434, 1992.

Albano G.D. et al. Adverse effects of anabolic-androgenic steroids: A literature review. *Healthcare.* 9:2021.

Arvary D. et al. Anabolic-androgenic steroids as a gateway to opioid dependence. *N Engl J Med.* 342:1532, 2000.

Baranska-Rybak W. et al. Severe acne fulminans following low-dose isotretinoin and testosterone use. *Cutis.* 103:E20, 2019.

Barrett R.L. et al. Anabolic steroids and craniofacial growth in the rat. *Angle Orthod.* 63:289, 1993.

Basaria S. et al. Adverse events associated with testosterone administration. *N Engl J Med.* 363:109, 2010.

Basile J.R. et al. Supraphysiological doses of performance enhancing anabolic-androgenic steroids exert direct toxic effects on neuron-like cells. *Front Cell Neurosci.* 7:69, 2013.

Bertozzi G. et al. Immunodeficiency as a side effect of anabolic androgenic steroid abuse: A case of necrotizing myofasciitis. *Forensic Sci Med Pathol.* 15:616, 2019.

Bobyleva V. et al. Concerning the mechanism of increased thermogenesis in rats treated with dehydroepiandrosterone. *J Bioenerg Biomembr.* 25:313, 1993.

Bonetti A. et al. Side effects of anabolic androgenic steroids abuse. *Int J Sports Med.* 29:679, 2008.

Bronson F.H. et al. Exposure to anabolic-androgenic steroids shortens life span of male mice. *Med Sci Sports Exerc.* 29:615, 1997.

Brusca M.I. et al. Anabolic steroids affect human periodontal health and microbiota. *Clin Oral Investig.* 18:1579, 2014.

Buttner A. et al. Side effects of anabolic androgenic steroids: Pathological findings and structure-activity relationships. *Handb Exp Pharmacol.* 459, 2010.

Calabrese L.H. et al. The effects of anabolic steroids and strength training on the human immune response. *Med Sci Sports Exerc.* 21:386, 1989.

Caraci F. et al. Neurotoxic properties of the anabolic androgenic steroids nandrolone and methandrostenolone in primary neuronal cultures. *J Neurosci Res.* 89:592, 2011.

Comhaire F. Hormone replacement therapy and longevity. *Andrologia.* 48:65, 2016.

D'Errico S. et al. Renal heat shock proteins over-expression due to anabolic androgenic steroids abuse. *Mini Rev Med Chem.* 11:446, 2011.

Darke S. et al. Sudden or unnatural deaths involving anabolic-androgenic steroids. *J Forensic Sci.* 59:1025, 2014.

Dickerman R.D. et al. The hiccup reflex arc and persistent hiccups with high-dose anabolic steroids: Is the brainstem the steroid-responsive locus? *Clin Neuropharmacol.* 24:62, 2001.

Dickerman R.D. et al. Peripheral neuropathy and testosterone. *Neurotoxicology.* 18:587, 1997.

Farzam K. et al. Sudden death in athletes. In. *Statpearls.* Treasure Island (FL)2019.

Feller A.A. et al. Medical complications of anabolic steroids. *Med Health R I.* 85:338, 2002.

Ferrandez M.D. et al. Anabolic steroids and lymphocyte function in sedentary and exercise-trained rats. *J Steroid Biochem Mol Biol.* 59:225, 1996.

Fortunato R.S. et al. Abuse of anabolic steroids and its impact on thyroid function. *Arq Bras Endocrinol Metabol.* 51:1417, 2007.

Friedl K.E. et al. Self-treatment of gynecomastia in bodybuilders who use anabolic steroids. *Phys Sportsmed.* 17:67, 1989.

Goldberg L. Adverse effects of anabolic steroids. *JAMA.* 276:257, 1996.

Graham S. et al. Recent developments in the toxicology of anabolic steroids. *Drug Saf.* 5:458, 1990.

Griffiths S. et al. Anabolic steroids: Lots of muscle in the short-term, potentially devastating health consequences in the long-term. *Drug Alcohol Rev.* 35:375, 2016.

Hashemi S.J. et al. A comparative survey of serum androgenic hormones levels between male patients with dermatophytosis and normal subjects. *Jpn J Infect Dis.* 57:60, 2004.

Henrion R. et al. HIV contamination after injections of anabolic steroids. *Presse Med.* 21:218, 1992.

Heydenreich G. Testosterone and anabolic steroids and acne fulminans. *Arch Dermatol.* 125:571, 1989.

Hickson R.C. et al. Adverse effects of anabolic steroids. *Med Toxicol Adverse Drug Exp.* 4:254, 1989.

Horwitz H. et al. Health consequences of androgenic anabolic steroid use. *J Intern Med.* 285:333, 2019.

Kara M. et al. Determination of DNA damage and telomerase activity in stanozolol-treated rats. *Exp Ther Med.* 13:614, 2017.

Karakida L.M. et al. Interaction of anabolic androgenic steroids and induced tooth movement in rats. *Braz Dent J.* 28:504, 2017.

Kibble M.W. et al. Adverse effects of anabolic steroids in athletes. *Clin Pharm.* 6:686, 1987.

Kimergard A. et al. Environments, risk and health harms: A qualitative investigation into the illicit use of anabolic steroids among people using harm reduction services in the UK. *BMJ Open.* 4:e005275, 2014.

Kiraly C.L. et al. Effect of androgenic and anabolic steroids on the sebaceous gland in power athletes. *Acta Derm Venereol.* 67:36, 1987.

Kiraly C.L. et al. Effect of testosterone and anabolic steroids on the size of sebaceous glands in power athletes. *Am J Dermatopathol.* 9:515, 1987.

Kraus S.L. et al. The dark side of beauty: Acne fulminans induced by anabolic steroids in a male bodybuilder. *Arch Dermatol.* 148:1210, 2012.

Lear J.T. et al. Anabolic steroids and psoriasis exacerbation. *Br J Dermatol.* 134:809, 1996.

Lindqvist Bagge A.S. et al. Somatic effects of AAS abuse: A 30-years follow-up study of male former power sports athletes. *J Sci Med Sport.* 20:814, 2017.

LoBue S.A. et al. Recurrent herpes zoster ophthalmicus preceded by anabolic steroids and high-dose l-arginine. *Case Rep Ophthalmol Med.* 2020:8861892, 2020.

Maravelias C. et al. Adverse effects of anabolic steroids in athletes. A constant threat. *Toxicol Lett.* 158:167, 2005.

Martins R.A. et al. Chromosome damage and cytotoxicity in oral mucosa cells after 2 months of exposure to anabolic steroids (Deca Durabolin and Winstrol) in weight lifting. *Steroids.* 75:952, 2010.

Melnik B. et al. Abuse of anabolic-androgenic steroids and bodybuilding acne: An underestimated health problem. *J Dtsch Dermatol Ges.* 5:110, 2007.

Merkle T. et al. Acne conglobata-like exacerbation of acne vulgaris following administration of anabolic steroids and vitamin b complex-containing preparations. *Hautarzt.* 41:280, 1990.

Namjoshi D.R. et al. Chronic exposure to androgenic-anabolic steroids exacerbates axonal injury and microgliosis in the chimera mouse model of repetitive concussion. *PLoS One.* 11:e0146540, 2016.

Orlandi M.A. et al. Gynecomastia in two young men with histories of prolonged use of anabolic androgenic steroids. *J Ultrasound.* 13:46, 2010.

Orlando R. et al. Nanomolar concentrations of anabolic-androgenic steroids amplify excitotoxic neuronal death in mixed mouse cortical cultures. *Brain Res.* 1165:21, 2007.

Pai R. et al. Mycobacterium fortuitum skin infection as a complication of anabolic steroids: A rare case report. *Ann R Coll Surg Engl.* 95:e12, 2013.

Park J.A. et al. Risk factors for acne development in the first 2 years after initiating masculinizing testosterone therapy among transgender men. *J Am Acad Dermatol.* 81:617, 2019.

Petersson A. et al. Morbidity and mortality in patients testing positively for the presence of anabolic androgenic steroids in connection with receiving medical care. A controlled retrospective cohort study. *Drug Alcohol Depend.* 81:215, 2006.

Petersson A. et al. Convulsions in users of anabolic androgenic steroids: Possible explanations. *J Clin Psychopharmacol.* 27:723, 2007.

Petersson A. et al. Toxicological findings and manner of death in autopsied users of anabolic androgenic steroids. *Drug Alcohol Depend.* 81:241, 2006.

Rastad J. et al. Gluteal infection in weightlifters after injection of anabolic steroids. *Lakartidningen.* 82:3407, 1985.

Ribas C.R. et al. Increments in virulence of candida albicans induced by androgenic anabolic steroids. *Steroids.* 152:108501, 2019.

Roselli C.E. The effect of anabolic-androgenic steroids on aromatase activity and androgen receptor binding in the rat preoptic area. *Brain Res.* 792:271, 1998.

Scott M.J., 3rd et al. Effects of anabolic-androgenic steroids on the pilosebaceous unit. *Cutis.* 50:113, 1992.

Scott M.J. et al. HIV infection associated with injections of anabolic steroids. *JAMA.* 262:207, 1989.

Solakovic S. et al. Hidden danger of irrational abusing illegal androgenic-anabolic steroids in recreational athletes age under 35 in Bosnia & Herzegovina. *Med Arch.* 69:200, 2015.

Strauss R.H. et al. Side effects of anabolic steroids in weight-trained men. *Phys Sportsmed.* 11:86, 1983.

Tabassom A. et al. Epistaxis (nose bleed). In. *Statpearls.* Treasure Island (FL)2020.

Thiblin I. et al. Cause and manner of death among users of anabolic androgenic steroids. *J Forensic Sci.* 45:16, 2000.

Tikka T. et al. Acute unilateral sensorineural hearing loss associated with anabolic steroids and polycythaemia: Case report. *J Laryngol Otol.* 130:309, 2016.

Torres-Bugarin O. et al. Anabolic androgenic steroids induce micronuclei in buccal mucosa cells of bodybuilders. *Br J Sports Med.* 41:592, 2007.

Tostes R.C. et al. Reactive oxygen species: Players in the cardiovascular effects of testosterone. *Am J Physiol Regul Integr Comp Physiol.* 310:R1, 2016.

Vorona E. et al. Adverse effects of doping with anabolic androgenic steroids in competitive athletics, recreational sports and bodybuilding. *Minerva Endocrinol.* 43:476, 2018.

Wollina U. et al. Side-effects of topical androgenic and anabolic substances and steroids. A short review. *Acta Dermatovenerol Alp Pannonica Adriat.* 16:117, 2007.
Yilmaz B. et al. Endocrinology of hirsutism: From androgens to androgen excess disorders. *Front Horm Res.* 53:108, 2019.

References: Anabolic Steroids and the Kidney

Acharjee B.K. et al. Enhanced hepatic and kidney cytochrome p-450 activities in nandrolone decanoate treated albino mice. *Drug Metab Lett.* 3:120, 2009.
Ahmad A. et al. Oxandrolone protects against the development of multiorgan failure, modulates the systemic inflammatory response and promotes wound healing during burn injury. *Burns.* 45:671, 2019.
Alkhunaizi A.M. et al. Acute bile nephropathy secondary to anabolic steroids. *Clin Nephrol.* 85:121, 2016.
Almukhtar S.E. et al. Acute kidney injury associated with androgenic steroids and nutritional supplements in bodybuilders. *Clin Kidney J.* 8:415, 2015.
Barton Pai A. et al. The effects of nandrolone decanoate on nutritional parameters in hemodialysis patients. *Clin Nephrol.* 58:38, 2002.
Basic-Jukic N. et al. How to prevent protein-energy wasting in patients with chronic kidney disease--position statement of the Croatian society of nephrology, dialysis and transplantation. *Acta Med Croatica.* 68:191, 2014.
Bordin D.M. et al. Understanding alterations on blood and biochemical parameters in athletes that use dietary supplements, steroids and illicit drugs. *Toxicology.* 376:75, 2017.

Bossola M. et al. Artificial nutritional support in chronic hemodialysis patients: A narrative review. *J Ren Nutr.* 20:213, 2010.

Brasil G.A. et al. Nandrolone decanoate induces cardiac and renal remodeling in female rats, without modification in physiological parameters: The role of ANP system. *Life Sci.* 137:65, 2015.

Bronson F.H. et al. Exposure to anabolic-androgenic steroids shortens life span of male mice. *Med Sci Sports Exerc.* 29:615, 1997.

Brunier G. An update on the pathogenesis, pathology and treatment of the anemia of chronic renal failure. *J CANNT.* 15, 1990.

Comar O.B. et al. The action of anabolic steroids in chronic renal insufficiency. *Minerva Urol.* 15:109, 1963.

D'Errico S. et al. Renal heat shock proteins over-expression due to anabolic androgenic steroids abuse. *Mini Rev Med Chem.* 11:446, 2011.

Daher E.F. et al. Acute kidney injury due to anabolic steroid and vitamin supplement abuse: Report of two cases and a literature review. *Int Urol Nephrol.* 41:717, 2009.

Davani-Davari D. et al. The potential effects of anabolic-androgenic steroids and growth hormone as commonly used sport supplements on the kidney: A systematic review. *BMC Nephrol.* 20:198, 2019.

Deshmukh N. et al. Potentially harmful advantage to athletes: A putative connection between UGT2b17 gene deletion polymorphism and renal disorders with prolonged use of anabolic androgenic steroids. *Subst Abuse Treat Prev Policy.* 5:7, 2010.

Dieckhoff J. et al. On the effect of anabolic metabolites on enzyme activities (LDH, MDH, GPT, GOT, ALD) in heart, liver and kidney tissues. *Z Kinderheilkd.* 90:200, 1964.

Dontas A.S. et al. Long-term effects of anabolic steroids on renal functions in the aged subject. *J Gerontol.* 22:268, 1967.

Dornelles G.L. et al. Biochemical and oxidative stress markers in the liver and kidneys of rats submitted to different protocols of anabolic steroids. *Mol Cell Biochem.* 425:181, 2017.

El-Reshaid W. et al. Complementary bodybuilding: A potential risk for permanent kidney disease. *Saudi J Kidney Dis Transpl.* 29:326, 2018.

Fisler A. et al. Bile cast nephropathy: The unknown dangers of online shopping. *Case Rep Nephrol Dial.* 8:98, 2018.

Flachi M. et al. FSGS collapsing variant during anabolic steroid abuse: Case report. *G Ital Nefrol.* 35:2018.

Flores A. et al. Severe cholestasis and bile acid nephropathy from anabolic steroids successfully treated with plasmapheresis. *ACG Case Rep J.* 3:133, 2016.

Frankenfeld S.P. et al. The anabolic androgenic steroid nandrolone decanoate disrupts redox homeostasis in liver, heart and kidney of male Wistar rats. *PLoS One.* 9:e102699, 2014.

Grimmer N.M. et al. Rhabdomyolysis secondary to clenbuterol use and exercise. *J Emerg Med.* 50:e71, 2016.

Grogan S. et al. Experiences of anabolic steroid use: In-depth interviews with men and women body builders. *J Health Psychol.* 11:845, 2006.

Gullett N.P. et al. Update on clinical trials of growth factors and anabolic steroids in cachexia and wasting. *Am J Clin Nutr.* 91:1143S, 2010.

Habscheid W. et al. Severe cholestasis with kidney

failure from anabolic steroids in a body builder. *Dtsch Med Wochenschr.* 124:1029, 1999.

Hausmann D.F. et al. Anabolic steroids in polytrauma patients. Influence on renal nitrogen and amino acid losses: A double-blind study. *JPEN J Parenter Enteral Nutr.* 14:111, 1990.

Heitzman R.J. The absorption, distribution and excretion of anabolic agents. *J Anim Sci.* 57:233, 1983.

Herlitz L.C. et al. Development of focal segmental glomerulosclerosis after anabolic steroid abuse. *J Am Soc Nephrol.* 21:163, 2010.

Hoseini L. et al. Nandrolone decanoate increases the volume but not the length of the proximal and distal convoluted tubules of the mouse kidney. *Micron.* 40:226, 2009.

Hudson J.I. et al. Glomerular filtration rate and supraphysiologic-dose anabolic-androgenic steroid use: A cross-sectional cohort study. *Am J Kidney Dis.* 2020.

Ikizler T.A. et al. Prevention and treatment of protein energy wasting in chronic kidney disease patients: A consensus statement by the International Society of Renal Nutrition and Metabolism. *Kidney Int.* 84:1096, 2013.

Ilhan E. et al. Acute myocardial infarction and renal infarction in a bodybuilder using anabolic steroids. *Turk Kardiyol Dern Ars.* 38:275, 2010.

Johansen K.L. et al. Anabolic effects of nandrolone decanoate in patients receiving dialysis: A randomized controlled trial. *JAMA.* 281:1275, 1999.

Johnson C.A. Use of androgens in patients with renal failure. *Semin Dial.* 13:36, 2000.

Jones R.W. et al. The effects of anabolic steroids on growth, body composition, and metabolism in boys with chronic renal failure on regular hemodialysis. *J Pediatr*. 97:559, 1980.

Kantarci U.H. et al. Evaluation of anabolic steroid induced renal damage with sonography in bodybuilders. *J Sports Med Phys Fitness*. 58:1681, 2018.

Kimergard A. et al. The composition of anabolic steroids from the illicit market is largely unknown: Implications for clinical case reports. *QJM*. 107:597, 2014.

Lindblom J. et al. Nandrolone treatment decreases the alpha1b-adrenoceptor mrna level in rat kidney, but not the density of alpha1b-adrenoceptors in cultured mdckd1 kidney cells. *Eur J Pharmacol*. 527:157, 2005.

Luciano R.L. et al. Bile acid nephropathy in a bodybuilder abusing an anabolic androgenic steroid. *Am J Kidney Dis*. 64:473, 2014.

Malin A. et al. Dialysis for severe rhabdomyolysis 7 days after multiple trauma. *Anaesthesist*. 61:224, 2012.

Maravelias C. et al. Adverse effects of anabolic steroids in athletes. A constant threat. *Toxicol Lett*. 158:167, 2005.

Milla Castellanos M. et al. Bile cast nephropathy associated with severe liver dysfunction caused by anabolic steroids. *Nefrologia*. 38:221, 2018.

Modlinski R. et al. The effect of anabolic steroids on the gastrointestinal system, kidneys, and adrenal glands. *Curr Sports Med Rep*. 5:104, 2006.

Nieschlag E. et al. Doping with anabolic androgenic steroids (AAS): Adverse effects on non-reproductive organs and functions. *Rev Endocr Metab Disord*. 16:199, 2015.

Parente Filho S.L.A. et al. Kidney disease associated with androgenic-anabolic steroids and vitamin supplements abuse: Be aware! *Nefrologia*. 2019.

Pendergraft W.F., 3rd et al. Nephrotoxic effects of

common and emerging drugs of abuse. *Clin J Am Soc Nephrol.* 9:1996, 2014.

Pinto F. et al. Doping and urologic tumors. *Urologia.* 77:92, 2010.

Robles-Diaz M. et al. Distinct phenotype of hepato-toxicity associated with illicit use of anabolic andro-genic steroids. *Aliment Pharmacol Ther.* 41:116, 2015.

Rosenfeld G.A. et al. Cholestatic jaundice, acute kidney injury and acute pancreatitis secondary to the recreational use of methandrostenolone: A case report. *J Med Case Rep.* 5:138, 2011.

Salem N.A. et al. The impact of nandrolone de-canoate abuse on experimental animal model: Hor-monal and biochemical assessment. *Steroids.* 153:108526, 2019.

Tarashande Foumani A. et al. Oxymetholone-induced acute renal failure: A case report. *Caspian J Intern Med.* 9:410, 2018.

Tsitsimpikou C. et al. Nephrotoxicity in rabbits after long-term nandrolone decanoate administration. *Toxicol Lett.* 259:21, 2016.

Turani H. et al. Hepatic lesions in patients on anabolic androgenic therapy. *Isr J Med Sci.* 19:332, 1983.

Uhlen S. et al. Nandrolone treatment decreases the level of rat kidney alpha(1b)-adrenoceptors. *Naunyn Schmiedebergs Arch Pharmacol.* 368:91, 2003.

Unai S. et al. Caution for anabolic androgenic steroid use: A case report of multiple organ dysfunction syn-drome. *Respir Care.* 58:e159, 2013.

References: Anabolic Steroids and the Liver

Bakker K. et al. Liver lesions due to long-term use of

anabolic steroids and oral contraceptives. *Ned Tijdschr Geneeskd.* 120:2214, 1976.

Balgoma D. et al. Anabolic androgenic steroids exert a selective remodeling of the plasma lipidome that mirrors the decrease of the de novo lipogenesis in the liver. *Metabolomics.* 16:12, 2020.

Boks M.N. et al. A jaundiced bodybuilder cholestatic hepatitis as side effect of injectable anabolic-androgenic steroids. *J Sports Sci.* 35:2262, 2017.

Booth J. et al. The effect of anabolic steroids on drug metabolism by microsomal enzymes in rat liver. *J Pharmacol Exp Ther.* 137:374, 1962.

Carmichael R.H. et al. Effect of anabolic steroids on liver function tests in rabbits. *Proc Soc Exp Biol Med.* 113:1006, 1963.

Clark B.M. et al. Dilated cardiomyopathy and acute liver injury associated with combined use of ephedra, gamma-hydroxybutyrate, and anabolic steroids. *Pharmacotherapy.* 25:756, 2005.

Creagh T.M. et al. Hepatic tumours induced by anabolic steroids in an athlete. *J Clin Pathol.* 41:441, 1988.

Dornelles G.L. et al. Biochemical and oxidative stress markers in the liver and kidneys of rats submitted to different protocols of anabolic steroids. *Mol Cell Biochem.* 425:181, 2017.

El Sherrif Y. et al. Hepatotoxicity from anabolic androgenic steroids marketed as dietary supplements: Contribution from ATP8b1/AABCB11 mutations? *Liver Int.* 33:1266, 2013.

Elsharkawy A.M. et al. Cholestasis in young men after taking anabolic steroids. *Praxis.* 101:661, 2012.

Falk H. et al. Hepatic angiosarcoma associated with androgenic-anabolic steroids. *Lancet.* 2:1120, 1979.

Giannitrapani L. et al. Sex hormones and risk of liver tumor. *Ann N Y Acad Sci.* 1089:228, 2006.

Goldman B. Liver carcinoma in an athlete taking anabolic steroids. *J Am Osteopath Assoc.* 85:56, 1985.

Gragera R. et al. Ultrastructural changes induced by anabolic steroids in liver of trained rats. *Histol Histopathol.* 8:449, 1993.

Hartgens F. et al. Body composition, cardiovascular risk factors and liver function in long-term androgenic-anabolic steroids using bodybuilders three months after drug withdrawal. *Int J Sports Med.* 17:429, 1996.

Hedstrom M. et al. Positive effects of anabolic steroids, vitamin D and calcium on muscle mass, bone mineral density and clinical function after a hip fracture. A randomised study of 63 women. *J Bone Joint Surg Br.* 84:497, 2002.

Ishak K.G. Hepatic lesions caused by anabolic and contraceptive steroids. *Semin Liver Dis.* 1:116, 1981.

Ishak K.G. et al. Hepatotoxic effects of the anabolic/androgenic steroids. *Semin Liver Dis.* 7:230, 1987.

Kuipers H. et al. Influence of anabolic steroids on body composition, blood pressure, lipid profile and liver functions in body builders. *Int J Sports Med.* 12:413, 1991.

Lax E.R. et al. Effect of androgenic, oestrogenic, anabolic, progestational and catatoxic steroids on the kidney, adrenal and liver mass of the rat. *Z Versuchstierkd.* 26:99, 1984.

Lenders J.W. et al. Deleterious effects of anabolic steroids on serum lipoproteins, blood pressure, and liver function in amateur body builders. *Int J Sports Med.* 9:19, 1988.

Luciano R.L. et al. Bile acid nephropathy in a bodybuilder abusing an anabolic androgenic steroid. *Am J Kidney Dis.* 64:473, 2014.

Magee C.D. et al. Mission compromised? Drug-induced liver injury from prohormone supplements containing anabolic-androgenic steroids in two deployed u.S. Service members. *Mil Med.* 181:e1169, 2016.

Marcacuzco Quinto A.A. et al. Spontaneous hepatic rupture associated with the use of anabolic steroids. *Cir Esp.* 92:570, 2014.

Marquardt G.H. et al. Effect of anabolic steroids on liver function tests and creatine excretion. *JAMA.* 175:851, 1961.

Marquardt G.H. et al. Failure of non-17-alkylated anabolic steroids to produce abnormal liver function tests. *J Clin Endocrinol Metab.* 24:1334, 1964.

Mendenhall C.L. Augmented release of hepatic triglycerides with anabolic steroids in patients with fatty liver. *Am J Dig Dis.* 19:122, 1974.

Milla Castellanos M. et al. Bile cast nephropathy associated with severe liver dysfunction caused by anabolic steroids. *Nefrologia.* 38:221, 2018.

Molano F. et al. Rat liver lysosomal and mitochondrial activities are modified by anabolic-androgenic steroids. *Med Sci Sports Exerc.* 31:243, 1999.

Navarro V.J. et al. Liver injury from herbal and dietary supplements. *Hepatology.* 65:363, 2017.

Neri M. et al. Anabolic androgenic steroids abuse and liver toxicity. *Mini Rev Med Chem.* 11:430, 2011.

Nieschlag E. et al. Doping with anabolic androgenic steroids (AAS): Adverse effects on non-reproductive organs and functions. *Rev Endocr Metab Disord.* 16:199, 2015.

Orlandi F. et al. The action of some anabolic steroids

on the structure and the function of human liver cell. *Tijdschr Gastroenterol.* 7:109, 1964.

Perezagua-Clamagirand C. et al. A clinical and experimental study of the effects of some anabolic steroids on hepatic structure and function. *Arch Farmacol Toxicol.* 1:77, 1975.

Romano A. et al. An unusual case of left hepatectomy for focal nodular hyperplasia (FNH) linked to the use of anabolic androgenic steroids (AASS). *Int J Surg Case Rep.* 30:169, 2017.

Saad Al-Dhuayan I. Possible protective role of whey protein on the rat's liver tissues treated with nandrolone decanoate. *Pak J Biol Sci.* 21:262, 2018.

Saborido A. et al. Effect of training and anabolic-androgenic steroids on drug metabolism in rat liver. *Med Sci Sports Exerc.* 25:815, 1993.

Sanchez-Osorio M. et al. Anabolic-androgenic steroids and liver injury. *Liver Int.* 28:278, 2008.

Santos J.D.B. et al. Food-drug interaction: Anabolic steroids aggravate hepatic lipotoxicity and nonalcoholic fatty liver disease induced by trans fatty acids. *Food Chem Toxicol.* 116:360, 2018.

Schwingel P.A. et al. Anabolic-androgenic steroids: A possible new risk factor of toxicant-associated fatty liver disease. *Liver Int.* 31:348, 2011.

Schwingel P.A. et al. Recreational anabolic-androgenic steroid use associated with liver injuries among Brazilian young men. *Subst Use Misuse.* 50:1490, 2015.

Silva Ruiz M.D.P. et al. Canalicular cholestasis induced by anabolic steroids. *Rev Esp Enferm Dig.* 109:735, 2017.

Smit D.L. et al. Spontaneous haemorrhage of hepatic adenoma in a patient addicted to anabolic steroids. *Neth J Med.* 77:261, 2019.

Smit D.L. et al. Spontaneous haemorrhage of hepatic

adenoma in a patient addicted to anabolic steroids. *Neth J Med.* 77:261, 2019.

Soe K.L. et al. Liver pathology associated with the use of anabolic-androgenic steroids. *Liver.* 12:73, 1992.

Solimini R. et al. Hepatotoxicity associated with illicit use of anabolic androgenic steroids in doping. *Eur Rev Med Pharmacol Sci.* 21:7, 2017.

Stang-Voss C. et al. Structural alterations of liver parenchyma induced by anabolic steroids. *Int J Sports Med.* 2:101, 1981.

Woodward C. et al. Hepatocellular carcinoma in body builders; an emerging rare but serious complication of androgenic anabolic steroid use. *Ann Hepatobiliary Pancreat Surg.* 23:174, 2019.

References: Anabolic Steroids and Muscle Disorders

Abu-Shakra S. et al. Anabolic steroids induce injury and apoptosis of differentiated skeletal muscle. *J Neurosci Res.* 47:186, 1997.

Abu-Shakra S.R. et al. Anabolic steroids induce skeletal muscle injury and immediate early gene expression through a receptor-independent mechanism. *Ann N Y Acad Sci.* 761:395, 1995.

Farkash U. et al. Rhabdomyolysis of the deltoid muscle in a bodybuilder using anabolic-androgenic steroids: A case report. *J Athl Train.* 44:98, 2009.

Filho N.S. et al. Pyomyositis in athletes after the use of anabolic steroids - case reports. *Rev Bras Ortop.* 46:97, 2011.

Fiore C.E. et al. The effects of muscle-building exercise on forearm bone mineral content and osteoblast activity in drug-free and anabolic steroids self-administering young men. *Bone Miner.* 13:77, 1991.

Frankle M.A. Association of anabolic steroids and avascular necrosis of femoral heads. *Am J Sports Med.* 20:488, 1992.

Freeman B.J. et al. Spontaneous rupture of the anterior cruciate ligament after anabolic steroids. *Br J Sports Med.* 29:274, 1995.

Gallagher J.A. et al. Effects of glucocorticoids and anabolic steroids on cells derived from human skeletal and articular tissues in vitro. *Adv Exp Med Biol.* 171:279, 1984.

Gerber C. et al. Anabolic steroids reduce muscle degeneration associated with rotator cuff tendon release in sheep. *Am J Sports Med.* 43:2393, 2015.

Gerber C. et al. Anabolic steroids reduce muscle damage caused by rotator cuff tendon release in an experimental study in rabbits. *J Bone Joint Surg Am.* 93:2189, 2011.

Gerber C. et al. Rotator cuff muscles lose responsiveness to anabolic steroids after tendon tear and musculotendinous retraction: An experimental study in sheep. *Am J Sports Med.* 40:2454, 2012.

Gharahdaghi N. et al. Testosterone therapy induces molecular programming augmenting physiological adaptations to resistance exercise in older men. *J Cachexia Sarcopenia Muscle.* 10:1276, 2019.

Guzzoni V. et al. Tendon remodeling in response to resistance training, anabolic androgenic steroids and aging. *Cells.* 7:2018.

Hageloch W. et al. Rhabdomyolysis in a bodybuilder using anabolic steroids. *Sportverletz Sportschaden.* 2:122, 1988.

Horn S. et al. Self-reported anabolic-androgenic

steroids use and musculoskeletal injuries: Findings from the Center for the Study of Retired Athletes health survey of retired NFL players. *Am J Phys Med Rehabil.* 88:192, 2009.

Husen M. et al. Doping in elite and popular sport : What orthopedic and trauma surgeons should know. *Orthopade.* 48:711, 2019.

Inhofe P.D. et al. The effects of anabolic steroids on rat tendon. An ultrastructural, biomechanical, and biochemical analysis. *Am J Sports Med.* 23:227, 1995.

Isenberg J. et al. Successive ruptures of patellar and Achilles tendons. Anabolic steroids in competitive sports. *Unfallchirurg.* 111:46, 2008.

Jones I.A. et al. Anabolic steroids and tendons: A review of their mechanical, structural, and biologic effects. *J Orthop Res.* 36:2830, 2018.

Kanayama G. et al. Ruptured tendons in anabolic-androgenic steroid users: A cross-sectional cohort study. *Am J Sports Med.* 43:2638, 2015.

Karpakka J.A. et al. The effects of anabolic steroids on collagen synthesis in rat skeletal muscle and tendon. A preliminary report. *Am J Sports Med.* 20:262, 1992.

Kramhoft M. et al. Spontaneous rupture of the extensor pollicis longus tendon after anabolic steroids. *J Hand Surg Br.* 11:87, 1986.

Laseter J.T. et al. Anabolic steroid-induced tendon pathology: A review of the literature. *Med Sci Sports Exerc.* 23:1, 1991.

Liow R.Y. et al. Bilateral rupture of the quadriceps tendon associated with anabolic steroids. *Br J Sports Med.* 29:77, 1995.

Marqueti R.C. et al. Androgenic-anabolic steroids associated with mechanical loading inhibit matrix metallopeptidase activity and affect the remodeling of the

Achilles tendon in rats. *Am J Sports Med.* 34:1274, 2006.

Marqueti R.C. et al. Tendon structural adaptations to load exercise are inhibited by anabolic androgenic steroids. *Scand J Med Sci Sports.* 24:e39, 2014.

Marqueti R.C. et al. Matrix metallopeptidase 2 activity in tendon regions: Effects of mechanical loading exercise associated to anabolic-androgenic steroids. *Eur J Appl Physiol.* 104:1087, 2008.

Marz J. et al. Pectoralis major tendon rupture and anabolic steroids in anamnesis--a case review. *Rozhl Chir.* 87:380, 2008.

Michna H. Tendon injuries induced by exercise and anabolic steroids in experimental mice. *Int Orthop.* 11:157, 1987.

Miles J.W. et al. The effect of anabolic steroids on the biomechanical and histological properties of rat tendon. *J Bone Joint Surg Am.* 74:411, 1992.

Parssinen M. et al. The effect of supraphysiological doses of anabolic androgenic steroids on collagen metabolism. *Int J Sports Med.* 21:406, 2000.

Saad F. et al. Testosterone deficiency and testosterone treatment in older men. *Gerontology.* 63:144, 2017.

Schultzel M.M. et al. Bilateral deltoid myositis ossificans in a weightlifter using anabolic steroids. *Orthopedics.* 37:e844, 2014.

Seynnes O.R. et al. Effect of androgenic-anabolic steroids and heavy strength training on patellar tendon morphological and mechanical properties. *J Appl Physiol (1985).* 115:84, 2013.

Talaat M. et al. Histologic and histochemical study of effects of anabolic steroids on the female larynx. *Ann Otol Rhinol Laryngol.* 96:468, 1987.

Tsitsilonis S. et al. Anabolic androgenic steroids reverse the beneficial effect of exercise on tendon biomechanics: An experimental study. *Foot Ankle Surg.* 20:94, 2014.

Visuri T. et al. Bilateral distal biceps tendon avulsions with use of anabolic steroids. *Med Sci Sports Exerc.* 26:941, 1994.

Weinreb I. et al. Factitial soft tissue pseudotumor due to injection of anabolic steroids: A report of 3 cases in 2 patients. *Hum Pathol.* 41:452, 2010.

Wood T.O. et al. The effect of exercise and anabolic steroids on the mechanical properties and crimp morphology of the rat tendon. *Am J Sports Med.* 16:153, 1988.

Yu-Yahiro J.A. et al. Morphologic and histologic abnormalities in female and male rats treated with anabolic steroids. *Am J Sports Med.* 17:686, 1989.

References: Anabolic Steroids and the Law

Aamo T.O. et al. The doping rules--a set of rules in good Olympic spirit? *Tidsskr Nor Laegeforen.* 115:2120, 1995.

Alladio E. et al. Application of multivariate statistics to the steroidal module of the athlete biological passport: A proof of concept study. *Anal Chim Acta.* 922:19, 2016.

Allen H. Anti-doping policy, therapeutic use. *Sports Med.* 49:659, 2019.

Amos A. et al. Drugs in sport: The legal issues. *Sport in Society.* 12:356, 2009.

Beauregard S.-E. Secrets of the dead: Doping for gold. *Booklist.* 105:118, 2008.

Beran R.G. Analysis - what is legal medicine? *J Forensic Leg Med.* 15:158, 2008.

Berge K.H. et al. The subversion of urine drug testing. *Minn Med.* 93:45, 2010.

Borry P. et al. Geolocalisation of athletes for out-of-competition drug testing: Ethical considerations. Position statement by the WADA ethics panel. *Br J Sports Med.* 52:456, 2018.

Boudreau F. et al. Ben Johnson and the use of steroids in sport: Sociological and ethical considerations. *Can J Sport Sci.* 16:88, 1991.

Bourdon R. Ethical and analytical problems in man and greater mammals. *Ann Pharm Fr.* 49:67, 1991.

Charlish P. Drugs in sport. *Legal Information Management.* 12:109, 2012.

Christophersen A.S. et al. Drug analysis for control purposes in forensic toxicology, workplace testing, sports medicine and related areas. *Pharmacol Toxicol.* 74:202, 1994.

Cook J. Doping and free speech. *Entertain Sport Law J.* 5: 2007.

Cowan D.A. et al. Doping in sport: Misuse, analytical tests, and legal aspects. *Clin Chem.* 43:1110, 1997.

Crawley F.P. et al. Health, integrity, and doping in sports for children and young adults. A resolution of the European Academy of Paediatrics. *Eur J Pediatr.* 176:825, 2017.

Deventer K. et al. Prevalence of legal and illegal stimulating agents in sports. *Anal Bioanal Chem.* 401:421, 2011.

Devriendt T. et al. The athlete biological passport: Challenges and possibilities. *INT J Sport Pol.* 11:315, 2019.

Devriendt T. et al. Do athletes have a right to access

data in their athlete biological passport? *Drug Test Anal.* 10:802, 2018.

Dodge T. et al. Judgments about illegal performance-enhancing substances: Reasoned, reactive, or both? *J Health Psychol.* 18:962, 2013.

Drug Enforcement Administration D.O.J. Classification of three steroids as schedule III anabolic steroids under the controlled substances act. Final rule. *Fed Regist.* 74:63603, 2009.

Drug Enforcement Administration D.O.J. Classification of two steroids, prostanozol and methasterone, as schedule III anabolic steroids under the Controlled Substance Act. Final rule. *Fed Regist.* 77:44456, 2012.

Ekmekci P.E. Physicians' ethical dilemmas in the context of anti-doping practices. *Ann Sports Med Res.* 3:2016.

Fink J. et al. Anabolic-androgenic steroids: Procurement and administration practices of doping athletes. *Phys Sportsmed.* 47:10, 2019.

Frude E. et al. A focused netnographic study exploring experiences associated with counterfeit and contaminated anabolic-androgenic steroids. *Harm Reduct J.* 17:42, 2020.

Garasic M.D. et al. Moral and social reasons to acknowledge the use of cognitive enhancers in competitive-selective contexts. *BMC Med Ethics.* 17:18, 2016.

Gilbert S. The biological passport. *Hastings Cent Rep.* 40:18, 2010.

Haas U. Is the fight against doping in sport a legal minefield like any other? *Med Sport Sci.* 62:22, 2017.

Glassman, K.M. Shedding their rights: The Fourth Amendment and suspicionless drug testing in public school students participating in extracurricular activities. Cath Univ Law Rev. 51: Rev 951, 2002.

Hailey N. A false start in the race against doping in sport: Concerns with cycling's biological passport. *Duke Law J.* 61:393, 2011.

Hanstad D.V. et al. Sport, health and drugs: A critical re-examination of some key issues and problems. *Perspect Public Health.* 129:174, 2009.

Hochstetler D.R. The ethics of doping and anti-doping: Redeeming the soul of sport? *Choice: Current Reviews for Academic Libraries.* 47:1732, 2010.

Kamber M. The fight against doping: International and national efforts as exemplified by the convention of the council of Europe and the doping regulations of the swiss national association for sports. *Schweiz Z Sportmed.* 38:101, 1990.

Karkazis K. et al. Tracking U.S. Professional athletes: The ethics of biometric technologies. *Am J Bioeth.* 17:45, 2017.

Kayser B. et al. The Olympics and harm reduction? *Harm Reduct J.* 9:33, 2012.

Kayser B. et al. Current anti-doping policy: A critical appraisal. *BMC Med Ethics.* 8:2, 2007.

Landry G.L. et al. Drug screening in the athletic setting. *Curr Probl Pediatr.* 24:344, 1994.

Laure P. Epidemiologic approach of doping in sport. A review. *J Sports Med Phys Fitness.* 37:218, 1997.

Lippi G. et al. Doping in competition or doping in sport? *Br Med Bull.* 86:95, 2008.

Lippi G. et al. Athlete's biological passport: To test or not to test? *Clin Chem Lab Med.* 49:1393, 2011.

Lundby C. et al. The evolving science of detection of 'blood doping'. *Br J Pharmacol.* 165:1306, 2012.

McEvoy D. Steroid nation. *Publishers Weekly.* 255:23, 2008.

McNamee M.J. et al. Juridical and ethical peculiarities in doping policy. *J Med Ethics.* 36:165, 2010.

Ng T.L. Dope testing in sports: Scientific and medico-legal issues. *Ann Acad Med Singapore.* 22:48, 1993.

Niggli O. How will the legal and sport environment influence a future code? *Med Sport Sci.* 62:34, 2017.

Nunes A.J. et al. Early warning of suspected doping from biological passport based on multivariate trends. *Int J Sports Med.* 2019.

Nuriev A. Non-intentional anti-doping rule violations: Does a new trend in evidence provision suffice? *Int Sport Law J.* 19: 222, 2019.

Parr M.K. et al. Sports-related issues and biochemistry of natural and synthetic anabolic substances. *Endocrinol Metab Clin North Am.* 39:45, 2010.

Paterson E.R. Testosterone dreams: Rejuvenation, aphrodisia, doping. *Choice: Current Reviews for Academic Libraries.* 45:1715, 2008.

Paterson E.R. A guide to the world anti-doping code: A fight for the spirit of sport. *Choice: Current Reviews for Academic Libraries.* 46:1979, 2009.

Patterson E.R. Testosterone dreams: Rejuvenation, aphrodisia, doping. *Choice: Current Reviews for Academic Libraries.* 42:2021, 2005.

Petroczi A. et al. A call for policy guidance on psychometric testing in doping control in sport. *Int J Drug Policy.* 26:1130, 2015.

Phillips D. Anabolic steroid legislation ACT 249 of 1989. *J Ark Med Soc.* 86:67, 1989.

Rowe R.K. The challenges of modern sport to ethics: From doping to cyborgs. *Choice: Current Reviews for Academic Libraries.* 51:851, 2014.

Sando B.G. Is it legal? Prescribing for the athlete. *Aust Fam Physician.* 28:549, 1999.

Saugy M. et al. Monitoring of biological markers indicative of doping: The athlete biological passport. *Br J Sports Med.* 48:827, 2014.

Schneider A.J. et al. Human genetic variation: New challenges and opportunities for doping control. *J Sports Sci.* 30:1117, 2012.

Segura J. Is anti-doping analysis so far from clinical, legal or forensic targets?: The added value of close relationships between related disciplines. *Drug Test Anal.* 1:479, 2009.

Shapiro M.H. The identity of identity: Moral and legal aspects of technological self-transformation. *Soc Philos Policy.* 22:308, 2005.

Slobodien H.D. The rights of every man and woman in the United States. *N J Med.* 93:15, 1996.

Smith A.C. et al. Why the war on drugs in sport will never be won. *Harm Reduct J.* 12:53, 2015.

Sobolevsky T. et al. Anti-doping analyses at the Sochi Olympic and Paralympic Games 2014. *Drug Test Anal.* 6:1087, 2014.

St Mary E.W. Legal and ethical dilemmas in drug management for team physicians and athletic trainers. *South Med J.* 91:421, 1998.

Valkenburg D. et al. Doping control, providing whereabouts and the importance of privacy for elite athletes. *Int J Drug Policy.* 25:212, 2014.

Verzeletti A. Medical malpractice and the professional legal responsibility of the sports physician. *J Law Med.* 21:179, 2013.

Weston M. The regulation of doping in the U.S. and international sports. In. *The Oxford Handbook of American Sports Law.* London: Oxford Handbooks; 2018.

Wheatcroft G. Tour de farce. *New York Times Book Review.* 45, 2012.

Wiesing U. Should performance-enhancing drugs in sport be legalized under medical supervision? *Sports Med.* 41:167, 2011.

Zelenkova I. et al. Redefining sport based on the Russian doping experience. *Curr Sports Med Rep.* 18:188, 2019.

Zenic N. et al. Religiousness as a factor of hesitation against doping behavior in college-age athletes. *J Relig Health.* 52:386, 2013.

Zorzoli M. The athlete biological passport from the perspective of an anti-doping organization. *Clin Chem Lab Med.* 49:1423, 2011.

References: Anabolic Steroids and Doping Control

Abushareeda W. et al. Gas chromatographic quadrupole time-of-flight full scan high resolution mass spectrometric screening of human urine in anti-doping analysis. *J Chromatogr B Analyt Technol Biomed Life Sci.* 1063:74, 2017.

Abushareeda W. et al. Comparison of gas chromatography/quadrupole time-of-flight and quadrupole orbitrap mass spectrometry in anti-doping analysis: I. Detection of anabolic-androgenic steroids. *Rapid Commun Mass Spectrom.* 32:2055, 2018.

Adhikary P.M. et al. The use of carbon skeleton chromatography for the detection of steroid drug metabolites: The metabolism of anabolic steroids in man. *Acta Endocrinol.* 67:721, 1971.

Albanese A.A. Newer methodology in the clinical investigation of anabolic steroids. *J New Drugs.* 5:208, 1965.

Albeiroti S. et al. The influence of small doses of

ethanol on the urinary testosterone to epitestosterone ratio in men and women. *Drug Test Anal.* 10:575, 2018.

Alladio E. et al. Application of multivariate statistics to the steroidal module of the athlete biological passport: A proof of concept study. *Anal Chim Acta.* 922:19, 2016.

Alquraini H. et al. Strategies that athletes use to avoid detection of androgenic-anabolic steroid doping and sanctions. *Mol Cell Endocrinol.* 464:28, 2018.

Athanasiadou I. et al. Hyperhydration using different hydration agents does not affect the haematological markers of the athlete biological passport in euhydrated volunteers. *J Sports Sci.* 1, 2020.

Ayotte C. Detecting the administration of endogenous anabolic androgenic steroids. *Handb Exp Pharmacol.* 77, 2010.

Balcells G. et al. Detection of stanozolol o- and n-sulfate metabolites and their evaluation as additional markers in doping control. *Drug Test Anal.* 9:1001, 2017.

Balcells G. et al. Screening for anabolic steroids in sports: Analytical strategy based on the detection of phase I and phase II intact urinary metabolites by liquid chromatography tandem mass spectrometry. *J Chromatogr A.* 1389:65, 2015.

Baranov P.A. et al. The potential use of complex derivatization procedures in comprehensive HPLC-MS/MS detection of anabolic steroids. *Drug Test Anal.* 2:475, 2010.

Baume N. et al. Antidoping programme and biological monitoring before and during the 2014 FIFA World Cup Brazil. *Br J Sports Med.* 49:614, 2015.

Beaumann S. Long-term detection of anabolic steroid metabolites in urine. *Agilent Technologies, Inc, Santa Clara, CA.* 2010.

Berneira L.M. et al. Application of differential scanning calorimetry in the analysis of apprehended formulations of anabolic androgenic steroids. *Forensic Sci Int.* 296:15, 2019.

Borjesson A. et al. Studies of athlete biological passport biomarkers and clinical parameters in male and female users of anabolic androgenic steroids and other doping agents. *Drug Test Anal.* 12:514, 2020.

Cohen P.A. et al. Analysis of ingredients of supplements in the National Institutes of Health supplement database marketed as containing a novel alternative to anabolic steroids. *JAMA Netw Open.* 3: e202818, 2020.

Causanilles A. et al. Wastewater-based tracing of doping use by the general population and amateur athletes. *Anal Bioanal Chem.* 410:1793, 2018.

Cha E. et al. Coupling of gas chromatography and electrospray ionization high resolution mass spectrometry for the analysis of anabolic steroids as trimethylsilyl derivatives in human urine. *Anal Chim Acta.* 964:123, 2017.

Cha E. et al. Relationships between structure, ionization profile and sensitivity of exogenous anabolic steroids under electrospray ionization and analysis in human urine using liquid chromatography-tandem mass spectrometry. *Biomed Chromatogr.* 30:555, 2016.

Christou G.A. et al. Indirect clinical markers for the detection of anabolic steroid abuse beyond the conventional doping control in athletes. *Eur J Sport Sci.* 19:1276, 2019.

de Albuquerque Cavalcanti G. et al. Non-targeted acquisition strategy for screening doping compounds based on GC-EI-hybrid quadrupole-orbitrap mass spectrometry: A focus on exogenous anabolic steroids. *Drug Test Anal.* 10:507, 2018.

De Cock K.J. et al. Detection and determination of anabolic steroids in nutritional supplements. *J Pharm Biomed Anal.* 25:843, 2001.

Devriendt T. et al. The athlete biological passport: Challenges and possibilities. *Int J Sport Pol Pol.* 11:315, 2019.

Dumestre-Toulet V. et al. Hair analysis of seven bodybuilders for anabolic steroids, ephedrine, and clenbuterol. *J Forensic Sci.* 47:211, 2002.

Dumont Q. et al. Improved steroids detection and evidence for their regiospecific decompositions using anion attachment mass spectrometry. *Anal Chem.* 88:3585, 2016.

Esquivel A. et al. Direct quantitation of endogenous steroid sulfates in human urine by liquid chromatography-electrospray tandem mass spectrometry. *Drug Test Anal.* 10:1734, 2018.

Forsdahl G. et al. Detection of testosterone esters in blood. *Drug Test Anal.* 7:983, 2015.

Fragkaki A.G. et al. Schemes of metabolic patterns of anabolic androgenic steroids for the estimation of metabolites of designer steroids in human urine. *J Steroid Biochem Mol Biol.* 115:44, 2009.

Frude E. et al. A focused netnographic study exploring experiences associated with counterfeit and contaminated anabolic-androgenic steroids. *Harm Reduct J.* 17:42, 2020.

Georgakopoulos C.G. et al. Prediction of gas chromatographic relative retention times of anabolic steroids. *Anal Chem.* 63:2025, 1991.

Graham M. et al. Anabolic steroid use patterns of use and detection of doping. *Sports Med.* 38:505, 2008.

Hadef Y. et al. Multivariate optimization of a derivatisation procedure for the simultaneous determination of nine anabolic steroids by gas chromatography coupled with mass spectrometry. *J Chromatogr A.* 1190:278, 2008.

Harrison L.M. et al. Effect of extended use of single anabolic steroids on urinary steroid excretion and metabolism. *J Chromatogr.* 489:121, 1989.

Hatton C.K. et al. Detection of androgenic anabolic steroids in urine. *Clin Lab Med.* 7:655, 1987.

He G. et al. Doping control analysis of 13 steroids and structural-like analytes in human urine using quadrupole-orbitrap LC-MS/MS with parallel reaction monitoring (PRM) mode. *Steroids.* 131:1, 2018.

Hemmersbach P. The probenecid-story - a success in the fight against doping through out-of-competition testing. *Drug Test Anal.* 2019.

Hill S.A. et al. Pharmacological effects and safety monitoring of anabolic androgenic steroid use: Differing perceptions between users and healthcare professionals. *Ther Adv Drug Saf.* 10:2042098619855291, 2019.

Iljukov S. et al. Association between implementation of the athlete biological passport and female elite runners' performance. *Int J Sports Physiol Perform.* 1, 2020.

Jardines D. et al. Longitudinal evaluation of the isotope ratio mass spectrometric data: Towards the 'isotopic module' of the athlete biological passport? *Drug Test Anal.* 8:1212, 2016.

Kim S.H. et al. Simultaneous ionization and analysis of 84 anabolic androgenic steroids in human urine using liquid chromatography-silver ion coordination ionspray/triple-quadrupole mass spectrometry. *Drug Test Anal.* 6:1174, 2014.

Kiss A. et al. Urinary signature of anabolic steroids and glucocorticoids in humans by lc-ms. *Talanta.* 83:1769, 2011.

Kotronoulas A. et al. Evaluation of markers out of the steroid profile for the screening of testosterone misuse. Part II: Intramuscular administration. *Drug Test Anal.* 10:849, 2018.

Mazzarino M. et al. Drug-drug interaction and doping: Effect of non-prohibited drugs on the urinary excretion profile of methandienone. *Drug Test Anal.* 10:1554, 2018.

Miller G.D. et al. Intranasal delivery of Natesto® testosterone gel and its effects on doping markers. *Drug Test Anal.* 8:1197, 2016.

Mullen J. et al. Sensitivity of doping biomarkers after administration of a single dose testosterone gel. *Drug Test Anal.* 10:839, 2018.

Mullen J.E. et al. Urinary steroid profile in females -- the impact of menstrual cycle and emergency contraceptives. *Drug Test Anal.* 9:1034, 2017.

Narducci W.A. et al. Anabolic steroids--a review of the clinical toxicology and diagnostic screening. *J Toxicol Clin Toxicol.* 28:287, 1990.

Novakova L. et al. Fast and sensitive supercritical fluid chromatography - tandem mass spectrometry multi-class screening method for the determination of doping agents in urine. *Anal Chim Acta.* 915:102, 2016.

Palermo A. et al. Non-targeted LC-MS based metabolomics analysis of the urinary steroidal profile. *Anal Chim Acta.* 964:112, 2017.

Piper T. et al. Epiandrosterone sulfate prolongs the detectability of testosterone, 4-androstenedione, and dihydrotestosterone misuse by means of carbon isotope ratio mass spectrometry. *Drug Test Anal.* 9:1695, 2017.

Piper T. et al. Genotype-dependent metabolism of exogenous testosterone - new biomarkers result in prolonged detectability. *Drug Test Anal.* 8:1163, 2016.

Piper T. et al. Revisiting the metabolism of 19-nortestosterone using isotope ratio and high resolution/high accuracy mass spectrometry. *J Steroid Biochem Mol Biol.* 162:80, 2016.

Piper T. et al. Applications of isotope ratio mass spectrometry in sports drug testing accounting for isotope fractionation in analysis of biological samples. *Methods Enzymol.* 596:403, 2017.

Pirola I. et al. Anabolic steroids purchased on the internet as a cause of prolonged hypogonadotropic hypogonadism. *Fertil Steril.* 94:2331 e1, 2010.

Pitarch-Motellon J. et al. Determination of selected endogenous anabolic androgenic steroids and ratios in urine by ultra-high performance liquid chromatography tandem mass spectrometry and isotope pattern deconvolution. *J Chromatogr A.* 1515:172, 2017.

Ponzetto F. et al. High-resolution mass spectrometry as an alternative detection method to tandem mass spectrometry for the analysis of endogenous steroids in serum. *J Chromatogr B Analyt Technol Biomed Life Sci.* 1052:34, 2017.

Ponzetto F. et al. Methods for doping detection. *Front Horm Res.* 47:153, 2016.

Ponzetto F. et al. Longitudinal monitoring of endogenous steroids in human serum by UHPLC-MS/MS as a tool to detect testosterone abuse in sports. *Anal Bioanal Chem.* 408:705, 2016.

Putz M. et al. Identification of trenbolone metabolites using hydrogen isotope ratio mass spectrometry and liquid chromatography/high accuracy/high resolution mass spectrometry for doping control analysis. *Front Chem.* 8:435, 2020.

Raro M. et al. Untargeted metabolomics in doping control: Detection of new markers of testosterone misuse by ultrahigh performance liquid chromatography coupled to high-resolution mass spectrometry. *Anal Chem.* 87:8373, 2015.

Raro M. et al. Potential of atmospheric pressure chemical ionization source in gas chromatography tandem mass spectrometry for the screening of urinary exogenous androgenic anabolic steroids. *Anal Chim Acta.* 906:128, 2016.

Rzeppa S. et al. Analysis of anabolic androgenic steroids as sulfate conjugates using high performance liquid chromatography coupled to tandem mass spectrometry. *Drug Test Anal.* 7:1030, 2015.

Schonfelder M. et al. Potential detection of low-dose transdermal testosterone administration in blood, urine, and saliva. *Drug Test Anal.* 8:1186, 2016.

Sessa F. et al. Anabolic androgenic steroids: Searching new molecular biomarkers. *Front Pharmacol.* 9:1321, 2018.

Shen M. et al. Physiological concentrations of anabolic steroids in human hair. *Forensic Sci Int.* 184:32, 2009.

Sobolevsky T. et al. Isotopically labeled boldenone as a better marker of derivatization efficiency for improved quality control in anti-doping analysis. *Drug Test Anal.* 11:336, 2019.

Strahm E. et al. Dose-dependent testosterone sensitivity of the steroidal passport and GC-C-IRMS analysis in relation to the UGT2b17 deletion polymorphism. *Drug Test Anal.* 7:1063, 2015.

Thevis M. et al. Detection of SARMs in doping control analysis. *Mol Cell Endocrinol.* 464:34, 2018.

Tudela E. et al. Urinary detection of conjugated and unconjugated anabolic steroids by dilute-and-shoot liquid chromatography-high resolution mass spectrometry. *Drug Test Anal.* 7:95, 2015.

Virus E.D. et al. High-temperature high-performance liquid chromatography on a porous graphitized carbon column coupled to an orbitrap mass spectrometer with atmospheric pressure photoionization for screening exogenous anabolic steroids in human urine. *Rapid Commun Mass Spectrom.* 29:1779, 2015.

WADA. Endogenous anabolic androgenic steroids measurement and reporting. *WADA Technical Document – TD2018EAAS.* 2018.

Wang Z. et al. A novel HPLC-MRM strategy to discover unknown and long-term metabolites of stanozolol for expanding analytical possibilities in doping-control. *J Chromatogr B Analyt Technol Biomed Life Sci.* 1040:250, 2017.

Weinand J. et al. Pancreatic islet hyperplasia: A potential marker for anabolic-androgenic steroid use. *Acad Forensic Pathol.* 8:777, 2018.

INDEX

Index

www.ingramcontent.com/pod-product-compliance
Lightning Source LLC
Chambersburg PA
CBHW072104270326
41931CB00010B/1457